Functional Foods as a New
Therapeutic Strategy

Functional Foods as a New Therapeutic Strategy

Editor

Ivan Cruz-Chamorro

MDPI • Basel • Beijing • Wuhan • Barcelona • Belgrade • Manchester • Tokyo • Cluj • Tianjin

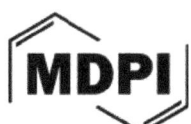

Editor
Ivan Cruz-Chamorro
Universidad de Sevilla
Spain

Editorial Office
MDPI
St. Alban-Anlage 66
4052 Basel, Switzerland

This is a reprint of articles from the Special Issue published online in the open access journal *Nutraceuticals* (ISSN 1661-3821) (available at: https://www.mdpi.com/journal/nutraceuticals/special_issues/FFoods).

For citation purposes, cite each article independently as indicated on the article page online and as indicated below:

LastName, A.A.; LastName, B.B.; LastName, C.C. Article Title. *Journal Name* **Year**, *Volume Number*, Page Range.

ISBN 978-3-0365-7708-1 (Hbk)
ISBN 978-3-0365-7709-8 (PDF)

Cover image courtesy of Ivan Cruz-Chamorro

© 2023 by the authors. Articles in this book are Open Access and distributed under the Creative Commons Attribution (CC BY) license, which allows users to download, copy and build upon published articles, as long as the author and publisher are properly credited, which ensures maximum dissemination and a wider impact of our publications.

The book as a whole is distributed by MDPI under the terms and conditions of the Creative Commons license CC BY-NC-ND.

Contents

About the Editor vii

Preface to "Functional Foods as a New Therapeutic Strategy" ix

Ivan Cruz-Chamorro
Functional Foods as a New Therapeutic Strategy
Reprinted from: *Nutraceuticals* 2023, 3, 18, doi:10.3390/nutraceuticals3020018 1

Madalina Neacsu, James S. Christie, Gary J. Duncan, Nicholas J. Vaughan and Wendy R. Russell
Buckwheat, Fava Bean and Hemp Flours Fortified with Anthocyanins and Other Bioactive Phytochemicals as Sustainable Ingredients for Functional Food Development
Reprinted from: *Nutraceuticals* 2022, 2, 11, doi:10.3390/nutraceuticals2030011 5

Gabriele Carullo, Umile Gianfranco Spizzirri, Rocco Malivindi, Vittoria Rago, Marisa Francesca Motta, Danilo Lofaro, et al.
Development of Quercetin-DHA Ester-Based Pectin Conjugates as New Functional Supplement: Effects on Cell Viability and Migration
Reprinted from: *Nutraceuticals* 2022, 2, 21, doi:10.3390/nutraceuticals2040021 17

Grégoire Bouillon, Olav Gåserød, Łukasz Krych, Josué L. Castro-Mejía, Witold Kot, Markku T. Saarinen, et al.
Modulating the Gut Microbiota with Alginate Oligosaccharides In Vitro
Reprinted from: *Nutraceuticals* 2023, 3, 3, doi:10.3390/nutraceuticals3010003 29

Kirsty M. Reynolds, Loris A. Juett, James Cobb, Carl J. Hulston, Stephen A. Mears and Lewis J. James
Apple Puree as a Natural Fructose Source Provides an Effective Alternative to Artificial Fructose Sources for Fuelling Endurance Cycling Performance in Males
Reprinted from: *Nutraceuticals* 2022, 2, 15, doi:10.3390/nutraceuticals2030015 43

João P. G. Passos, Carlisson R. Melo, Felipe M. A. Carvalho, Patricia Severino, Juliana C. Cardoso, John L. S. Cunha, et al.
Combined Therapy of Chitosan and Exercise Improves the Lipid Profile, Adipose Tissue and Hepatic Alterations in an In Vivo Model of Induced-Hyperlipidemia
Reprinted from: *Nutraceuticals* 2022, 2, 9, doi:10.3390/nutraceuticals2020009 57

Yurika Kitamura, Kosuke Nishi, Momoko Ishida, Sogo Nishimoto and Takuya Sugahara
Anti-Allergic Effect of Aqueous Extract of Coriander (*Coriandrum sativum* L.) Leaf in RBL-2H3 Cells and Cedar Pollinosis Model Mice
Reprinted from: *Nutraceuticals* 2022, 2, 13, doi:10.3390/nutraceuticals2030013 73

Christian Setz, Maria Fröba, Maximilian Große, Pia Rauch, Janina Auth, Alexander Steinkasserer, et al.
European Black Elderberry Fruit Extract Inhibits Replication of SARS-CoV-2 In Vitro
Reprinted from: *Nutraceuticals* 2023, 3, 7, doi:10.3390/nutraceuticals3010007 85

Tariq A. Alalwan, Duha Mohammed, Mariam Hasan, Domenico Sergi, Cinzia Ferraris, Clara Gasparri, et al.
Almond, Hazelnut, and Pistachio Skin: An Opportunity for Nutraceuticals
Reprinted from: *Nutraceuticals* 2022, 2, 23, doi:10.3390/nutraceuticals2040023 101

Matúš Kučka, Katarína Ražná, Ľubomír Harenčár and Terézia Kolarovičová
Plant Seed Mucilage—Great Potential for Sticky Matter
Reprinted from: *Nutraceuticals* **2022**, *2*, 19, doi:10.3390/nutraceuticals2040019 . . . . **113**

Seiichi Matsugo, Toshio Sakamoto, Koji Wakame, Yutaka Nakamura, Kenichi Watanabe and Tetsuya Konishi
Mushrooms as a Resource for Mibyou-Care Functional Food; The Role of Basidiomycetes-X (Shirayukidake) and Its Major Components
Reprinted from: *Nutraceuticals* **2022**, *2*, 10, doi:10.3390/nutraceuticals2030010 . . . . **131**

Lorenzo Zanella and Fabio Vianello
Potential of Microalgae as Functional Foods Applied to Mitochondria Protection and Healthy Aging Promotion
Reprinted from: *Nutraceuticals* **2023**, *3*, 10, doi:10.3390/nutraceuticals3010010 . . . . **149**

Taiki Miyazawa, Chizumi Abe, Gregor Carpentero Burdeos, Akira Matsumoto and Masako Toda
Food Antioxidants and Aging: Theory, Current Evidence and Perspectives
Reprinted from: *Nutraceuticals* **2022**, *2*, 14, doi:10.3390/nutraceuticals2030014 . . . . **183**

Prodromos Skenderidis, Stefanos Leontopoulos and Dimitrios Lampakis
Goji Berry: Health Promoting Properties
Reprinted from: *Nutraceuticals* **2022**, *2*, 3, doi:10.3390/nutraceuticals2010003 . . . . **207**

About the Editor

Ivan Cruz-Chamorro

Ivan Cruz-Chamorro (Ph.D.) is a post-doctoral researcher at the University of Seville, Spain. Since 2012, he has been a member of the Molecular Neuroimmunoendocrinology Laboratory of the Institute of Biomedicine of Seville (IBiS) and his workplace. In 2018, he discussed his doctoral thesis, "Assessment of the health effects of plant bioactive peptides: immunomodulatory, antioxidant, and metabolic effects", obtaining an outstanding cum laude rating. Ivan is involved in studying the biological effects (immunomodulators, antioxidants, lipid-lowering, etc.) of protein hydrolysates from several plant sources such as lupine, olive, and hemp. He directed a doctoral thesis in which the capacity of protein hydrolysate from lupine was explored in metabolic syndrome (MetS) and in the preclinical mouse model of hypercholesterolemia. Ivan collaborates with different international groups, and he is currently exploring the effects of different natural matrices on some diseases such as MetS, metabolic-associated fatty liver disease, and multiple sclerosis. Last, his future research objective is to explore the biological effects of these matrices on cancer models.

Preface to "Functional Foods as a New Therapeutic Strategy"

Dear Readers,

The subject of this book is the identification of new functional foods that are capable of acting on human health to improve it without the use of synthesized chemical compounds. This topic arises from the need to demonstrate, at a scientific level, the importance of these new compounds and their important applications.

The authors of the different articles are internationally recognized scientists, and they have been researching these issues for many years.

Thus, this book is not only directed at researchers but also the general public in order to expand knowledge on the potential application of different natural compounds.

These findings encourage us to continue investigations in this direction and confirm the importance of these studies.

Ivan Cruz-Chamorro
Editor

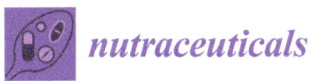

Editorial

Functional Foods as a New Therapeutic Strategy

Ivan Cruz-Chamorro [1,2]

[1] Departamento de Bioquímica Médica y Biología Molecular e Inmunología, Facultad de Medicina, Universidad de Sevilla, 41009 Seville, Spain; icruz-ibis@us.es
[2] Instituto de Biomedicina de Sevilla, IBiS/Hospital Universitario Virgen del Rocío/CSIC/Universidad de Sevilla, 41013 Seville, Spain

Recently, the use of nutraceuticals has drawn attention in the food industry due to their potential health benefits. Nutraceuticals are products that are produced from foods and sold in pills, powders, and other medicinal forms that have both nutritional value and health-promoting properties. They contain bioactive compounds that can prevent and treat various chronic diseases such as antioxidants and anti-inflammatory and antimicrobial agents.

This Special Issue, entitled "Functional Foods as a New Therapeutic Strategy", provides an overview of various functional ingredients that are used as nutraceuticals, including almond, hazelnut, and pistachio skin, mushrooms, buckwheat, fava bean, hemp flours, apple puree, and microalgae. These have been shown to bestow beneficial effects and could be used for therapeutic, hypoallergenic, or sporting purposes.

Thus, the use of plant-derived materials that are rich in bioactive compounds has the potential to promote health and prevent diseases [1]. Similarly, plant seed mucilage, which is typically discarded during food processing, has been shown to have a range of potential applications in the development of functional foods [2]. The use of these by-products not only offers a potential source of nutraceuticals but also helps to reduce waste in the food industry. In fact, fruit- and plant-based waste (including anthocyanins and phenolic acids) can be incorporated into buckwheat, fava bean, and hemp flour to improve their health-promoting properties [3].

Similarly, mushrooms are being investigated as a potential source of functional food ingredients, with some species showing promise for health promotion and disease prevention [4]. In addition, modified quercetin and pectin have been shown to have effects on cell viability and migration [5].

Another important aspect of nutraceutical research is the study of the gut microbiome and its interactions with dietary components. Thus, in this Special Issue, a study explores the potential of alginate oligosaccharides to modulate gut microbiota and promote health [6].

The use of microalgae as functional foods for mitochondrial protection and the promotion of healthy aging was also revised [7]. Thus, the bioactive compounds present in microalgae, such as carotenoids, phycocyanin, and polyunsaturated fatty acids, have antioxidant and anti-inflammatory properties that have protective effects against aging-related diseases [8]. Goji berry fruits have also demonstrated several beneficial effects on age-related diseases, such as diabetes, atherosclerosis, and cancer, principally due to their bioactive secondary metabolites [9].

On the one hand, functional food can be used to improve sport performance. In this sense, this Special Issue shows that carbohydrate consumption during exercise is important for enhancing endurance, and for this reason, currently, there exist several artificial fructose sources. However, food can also be a source, and is a healthier one. The performance of nine trained male cyclists was not altered regardless of whether natural apple puree (+maltodextrin) or artificial crystalline fructose was consumed. Other parameters, such as heart rate, blood glucose/lactate concentrations, and gastrointestinal symptoms, were

Citation: Cruz-Chamorro, I. Functional Foods as a New Therapeutic Strategy. *Nutraceuticals* **2023**, *3*, 231–233. https://doi.org/10.3390/nutraceuticals3020018

Received: 19 April 2023
Accepted: 21 April 2023
Published: 25 April 2023

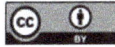

Copyright: © 2023 by the author. Licensee MDPI, Basel, Switzerland. This article is an open access article distributed under the terms and conditions of the Creative Commons Attribution (CC BY) license (https://creativecommons.org/licenses/by/4.0/).

not altered, showing that a natural fructose source is a valuable alternative to artificial sources [10].

On the other hand, the combination of a linear polysaccharide (chitosan) with physical exercise improved the lipid profile of high-fat diet-fed rats [11]. In fact, this synergism (chitosan + exercise), which lasted for eight weeks, reduced the body weight of the animals, as well as restoring the altered lipid profile (total cholesterol, triglycerides, LDL, and VLDL).

Furthermore, aqueous coriander (*Coriandrum sativum*) leaf extract (ACLE) possesses an anti-allergenic effect, inhibiting the degranulation of rat basophilic leukemia cells and suppressing the increase in intracellular Ca^{2+} that is responsible for this degranulation. Moreover, ACLE is capable of downregulating the phosphorylation of phosphatidylinositol 3-kinase and the tyrosine-protein kinase SYK, attenuating allergen-induced symptoms. Finally, its oral administration reduced the IgE serum level in a pollinosis mouse model [12].

In addition, buckwheat, fava bean, and hemp flours fortified with anthocyanins and other bioactive phytochemicals may have applications in the prevention and treatment of chronic diseases, moreover showing the importance of using sustainable and environmentally friendly practices in the food industry [3].

Of relevant interest is that European black elderberry fruit extract has been demonstrated to be capable of inhibiting the replication of SARS-CoV-2 in vitro [13].

In conclusion, the natural ingredients discussed in this Special Issue highlight the importance of incorporating them into functional food development, as well as of using sustainable and environmentally friendly practices in the food industry.

The continued exploration and generation of nutraceuticals will be critical in addressing the increasing prevalence of chronic diseases and promoting healthy aging.

As consumers continue to seek out natural and functional food products, this research will become increasingly important in the development of new and innovative products that meet their needs.

Funding: I.C.-C. was supported by a postdoctoral fellowship from the Andalusian Government Ministry of Economy, Knowledge, Business, and University (DOC_00587/2020).

Conflicts of Interest: The author declares no conflict of interest.

References

1. Alalwan, T.A.; Mohammed, D.; Hasan, M.; Sergi, D.; Ferraris, C.; Gasparri, C.; Rondanelli, M.; Perna, S. Almond, Hazelnut, and Pistachio Skin: An Opportunity for Nutraceuticals. *Nutraceuticals* **2022**, *2*, 300–310. [CrossRef]
2. Kučka, M.; Ražná, K.; Harenčár, Ľ.; Kolarovičová, T. Plant Seed Mucilage—Great Potential for Sticky Matter. *Nutraceuticals* **2022**, *2*, 253–269. [CrossRef]
3. Neacsu, M.; Christie, J.S.; Duncan, G.J.; Vaughan, N.J.; Russell, W.R. Buckwheat, Fava Bean and Hemp Flours Fortified with Anthocyanins and Other Bioactive Phytochemicals as Sustainable Ingredients for Functional Food Development. *Nutraceuticals* **2022**, *2*, 150–161. [CrossRef]
4. Matsugo, S.; Sakamoto, T.; Wakame, K.; Nakamura, Y.; Watanabe, K.; Konishi, T. Mushrooms as a resource for Mibyou-care functional food; the role of basidiomycetes-X (Shirayukidake) and its major components. *Nutraceuticals* **2022**, *2*, 132–149. [CrossRef]
5. Carullo, G.; Spizzirri, U.G.; Malivindi, R.; Rago, V.; Motta, M.F.; Lofaro, D.; Restuccia, D.; Aiello, F. Development of Quercetin-DHA Ester-Based Pectin Conjugates as New Functional Supplement: Effects on Cell Viability and Migration. *Nutraceuticals* **2022**, *2*, 278–288. [CrossRef]
6. Bouillon, G.; Gåserød, O.; Krych, Ł.; Castro-Mejía, J.L.; Kot, W.; Saarinen, M.T.; Ouwehand, A.C.; Nielsen, D.S.; Rattray, F.P. Modulating the Gut Microbiota with Alginate Oligosaccharides In Vitro. *Nutraceuticals* **2023**, *3*, 26–38. [CrossRef]
7. Zanella, L.; Vianello, F. Potential of Microalgae as Functional Foods Applied to Mitochondria Protection and Healthy Aging Promotion. *Nutraceuticals* **2023**, *3*, 119–152. [CrossRef]
8. Miyazawa, T.; Abe, C.; Burdeos, G.C.; Matsumoto, A.; Toda, M. Food antioxidants and aging: Theory, current evidence and perspectives. *Nutraceuticals* **2022**, *2*, 181–204. [CrossRef]
9. Skenderidis, P.; Leontopoulos, S.; Lampakis, D. Goji berry: Health promoting properties. *Nutraceuticals* **2022**, *2*, 32–48. [CrossRef]
10. Reynolds, K.M.; Juett, L.A.; Cobb, J.; Hulston, C.J.; Mears, S.A.; James, L.J. Apple Puree as a Natural Fructose Source Provides an Effective Alternative to Artificial Fructose Sources for Fuelling Endurance Cycling Performance in Males. *Nutraceuticals* **2022**, *2*, 205–217. [CrossRef]

11. Passos, J.P.; Melo, C.R.; Carvalho, F.M.; Severino, P.; Cardoso, J.C.; Cunha, J.L.; Cano, A.; Souto, E.B.; de Albuquerque-Júnior, R.L. Combined Therapy of Chitosan and Exercise Improves the Lipid Profile, Adipose Tissue and Hepatic Alterations in an In Vivo Model of Induced-Hyperlipidemia. *Nutraceuticals* **2022**, *2*, 116–131. [CrossRef]
12. Kitamura, Y.; Nishi, K.; Ishida, M.; Nishimoto, S.; Sugahara, T. Anti-Allergic Effect of Aqueous Extract of Coriander (Coriandrum sativum L.) Leaf in RBL-2H3 Cells and Cedar Pollinosis Model Mice. *Nutraceuticals* **2022**, *2*, 170–180. [CrossRef]
13. Setz, C.; Fröba, M.; Große, M.; Rauch, P.; Auth, J.; Steinkasserer, A.; Plattner, S.; Schubert, U. European Black Elderberry Fruit Extract Inhibits Replication of SARS-CoV-2 In Vitro. *Nutraceuticals* **2023**, *3*, 91–106. [CrossRef]

Disclaimer/Publisher's Note: The statements, opinions and data contained in all publications are solely those of the individual author(s) and contributor(s) and not of MDPI and/or the editor(s). MDPI and/or the editor(s) disclaim responsibility for any injury to people or property resulting from any ideas, methods, instructions or products referred to in the content.

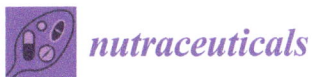

Article

Buckwheat, Fava Bean and Hemp Flours Fortified with Anthocyanins and Other Bioactive Phytochemicals as Sustainable Ingredients for Functional Food Development

Madalina Neacsu [1,*], James S. Christie [1,2], Gary J. Duncan [1], Nicholas J. Vaughan [1] and Wendy R. Russell [1]

[1] The Rowett Institute, University of Aberdeen, Aberdeen AB25 2ZD, UK; j.christie38@rgu.ac.uk (J.S.C.); gary.duncan@abdn.ac.uk (G.J.D.); nick.vaughan@abdn.ac.uk (N.J.V.); w.russell@abdn.ac.uk (W.R.R.)
[2] School of Pharmacy and Life Sciences, The Robert Gordon University, Aberdeen AB10 7QB, UK
* Correspondence: m.neacsu@abdn.ac.uk; Tel.: +44-1224438760

Abstract: Facing a climate emergency and an increasingly unhealthy population, functional foods should not only address health issues but must be prepared from sustainable ingredients while contributing to our sustainable development goals, such as tackling waste and promoting a healthy environment. High-protein crop flours, i.e., buckwheat, hemp and fava bean, are investigated as potential matrices to be fortified with key bioactive phytochemicals from soft fruits to explore potential waste valorization and to deliver sustainable functional food ingredients. Hemp flour provided the best matrix for anthocyanin fortification, adsorbing of 88.45 ± 0.88% anthocyanins and 69.77 mg/kg of additional phytochemicals. Buckwheat and fava bean absorbed 78.64 ± 3.15% and 50.46 ± 2.94% of anthocyanins 118.22 mg/kg and 103.88 mg/kg of additional phytochemicals, respectively. During the fortification, there was no detectable adsorption of the berry sugars to the flours, and the quantities of free sugars from the flours were also removed. One gram of fortified hemp flour provides the same amount of anthocyanins found in 20 g of fresh bilberries but has substantially less sugar. The optimum conditions for high protein flour fortification with anthocyanins was established and showed that it is a viable way to reduce and valorize potential agricultural waste, contributing to a circular and greener nutrition.

Keywords: buckwheat; fava bean; hemp; anthocyanin; flour fortification; functional food; berries; soft fruit; agricultural waste; bilberry

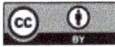

1. Introduction

Soft fruits are particularly prone to wastage and, in the case of strawberries alone, one in ten ends up as waste in the UK [1]. In 2015 alone, just over 9% of mature strawberries ended up as waste, as the product did not meet quality requirements, primarily because of fruit being misshapen [1]. It is essential that UK producers find higher value and novel uses for soft fruit waste, ultimately contributing to food waste reduction and sustainable food production. Anthocyanins are a major group of phytochemicals from soft fruits, shown to inhibit carbohydrate uptake from food, resulting in decreased postprandial blood glucose [2] and the inhibition of endogenous enzymes, including amylase, sucrase [3] and glucosidases [4], all enzymes associated with carbohydrate digestion. Supplementation with bilberry extract has been shown to modify the glycemic response in volunteers with type 2 diabetes mellitus (T2DM) [5], and wild bilberry-fortified soya flour reduced post prandial blood glucose levels in mice, along with weight gain [2]. As obesity and sustained high blood sugar levels are major risk factors in the development of T2DM [6], it is likely that products rich in dietary anthocyanin could contribute towards decreasing the incidence of this condition, delivering economically desirable preventative nutritional therapies. Revalorizing soft fruit bioactives and reintroducing them back into foods could deliver solutions to aid metabolically compromised individual and help reduce soft fruit agricultural waste.

High-protein crops, such as hemp, buckwheat and fava bean, besides having the potential to be grown sustainably in certain climates, could constitute key ingredients of a healthy, sustainable diet. We have shown that hemp and buckwheat flours are valuable sources of dietary amino acids, beneficially modulating gastrointestinal hormones and promoting satiety in healthy volunteers [7]. Foods prepared from buckwheat showed health benefits, attenuating insulin resistance and improving lipid profiles in patients with type 2 diabetes [8]. Buckwheat contains proanthocyanidins, which can inhibit digestive enzymes [9] and D-chiro-inositol, which can function as a mediator for anti-hyperinsulinemia [10,11]. Hemp flour is also a rich source of dietary fiber, around 25% [12], which could exert a prebiotic effect [13] and lower blood cholesterol [14].

Modern functional foods should not only provide a proven health benefit but should contribute to our sustainable development goals by finding solutions to tackle agricultural waste and contribute to a healthy and green environment. In the present paper, buckwheat, hemp and fava bean flours are investigated for their capacity to adsorb bioactive phytochemicals from bilberries, establishing the optimum conditions to enrich the flours with anthocyanins, while retaining no detectable sugar content from the soft fruits. This anthocyanin-rich food could represent a viable candidate to be incorporated into nutritional therapies for T2DM management. While the main aim of the work is to deliver the development of a functional food ingredient concept, this methodology could also be used to provide alternative solutions to tackle fruit and plant-based waste in general by revalorizing bioactive phytochemicals (anthocyanin). This work discusses innovative, climate-friendly, healthy and sustainable food ingredients to meet consumers' needs, while could also be addressing critical issues regarding agricultural waste.

2. Materials and Methods

Plant materials: Wild bilberries (*Vaccinium* sp.) were picked from the Tyrebagger Forest in Aberdeen, Scotland and stored at −80 °C. The berries were freeze dried (Labconco; Kansas City, MO, USA), freeze milled (Spex sample prep 6800; Munich, Germany) and stored at room temperature in desiccators under vacuum with exclusion of light. The hemp flour was purchased from Yorkshire Hemp (Driffield, UK), fava bean flour from Barry Farm (Cridersville, OH, USA) and buckwheat flour from Arrowhead Mills (Boulder, CO, USA). All flours were stored at room temperature with the exclusion of light, following the manufacturer's recommendation storage conditions.

Standards and reagents: Standards for the anthocyanin aglycones (anthocyanins), delphinidin (>95%), cyanidin (>95%), pelargonidin (undeclared purity), peonidin (>96.5%), were all purchased from Sigma-Aldrich (Dorset, UK) and malvidin (>95%) from Phytolab, Germany. The aglycone standard, petunidin, was purchased from ChemFaces (Hubei, China) at a purity of >95%. The anthocyanin glycoside (anthocyanidin) standards; delphinidin 3-glucoside (>97%), cyanidin 3-glucoside (>95%), cyanidin 3-galactoside (>95%), petunidin 3-glucoside (>95%), peonidin 3-glucoside (>95%), pelargonidin 3-glcusoside (>97%) and malvidin 3-glucoside (>95%), were all purchased from Sigma-Aldrich (Dorset, UK). All the phenolic standards were purchased from Sigma-Aldrich (Gillingham, UK), Phytolab, Germany or synthesized as described previously [15,16]. General reagents were purchased from Sigma-Aldrich (Dorset, UK) and Fischer Scientific (Loughborough, UK).

A schematic summary of the succession of procedures used in the experimental protocol is presented in the Figure 1.

Flour fortification with wild bilberry phytochemicals: The freeze-dried wild bilberries were used as a source of anthocyanins and other phenolics to enrich the buckwheat, fava bean and hemp flour. The freeze-dried berry powders were suspended at three different concentrations of 0.1 (A), 0.07 (B) and 0.04 g/mL (C), in citric acid (4.75 mM, pH 3.5). Suspensions were placed in an ultrasound bath for 5 min and then intermittently mixed at room temperature for 1 h. The supernatant was separated by centrifugation (5 min;

3220× g; 4 °C). This extract was used for the flour fortification experiments. Three different quantities of each flour, 1 g, 0.5 g and 0.2 g, respectively (n = 3) were suspended in the extracts prepared above (5 mL). The suspensions were then thoroughly mixed at room temperature for 5 min. The supernatants were separated by centrifugation (5 min; 3220× g; 4 °C), filtered (0.2 µm) and immediately analyzed.

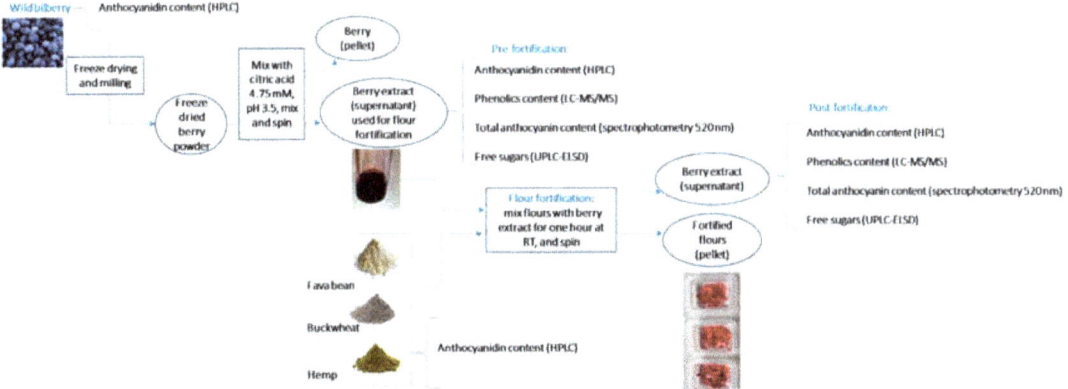

Figure 1. Overview of the experimental procedures used for the fortification of buckwheat, fava bean and hemp flours, highlighting the measurements (and methodologies) used in the experimental protocol.

The flour fortification (the amounts of anthocyanins and other phenolics added to the flour) was measured by comparing the total anthocyanin content (measured by UV-VIS spectrophotometry), the individual anthocyanins (measured by HPLC-DAD), other phenolics (measured by LC-MS/MS) and sugar content (measured by UPLC-ELSD) in the wild bilberry extracts (pre-fortification) and the resulting supernatants (post-fortification).

Estimation of total anthocyanins adsorbed on the flours: Total anthocyanin content was estimated by measuring the absorption between 400 nm and 700 nm for the extracts (pre-fortification) and resultant supernatants (post-fortification) using a µQuant 7271000 plate reader Biotek Instrument (Potton, UK). Subsequent absorption measurements were made at the λmax (520 nm). The semi-quantification for total anthocyanin glycoside content was performed using the cyanidin 3-glucoside standard.

Determination of individual anthocyanidin content from the bilberries, buckwheat, fava bean, hemp flours and anthocyanin adsorbed on the flours: To measure the anthocyanidin content of the bilberries and flours was used the extraction and hydrolysis methods adapted from [17]. Briefly, samples (n = 3) of wild bilberry (0.05 g) and buckwheat, fava bean and hemp flour (1 g) were extracted with methanol:water:hydrochloric acid (ratio of 50:33:17; $v/v/v$; 3 mL) three times, and the supernatants and the pellet combined and hydrolyzed at 100 °C for 60 min. Hydrolyzed samples were then immediately cooled to room temperature, filtered using 0.2 µm filters and analyzed by HPLC.

The quantification of the anthocyanins and anthocyanidins was performed using a 1260 Infinity HPLC from Agilent (Wokingham, UK) and a Synergi 4 µm Polar-RP 80A (250 × 4.6 mm) column with a Polar-RP 4 × 3 mm pre-column from Phenomenex (Macclesfield, UK). The DAD spectra were recorded between 200 and 700 nm and the chromatograms were monitored at 530 nm for the detection of the anthocyanidins and 520 nm for the glycoside forms (anthocyanins). For the HPLC separations the following solvents were used: A: formic acid (2.125%) and B: acetonitrile/methanol (85:15, v/v).

The HPLC method for anthocyanidin analysis was adapted from Zhang, Z. et al., (2004) [17]. The solvent program was isocratic 18% B for 40 min. The flow was constant at 1 mL/min and the column temperature was held at 35 °C. The anthocyanins content from the fortification extracts was determined directly in the extracts as prepared above for fortification using the HPLC method analysis adapted from [18]. The column temperature was constant at 28 °C using a solvent and flow rate gradient program.

The separation and quantification of anthocyanins was performed using external standardization with delphinidin (r^2 = 0.998, LOD = 8.52 µg/mL), cyanidin (r^2 = 0.997, LOD = 11.31 µg/mL), petunidin (r^2 = 0.999, LOD = 5.64 µg/mL), pelargonidin (r^2 = 0.997, LOD = 12.63 µg/mL), peonidin (r^2 = 0.999, LOD = 10.57 µg/mL), malvidin (r^2 = 0.99, LOD = 6.09 µg/mL), delphinidin 3-glucoside (r^2 = 0.997, LOD = 14.78 µg/mL), cyanidin 3-glucoside (r^2 = 0.994, LOD = 35.76 µg/mL), cyanidin 3-galactoside (r^2 = 0.997, LOD = 19.89 µg/mL), peonidin 3-glucoside (r^2 = 0.999, LOD = 2.36 µg/mL), pelargonidin 3-glucoside (r^2 = 0.999, LOD = 3.05 µg/mL) and malvidin 3-glucoside (r^2 = 0.999, LOD = 3.00 µg/mL).

LC-MS/MS analysis of other phenolics adsorbed on the flours: The wild bilberry aqueous extracts (0.1 g/mL) and the solution obtained after the flour fortification (0.04 g flour to each mL extract as described above) were collected and freeze dried. Freeze-dried samples (approx. 0.1 g dry weight; n = 3) were suspended in hydrochloric acid (2 M; 3 mL) and incubated at 90 °C for one hour with intermittent mixing. They were then cooled to room temperature and extracted with ethyl acetate three times, the organic layers were combined, filtered through sodium sulphate (anhydrous), the solvent was evaporated and the residue was dissolved in methanol/water (50:50, v/v; 0.5 mL) for LC-MS/MS analysis using internal standard for negative mode mass spectrometry ^{13}C benzoic acid at 2 µg/mL and, respectively, 2-amino-3,4,7,8-tetramethylimidazo(4,5-f)quinoxaline at 0.5 µg/mL, for positive mode mass spectrometry.

The LC-MS/MS analysis methods used for phenolics analysis was performed as previously published [19–21] and quantified using multiple reaction monitoring and internal standardization. The liquid chromatography separation of the metabolites was performed on an Agilent 1100 LC-MS system (Agilent Technologies, Wokingham, UK) using a Zorbax Eclipse 5 µm, 150 mm × 4.6 mm C18 column (Agilent Technologies). For all the phenolics quantifications the standard calibrations were over a concentration interval of 2 µg/mL to 10 ng/mL. The threshold used for quantification was a signal to noise ratio of 3 to 1. All the ion transitions for each of the metabolites were determined based upon their molecular ion and a strong fragment ion and their voltage parameters; their declustering potential, collision energy and cell entrance/exit potentials were optimized individually for each metabolite and have been previously described [18,19].

UPLC-ELSD quantification of mono- and disaccharides from wild bilberry fortification extracts: The separation and quantification of sugars used external standardization with fructose (r^2 = 0.999, LOD = 0.65 mg/mL), glucose (r^2 = 0.997, LOD = 0.70 mg/mL) and sucrose (r^2 = 0.996, LOD = 0.41 mg/mL). The instrument used was a Waters Acquity UPLC (Elstree, UK) equipped with an Acquity UPLC BEH Amide column (Elstree, UK) (1.7 µm 2.1 × 100 mm). Gradient elution starting with 100% mobile phase A (80% acetonitrile in water with 0.2% triethylamine), decreasing to 60% A and 40% B (30% acetonitrile in water with 0.2% triethylamine) over 10 min, followed by a 30-min isocratic elution at 100% A. Flow rate and temperature were constant at 0.12 mL/min and 23 °C, respectively. The ELSD detector used a gain of 200 and pressure at 40 psi.

Statistical analysis: All the data were averaged from three technical replicates of samples and are reported as means and standard deviation. The differences between concentrations of various macronutrients and phytochemicals between various plant materials from this study was assessed by two-sided post hoc t-tests, with p values less than 0.05 ($p < 0.05$) indicating significance. Microsoft® Excel® for Office 365 (Microsoft Corporation, Redmond, WA, USA) was used for statistical analyses.

3. Results

3.1. Anthocyanidin Content of Wild Bilberry, Buckwheat, Fava Bean and Hemp Flours

Bilberry samples were found to be rich in five of the six anthocyanidins measured; delphinidin (10.87 ± 1.57 g/kg dry weight), cyanidin (14.13 ± 1.47 g/kg dry weight), petunidin (3.18 ± 0.29 g/kg dry weight), peonidin (2.8 ± 0.21 g/kg dry weight) and malvidin (34.33 ± 2.94 g/kg dry weight). Pelargonidin was the only aglycone that was not detected. Cyanidin and pelargonidin were detected in buckwheat flour with concentrations of 170.83 ± 9.16 and 227.43 ± 11.01 mg/kg dry weight, respectively. Delphinidin and cyanidin were detected in fava bean flour at concentrations of 4.1 ± 0.31 and 2.23 ± 0.23 mg/kg dry weight, respectively. Cyanidin was the only anthocyanidin detected in hemp flour at a concentration of 5.77 ± 1.72 mg/kg.

3.2. Bilberry Anthocyanins Adsorbed by the Buckwheat, Fava Bean and Hemp Flour

The optimum conditions for fortifications (defined as highest anthocyanins quantity adsorbed by a minimum amount of flour) were 0.1 g/mL freeze-dried wild bilberry at a ratio of flour to extract of 0.04 g flour to each mL extract. By increasing the concentration and volume of the aqueous extract, the anthocyanin fortification of the flours was increased with hemp flour adsorbing the highest quantities of bilberry anthocyanins. This translates to 95.69 ± 12.47 mg of total anthocyanins per g of buckwheat flour, representing 78.64 ± 3.15% anthocyanins removed from the extracts or attached to the flour (Table 1); 88.86 ± 8.44 mg of total anthocyanins per g of fava bean flour (50.46 ± 2.94% anthocyanins removed from the bilberry extract) and 101.64 ± 1.57 of total anthocyanins per g of hemp flour (88.45 ± 0.88% anthocyanins removed from the bilberry extract), as can be seen in Table 1. This paper's results are in agreement with other researchers' work where high protein flours, such as soybean, adsorbed anthocyanins in a similar range of concentrations and amounts [22].

Table 1. Total berry anthocyanins (mg of total anthocyanins per g of flour) adsorbed by the buckwheat, fava bean and hemp flour.

Flour	Aqueous Wild Bilberry Extracts		
	A *	B *	C *
Buckwheat			
0.2 g/mL extract	24.93 ± 0.72 (97.02 ± 0.69)	10.07 ± 0.55 (94.56 ± 1.98)	5.26 ± 0.87 (92.91 ± 1.53)
0.1 g/mL extract	48.11 ± 2.19 (92.93 ± 1.6)	19.5 ± 1.08 (92 ± 1.76)	10.31 ± 1.67 (91 ± 1.38)
0.04 g/mL extract	**95.69 ± 12.47 (78.64 ± 3.15)**	26.23 ± 4.39 (48.64 ± 8.69)	14.27 ± 4.6 (8.56 ± 5.14)
Fava bean			
0.2 g/mL extract	24.43 ± 3.46 (91.26 ± 0.34)	10.76 ± 0.43 (85.04 ± 0.18)	12.91 ± 0.99 (90.85 ± 0.4)
0.1 g/mL extract	41.68 ± 6.51 (76.69 ± 2.9)	19.32 ± 0.66 (75.97 ± 1.05)	25.4 ± 1.99 (88.67 ± 0.66)
0.04 g/mL extract	**88.86 ± 8.44 (50.46 ± 2.94)**	24 ± 6.73 (37.02 ± 8.93)	31.58 ± 4.54 (52.55 ± 2.02)
Hemp			
0.2 g/mL extract	23.05 ± 0.95 (94.33 ± 0.4)	8.66 ± 0.89 (90.72 ± 1.01)	7.04 ± 0.4 (92.1 ± 0.93)
0.1 g/mL extract	44.92 ± 2.1 (91.83 ± 0.28)	16.48 ± 1.7 (86.67 ± 1.07)	14.07 ± 0.89 (91.6 ± 1.25)
0.04 g/mL extract	**101.64 ± 1.57 (88.45 ± 0.88)**	36.29 ± 6.28 (78.95 ± 3.61)	20.2 ± 0.62 (60.75 ± 0.65)

Values given are mean ± standard deviation (n = 3) in mg of total anthocyanins per g of flour. The values in parenthesis represent total anthocyanin quantities (%) removed from the extracts or attached to the flours. Total anthocyanins quantities were determined spectrophotometrically, the values are expressed in cyanidin 3-glucoside relative units. * Represents concentrations of bilberry extracts in aqueous solution at pH 3.5 citric acid prepared by suspending freeze-dried wild bilberry powder at concentrations of 0.1 g/mL (A), 0.07 g/mL (B) and 0.04 g/mL (C).

The decrease in the mass of flour per volume of juice increased the mass of anthocyanins ($p < 0.05$) bound to the flour. This increase in juice to flour ratio leaded to less efficient removal of polyphenols from juices. However, the main purpose of this work this is the enrichment of the flours and, for commercial applications, the non-absorbed polyphenols could represent a considerable expense. Similarly, increasing the concentration of the bilberry juice shows significant increases in the level of enrichment ($p < 0.01$) of each flour without affecting the level of non-absorbed anthocyanins. It is possible that further increases in concentration or volume could further increase the quality of enrichment but given the non-absorbed polyphenols already seen, this may not be practical or economically viable. The optimum condition of anthocyanin enrichment for all three flours with bilberry extracts was by suspending 0.04 g flour in 1 mL juice of concentration A (0.1 g/mL bilberry powder in citric acid pH 3.5).

The profile of the individual anthocyanins before and after fortification, using the optimum fortification conditions, was quantified by HPLC-DAD and are presented in Figure 2. The results showed a significant ($p < 0.001$) fortification with the major anthocyanins, identified as delphinidin-3-glucoside, cyanidin-3-galactoside, cyanidin-3-glucoside, peonidin-3-glucoside and malvidin-3-glucoside. It appeared that several additional anthocyanin glycosides were also observed in the HPLC chromatogram, but these could not be identified, as standards were not available. In all the cases, the fortification efficiency was higher for delphinidin-3-glucoside and cyanidin-3-galactoside at concentrations of 64.52 ± 1.57% and 65.55 ± 0.74% for buckwheat, 55.25 ± 0.33% and 50.25 ± 0.35% for fava bean and 68.29 ± 2.31% and 71.06 ± 0.79% for hemp flour, respectively (Table 2). Malvidin-3-glucoside was least efficiently adsorbed by the flours at concentrations of 46.94 ± 0.44%, 33.93 ± 0.42% and 53.83 ± 0.9% for buckwheat, fava bean and hemp flour, respectively (Table 2).

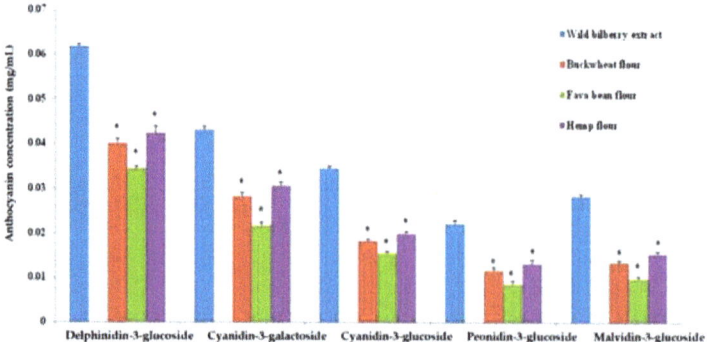

Figure 2. The adsorption of anthocyanin on the flours, as indicated by the amount (mg/mL) removed from aqueous wild bilberry extract (0.1 g/mL) with citric acid (pH 3.5). The first bar in each set (blue color) represents the concentration of individual anthocyanin in the initial wild bilberry extract used for the fortification of the flours. The subsequent bars represent individual concentration of anthocyanin adsorbed on each of the flours after fortification. For fortification, 0.04 g of flour was used for each mL of berry extract, where (*) represents significant reduction in the extract concentration of individual anthocyanin (or adsorption of individual anthocyanin on the flours from the extract) after the flour fortification ($p > 0.0001$).

Table 2. Individual anthocyanin adsorption (%) on the flours from wild bilberry extracts.

Flour	Flours Anthocyanins Fortification (%)				
	Delphinidin-3-Glucoside	Cyanidin-3-Glucoside	Cyanidin-3-Galactoside	Peonidin-3-Glucoside	Malvidin-3-Glucoside
Buckwheat	64.52 ± 1.57	65.55 ± 0.74	52.65 ± 0.2	51.53 ± 0.51	46.94 ± 0.44
Fava bean	55.25 ± 0.33	50.25 ± 0.35	44.53 ± 0.3	37.46 ± 0.51	33.93 ± 0.42
Hemp	68.29 ± 2.31	71.06 ± 0.79	57.68 ± 0.78	58.62 ± 1.51	53.83 ± 0.9

Values given are mean ± standard deviation (n = 3) as % of individual anthocyanins adsorbed on the flours from the wild bilberry extracts. Flour fortification was performed using aqueous wild bilberry extract (0.1 g/mL). For each mL of extract, 0.04 g flour was used for the fortification.

3.3. Other Phenolics from Wild Bilberries Adsorbed on the Flours

The quantity of several phenolics adsorbed by the flours was calculated by the difference between the amount in the wild bilberry extract before and after the fortification (Figure 3). The wild bilberry extract was found to be rich in phenolic acids including chlorogenic (40.03 ± 7.47 mg/kg), caffeic (28.76 ± 5.51 mg/kg), p-coumaric (28.23 ± 6.18 mg/kg), protocatechuic (11.38 ± 2.63 mg/kg), and vanillic acid (7.83 ± 1.64 mg/kg); and in flavonoids; quercetin (31.52 ± 5.31 mg/kg), myricetin (20.09 ± 4.6 mg/kg), and isorhamnetin (3.97 ± 0.94 mg/kg), (Figure 3).

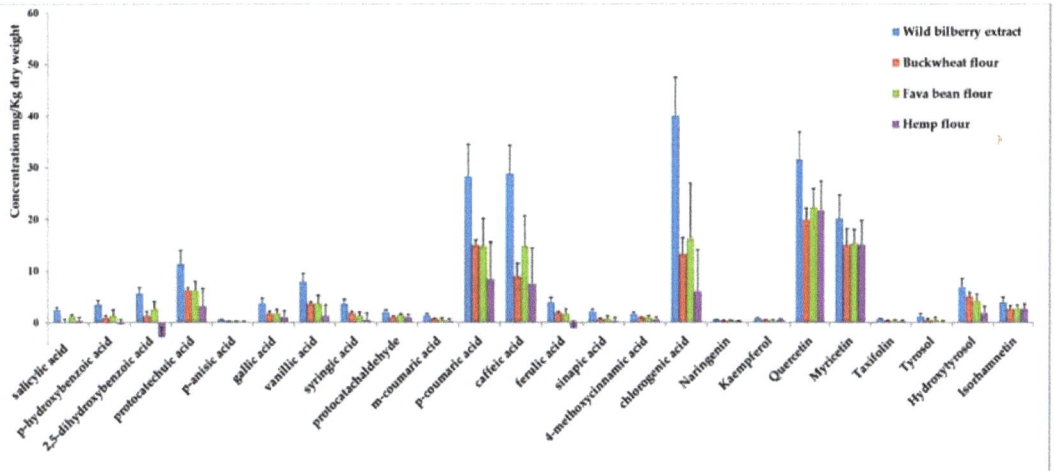

Figure 3. The main phenolics quantified in the initial aqueous wild bilberry extract (0.1 g/mL prepared in citric acid pH 3.5) used for the flour fortification (blue bars) and the adsorption of individual phenolic molecules (mg/kg dry weight) from the initial extract on the buckwheat flour (red bars) on fava bean flour (green bars) and hemp flour (purple bars). For the fortification, 0.04 g from each flour for each mL of wild bilberry extract was used.

From the flavonoids present in the initial extract used for the flour fortification, myricetin had the best adsorption on the fava bean flour 77.68 ± 12.6%, (corresponding to 15.07 ± 3.09 mg/kg dry weight from the initial extract), followed by isorhamnetin and quercetin with 71.93 ± 15.16% and 71.85 ± 15.97% adsorbed from the initial extract (corresponding to 2.82 ± 0.64 mg/kg and 22.27 ± 3.60 mg/kg dry weight from the initial extract), respectively (Figure 3). From the phenolic acids present in the initial extract used for flour fortification, protocatechuic acid had the best adsorption on the fava bean flour with 56.75 ± 24.52%, (corresponding to 6.12 ± 1.84 mg/kg dry weight from initial extract) being adsorbed. This was followed by p-coumaric and caffeic acid with 55.37 ± 26.95% and 54.54 ± 27.36% being adsorbed from the initial extract (corresponding to 14.77 ± 5.34 mg/kg and 17.87 ± 5.74 mg/kg dry weight from initial extract), respectively. Chlorogenic acid, which was the richest by weight on the fortified fava bean flour with 16.18 ± 10.71 mg/kg dry weight from the initial extract being adsorbed, representing 42.60 ± 30.60% adsorbed on the buckwheat flour, 78.61% on fava bean flour and 75.37% on hemp flour (Figure 3). Some phenolic acids, such as 2,3-dihydroxybenzoic acid in buckwheat and p-hydroxybenzoic, 2,5-dihydroxybenzoic and ferulic acid in hemp, were released from the flours into extracts during the fortification process (Figure 3). Overall, the flavonoids were better adsorbed compared to the phenolic acids, and from approximately 218 mg/kg total phenolics measured in the wild bilberry extract, 118 mg, 103 mg and 70 mg were adsorbed by the fava bean, buckwheat and hemp flours, respectively.

3.4. Sugar Content Following the Flour Fortification with Wild Bilberry

The free sugar content of the aqueous wild bilberry extracts (pre-fortification) and the remaining supernatants (post-fortification) were determined using UPLC-ELSD (Figure 4). None of the flours retained any of the sugars present in the aqueous bilberry extracts and the important quantities of the sugars were extracted from the flours during the fortification process (Figure 4). The total sugar content (representing the sum of fructose, glucose and sucrose) was measured before and after flour fortification. Comparing the initial extract before fortification with the extract recovered after the flour fortification, there was an increase in total sugar content varying from as little as 2.1% for the buckwheat fortification of 0.04 g flour to 1 mL of Extract B up to 55% after hemp fortification of 0.2 g flour with 1 mL of Extract B (prepared by adding 0.07 g wild bilberry powder to 1 mL citric acid pH 3.5).

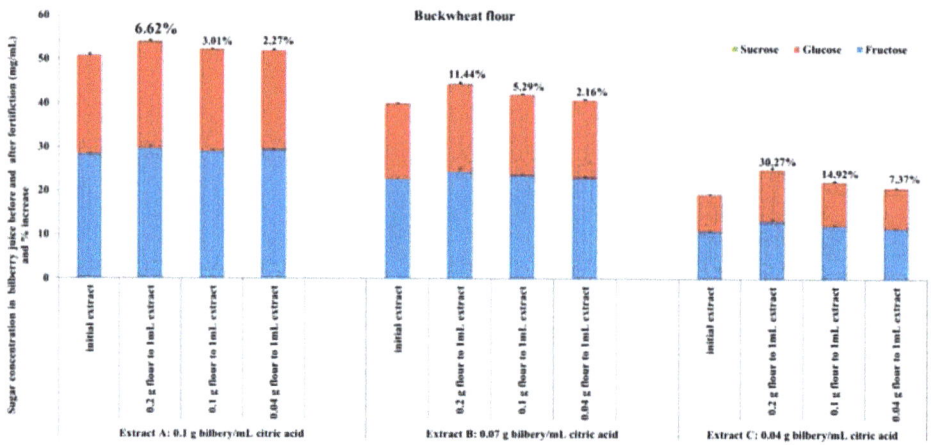

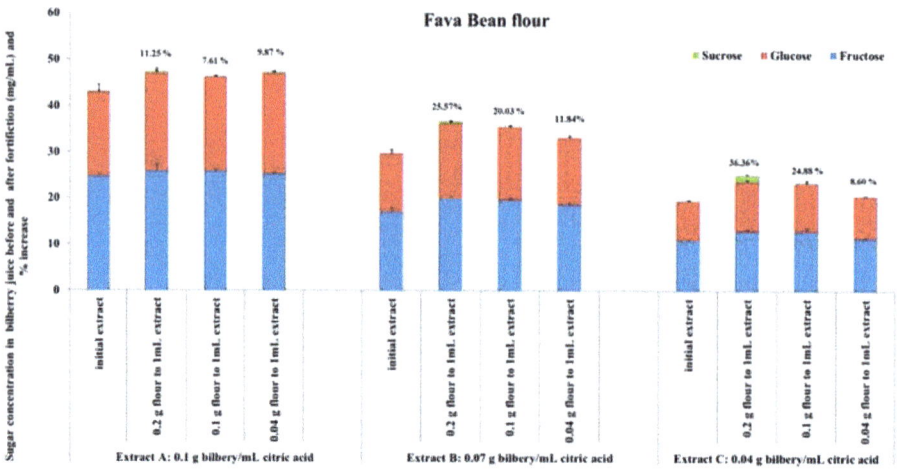

Figure 4. *Cont.*

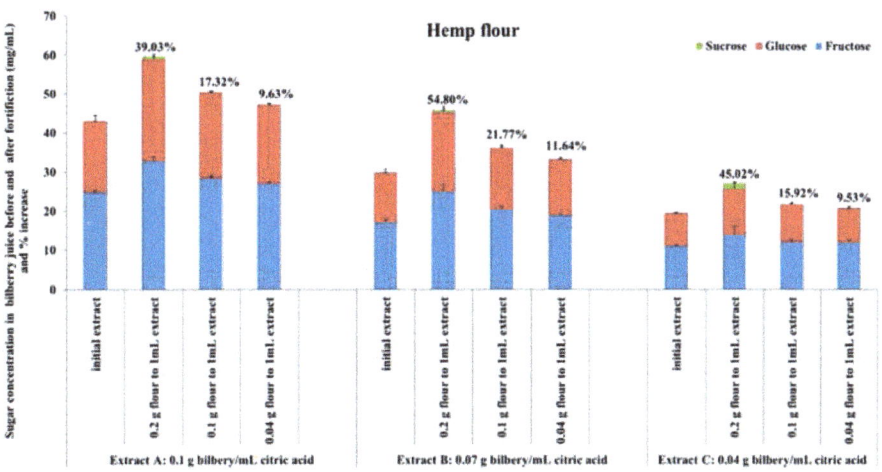

Figure 4. The sugar (glucose, sucrose and fructose) content of the bilberry extracts prepared at concentrations of 0.1 g/mL (Extract A), 0.07 g/mL (Extract B) and 0.04 g/mL (Extract C) before (initial extract) and after flour fortification, using flour to extract ratio of 1 to 5 (0.2 g flour to 1 mL extract), 1 to 10 (0.1 g flour to 1 mL extract) and 1 to 25 (0.04 g flour to 1 mL extract) for each concentration of extract presented above, respectively. The values in the top of each chart represent the total sugar increment (in %) from the initial bilberry extract after the flour fortification.

4. Discussion

As buckwheat, fava bean and hemp fortified flours retained the characteristic color of anthocyanins, it is likely that they are adsorbed, rather than covalently bound. In this context, it could be hypothesized that the compounds present in the flours act as co-pigments for bilberry-derived anthocyanins. It has been shown that most common co-pigments are flavonoids, phenolic acids, alkaloids, amino acids and organic acids [23]. Our previous research [7,12] reported buckwheat, fava bean and hemp flours as rich sources of bound phenolics acids, such as sinapic acid, ferulic acid caffeic acid and amino acids, including proline and arginine, which are all known efficient co-pigments [23–25]. Furthermore, the optimum conditions used for the flour fortification (pH 3.5 aqueous solution) are also favorable for co-pigmentation [23,26,27].

Using the optimized conditions for fortification, hemp adsorbed the highest quantities of anthocyanins from wild bilberries. Hemp was the best matrix for fortification with each gram of the fortified hemp flour potentially delivering the equivalent of anthocyanins present in 20 g of fresh berries. This is particularly important considering that anthocyanins have been extensively studied for their health benefits, including the prevention of cardiovascular disease [28–30], anti-cancer properties [31–33] and to benefit people living with type 2 diabetes mellitus [34–36]. Furthermore, buckwheat and hemp flours beneficially modulated gastrointestinal hormones and promoted satiety in healthy volunteers [7]. Therefore, these fortified flours could represent attractive functional foods for prevention and aid of several non-communicable disorders and for weight management in nutritional therapies. The additional phenolics adsorbed during the fortification, including phenolic acids (caffeic, p-coumaric and chlorogenic) and flavonoids (quercetin and myricetin) potentially confer additional health benefits to the final product, complementing to the nutritional value, shelf life and food reformulation versatility.

From 2.5 kg of dried bilberries, 1.88 kg of dried extract for flour fortification can be produced. Considering that 57% of bilberry extract is used for buckwheat fortification, 49% for fava bean fortification and 54% for hemp fortification, the resulting extract could be reused for further flour fortification, delivering a more economically viable process. Moreover, all the conditions and materials used in this process, such as water, citric acid, bilberry fruits, buckwheat, fava bean and hemp, are very accessible and could easily be scaled-up for commercial production.

Functional food ingredients rich in anthocyanins (and, importantly, with no free sugars) could represent a key component in the nutritional therapies for T2DM management for people at risk developing T2DM and people living with the disease. This due to the beneficial health attributes related to the regulation of sugar metabolism, as presented earlier in this paper. Moreover, there is strong scientific evidence from animal and human clinical studies describing the beneficial impact of anthocyanins on cardiovascular and neurodegenerative diseases, as has been recently reviewed by Mattioli et al. [34]. Additionally, the anthocyanin-rich ingredients as food components could also be beneficial to the food itself; it can protect the food from damage caused during baking, while improving its antioxidant capacity, this being superior to even synthetic additives [37]. Moreover, in products such as kefir, yoghurt, and other beverages, anthocyanins have been found to have high stability during storage and improve the color of processed foods, representing a viable alternative to synthetic colorants as highlighted in a recent review on food product fortification with anthocyanins carried out by Echegaray et al. [37].

Therefore, the health and food applications of anthocyanins-rich ingredients could be numerous, and the projections of the functional food market are very healthy; they were valued at USD 98.9 billion in 2021 and are projected to reach USD 137.1 billion by 2026 [38].

For this work, anthocyanin-rich plant material (soft fruits such as bilberry) was used to deliver a sustainable functional food ingredient concept design for T2DM management. However, this concept could also be used to valorize plant bioactives from agricultural/food waste/by-products [39]. Therefore, they could represent an alternative solution to tackling soft fruit waste by bioactive revalorization. The wild bilberries are also naturally high in readily available (free) sugars and much of these were removed during the flour's fortification process, reducing the glycemic load of the fortified food while adding key bioactives with known health benefits. This finding is of particular interest as anthocyanins are being extensively researched as potential natural remedies for diabetes [40]. Moreover, they could also represent a solution for sugars recovery from fruit waste and various agricultural by-products at the same time. Follow up research is necessary to prove the functionality of these fortifies flours in human dietary studies.

5. Conclusions

The current work has successfully established the optimum conditions for the fortification of buckwheat, fava bean and hemp flours with additional bioactives (including anthocyanins, phenolic acids and other flavonoids) relevant for the prevention and maintenance of conditions such as type 2 diabetes mellitus. The flours did not retain any of the free sugars in bilberry and additional sugars present in the flours were removed during the fortification process.

This paper discussed food ingredients naturally rich in protein, dietary fiber, micronutrients and bioactive phytochemicals. Being low in free sugars, there is huge potential for these ingredients to be used by the food and drink industry, especially as active functional ingredient for low glycemic food formulations. Additional work would also be necessary for further product development and to test their efficacy in sugar and/or lipid modulation in human dietary intervention studies before their recommendation in any nutritional therapy. The development of specialized food with potential health-promoting benefits using sustainable food sources will ultimately create the demand for the cultivation of these healthy and sustainable crops and deliver innovative ways to utilize potential agricultural waste streams and co-products.

Author Contributions: Conceptualization, M.N. and W.R.R.; methodology, M.N., W.R.R. and J.S.C.; formal analysis, J.S.C., N.J.V. and G.J.D.; data curation, M.N., J.S.C. and G.J.D.; writing—original draft preparation, M.N. and W.R.R.; writing—review and editing, M.N. and W.R.R.; visualization, M.N. and W.R.R.; supervision, M.N. and W.R.R. All authors have read and agreed to the published version of the manuscript.

Funding: This research was funded by the Scottish government's Rural and Environment Science and Analytical Services Division (RESAS).

Institutional Review Board Statement: Not applicable.

Informed Consent Statement: Not applicable.

Data Availability Statement: Not applicable.

Acknowledgments: The authors acknowledge Viv Buchan from the Analytical Department, The Rowett Institute, University of Aberdeen, for her help with the sugar content determinations.

Conflicts of Interest: The authors declare no conflict of interest.

References

1. Sheane, R.; McCosker, C.; Lillywhite, R. *Food Waste in Primary Production—A Preliminary Study on Strawberries and Lettuce*; Wrap report; Wrap: Banbury, UK, 2017; Available online: https://wrap.org.uk/sites/default/files/2020-10/WRAP-Food_waste_in_primary_production_report.pdf (accessed on 12 May 2022).
2. Roopchand, D.E.; Kuhn, P.; Rojo, L.E.; Lila, M.A.; Raskin, I. Blueberry polyphenol-enriched soybean flour reduces hyperglycemia; body weight gain and serum cholesterol in mice. *Pharmacol. Res.* **2013**, *69*, 59–67. [CrossRef] [PubMed]
3. Akkarachiyasit, S.; Charoenlertkul, P.; Yibchok-anun, S.; Adisakwattana, S. Inhibitor activities of cyanidin and it glycoside and synergistic effect with acarabose against intestinnal α-GLucosidase and pancreatic α-amylase. *Int. J. Mol. Sci.* **2010**, *119*, 3387–3396.
4. Matsui, T.; Ueda, T.; Oki, T.; Sugita, K.; Terahara, N.; Matsumoto, K. α-Glucosidase inhibitory action of natural acylated anthocyanins. 1. Survey of natural pigments with potent inhibitory activity. *J. Agric. Food Chem.* **2001**, *494*, 1948–1951. [CrossRef]
5. Hoggard, N.; Cruickshank, M.; Moar, K.M.; Bestwick, C.; Holst, J.J.; Russell, W.; Horgan, G. A single supplement of a standardised bilberry (*Vaccinium myrtillus* L.) extract (36% wet weight anthocyanins) modifies glycaemic response in individuals with type 2 diabetes controlled by diet and lifestyle. *J. Nutr. Sci.* **2013**, *2*, e22. [CrossRef] [PubMed]
6. Lyssenko, V.; Jonsson, A.; Almgern, P.; Pulizzi, N.; Isomaa, B.; Tuomi, T.; Berglund, G.; Altshuler, D.; Nilsson, P.; Groop, L. Clinical risk factors, DNA variants, and the development of type 2 diabetes. *N. Engl. J. Med.* **2008**, *359*, 2220–2232. [CrossRef]
7. Neacsu, M.; Vaughan, N.J.; Multari, S.; Haljas, E.; Scobbie, L.; Duncan, G.J.; Cantlay, L.; Fyfe, C.; Anderson, S.; Horgan, G.; et al. Hemp and buckwheat are valuable sources of dietary amino acids, beneficially modulating gastrointestinal hormones and promoting satiety in healthy volunteers. *Eur. J. Nutr.* **2022**, *61*, 1057–1072. [CrossRef]
8. Qiu, J.; Liu, Y.; Yue, Y.; Qin, Y.; Li, Z. Dietary tartary buckwheat intake attenuates insulin resistance and improves lipid profiles in patients with type 2 diabetes: A randomized controlled trial. *Nutr. Res.* **2016**, *36*, 1392–1401. [CrossRef]
9. Lee, Y.A.; Cho, E.J.; Tanaka, T.; Yokozawa, T. Inhibitory activities of proanthocyanidins from persimmon against oxidative stress and digestive enzymes related to diabetes. *J. Nutr. Sci. Vitaminol.* **2007**, *53*, 287–292. [CrossRef]
10. Kawa, J.M.; Przybylski, R.; Taylor, C.G. Urinary *chiro*-inositol and *myo*-inositol excretion is elevated in the diabetic db/db mouse and streptozotocin diabetic rat. *Exp. Biol. Med.* **2003**, *228*, 907–914. [CrossRef]
11. Yao, Y.; Shan, F.; Bian, J.; Chen, F.; Wang, M.; Ren, G. D-*chiro*-Inositol-enriched tartary buckwheat bran extract lowers the blood glucose level in KK-Ay mice. *J. Agric. Food Chem.* **2008**, *56*, 10027–10031. [CrossRef]
12. Multari, S.; Neacsu, M.; Scobbie, L.; Cantlay, L.; Duncan, G.; Vaughan, N.; Stewart, D.; Russell, W.R. Nutritional and Phytochemical Content of High-Protein Crops. *J. Agric. Food Chem.* **2016**, *64*, 7800–7811. [CrossRef] [PubMed]
13. Kapravelou, G.; Martínez, R.; Andrade, A.M.; Sánchez, C.; Chaves, C.L.; López-Jurado, M.; Aranda, P.; Cantarero, S.; Arrebola, F.; Fernández-Segura, E.; et al. Health promoting effects of Lupin (Lupinus albus var. multolupa) protein hydrolyzate and insoluble fiber in a diet-induced animal experimental model of hypercholesterolemia. *Food Res. Int.* **2013**, *54*, 1471–1481. [CrossRef]
14. Kristensen, M.; Jensen, M.G.; Aarestrup, J.; Petersen, K.E.N.; Sondergaard, L.; Mikkelsen, M.S.; Astrup, A. Flaxseed dietary fibers lower cholesterol and increase fecal fat excretion, but magnitude of effect depend on food type. *Nutr. Metab.* **2012**, *9*, 8. [CrossRef] [PubMed]
15. Russell, W.R.; Burkitt, M.J.; Forrester, A.R.; Chesson, A. Oxidative coupling during lignin polymerization is determined by unpaired electron delocalization within parent phenylpropanoid radicals. *Arch. Biochem. Biophys.* **1996**, *332*, 357–366. [CrossRef]
16. Russell, W.R.; Burkitt, M.J.; Scobbie, L.; Chesson, A. Radical formation and coupling of hydroxycinnamic acids containing 1, 2-dihydroxy substituents. *Bioorg. Chem.* **2003**, *31*, 206–215. [CrossRef]
17. Zhang, Z.; Kou, X.; Fugal, K.; Mclaughlin, J. Comparison of HPLC methods for determination of anthocyanins and anthocyanidins in bilberry extracts. *J. Agric. Food Chem.* **2004**, *52*, 688–691. [CrossRef]

18. Lätti, A.K.; Riihinen, K.R.; Kainulainen, P.S. Analysis of anthocyanin variation in wild populations of bilberry (*Vaccinium myrtillus* L.) in Finland. *J. Agric. Food Chem.* **2008**, *56*, 190–503. [CrossRef]
19. Russell, W.R.; Gratz, S.W.; Duncan, S.H.; Holtrop, G.; Ince, J.; Scobbie, L.; Duncan, G.; Johnstone, A.M.; Lobley, G.E.; Wallace, R.J.; et al. High-protein, reduced-carbohydrate weight-loss diets promote metabolite profiles likely to be detrimental to colonic health. *Am. J. Clin. Nutr.* **2011**, *93*, 1062–1072. [CrossRef]
20. Neacsu, M.; McMonagle, J.; Fletcher, R.J.; Scobbie, L.; Duncan, G.J.; Cantlay, L.; De Roos, B.; Duthie, G.G.; Russell, W.R. Bound phytophenols from ready-to-eat cereals; comparison with other plant-based foods. *Food Chem.* **2013**, *141*, 2880–2886. [CrossRef]
21. Neacsu, M.; Vaughan, N.J.; Raikos, V.; Multari, S.; Duncan, G.J.; Duthie, G.G.; Russell, W.R. Phytochemical profile of food plant powders: Their potential role in healthier food reformulations. *Food Chem.* **2015**, *179*, 159–169. [CrossRef]
22. Roopchand, D.E.; Grace, M.H.; Kuhn, P.; Cheng, D.M.; Plundrich, N.; Poulev, A.; Howell, A.; Fridlender, B.; Lila, M.A.; Raskin, I. Efficient sorption of polyphenols to soybean flour enables natural fortification of foods. *Food Chem.* **2012**, *131*, 1193–1200. [CrossRef] [PubMed]
23. Brouillard, R.; Mazza, G.; Saad, Z.; Albrecht-Gary, A.M.; Cheminat, A. The co-pigmentation reaction of anthocyanins: A microprobe for the structural study of aqueous solutions. *J. Am. Chem Soc.* **1989**, *111*, 2604–2610. [CrossRef]
24. Asen, S.; Stewart, R.N.; Norris, K.H. Copigmentation of anthocyanins in plant tissues and its effect on color. *Phytochemistry* **1972**, *11*, 1139–1144. [CrossRef]
25. Markovic, J.M.D.; Petranovic, N.A.; Baranac, J.M. A spectrophotometric study of the copigmentation of malvin with caffeic and ferulic acids. *J. Agric. Food Chem.* **2000**, *48*, 5530–5536. [CrossRef] [PubMed]
26. Williams, M.; Hrazdina, G. Anthocyanins as food colorants: Effect of pH on the formation of anthocyanin-rutin complexes. *J. Food Sci.* **1979**, *44*, 66–68. [CrossRef]
27. Brouillard, R.; Wigand, M.C.; Dangles, O.; Cheminat, A. The pH and solvent effects on the copigmentation reaction of malvin with polyphenols, purine and pyrimidine derivatives. *J. Chem. Soc.* **1991**, *2*, 1235–1241. [CrossRef]
28. Rechner, A.R.; Kroner, C. Anthocyanins and colonic metabolites of dietary polyphenols inhibit platelet function. *Thromb. Res.* **2005**, *116*, 327–334. [CrossRef]
29. Alvarez-Suarez, J.M.; Giampieri, F.; Tulipani, S.; Casoli, T.; Di Stefano, G.; González-Paramás, A.M.; Santos-Buelga, C.; Busco, F.; Quiles, J.L.; Cordero, M.D.; et al. One-month strawberry-rich anthocyanin supplementation ameliorates cardiovascular risk, oxidative stress markers and platelet activation in humans. *J. Nutr. Biochem.* **2014**, *25*, 289–294. [CrossRef]
30. Toufektsian, M.C.; De Lorgeril, M.; Nagy, N.; Salen, P.; Donati, M.B.; Giordano, L.; Mock, H.P.; Peterek, S.; Matros, A.; Petroni, K. Chronic dietary intake of plant-derived anthocyanins protects the rat heart against ischemia-reperfusion injury. *J. Nutr.* **2008**, *138*, 747–752. [CrossRef]
31. Wang, L.S.; Hecht, S.S.; Carmella, S.G.; Yu, N.; Larue, B.; Henry, C.; Mcintyre, C.; Rocha, C.; Lechner, J.F.; Stoner, G.D. Anthocyanins in black raspberries prevent esophagul tumours in rats. *Cancer Prev. Res.* **2009**, *2*, 84–93. [CrossRef]
32. Malik, M.; Zhao, C.; Schoene, N.; Guisti, M.M.; Moyer, M.; Magnuson, B.A. Anthocyanin-rich extract from Aronia meloncarpa E. induces a cell cycle block in colon cancer but not normal colonic cells. *Nutr. Cancer* **2003**, *46*, 186–196. [CrossRef] [PubMed]
33. Lin, B.W.; Gong, C.C.; Song, H.F.; Cui, Y.Y. Effects of anthocyanins on the prevention and treatment of cancer. *Br. J. Pharmacol.* **2017**, *174*, 1226–1243. [CrossRef] [PubMed]
34. Mattioli, R.; Francioso, A.; Mosca, L.; Silva, P. Anthocyanins: A Comprehensive Review of Their Chemical Properties and Health Effects on Cardiovascular and Neurodegenerative Diseases. *Molecules* **2020**, *25*, 3809. [CrossRef] [PubMed]
35. Alnajjar, M.; Barik, S.K.; Bestwick, C.; Campbell, F.; Cruickshank, M.; Farquharson, F.; Holtrop, G.; Horgan, G.; Louis, P.; Moar, K.M.; et al. Anthocyanin-enriched Bilberry extract attenuates glycaemic response in overweight volunteers without changes in insulin. *J. Funct. Foods* **2020**, *64*, 103597. [CrossRef]
36. Barik, S.K.; Dehury, B.; Russell, W.R.; Moar, K.; Cruickshabk, M.; Scobbie, L.; Hoggard, N. Analysis of polyphenolic metabolites from in vitro gastrointestinal digested soft fruit extracts identify malvidin-3-glucoside as an inhibitor of PTP1B. *Biochem. Pharmacol.* **2020**, *178*, 114109. [CrossRef]
37. Echegaray, N.; Munekata, P.E.S.; Gullón, P.; Dzuvor, K.K.O.; Gullón, B.; Kubi, F.; Lorenzo, J.M. Recent advances in food products fortification with anthocyanins. *Crit. Rev. Food Sci. Nutr.* **2022**, *62*, 1553–1567. [CrossRef]
38. Functional Food Ingredients Market by Type & Application—Global Forecast 2026. Functional Food Ingredients Market. Markets and Markets. 2021. Available online: https://www.marketsandmarkets.com/Market-Reports/functional-food-ingredients-market-9242020.html (accessed on 28 April 2022).
39. Nayak, A.; Bhushan, B. An overview of the recent trends on the waste valorization techniques for food wastes. *J. Environ. Manag.* **2019**, *233*, 352–370. [CrossRef]
40. Różańska, D.; Regulska-Ilow, B. The significance of anthocyanins in the prevention and treatment of type 2 diabetes. *Adv. Clin. Exp. Med.* **2018**, *27*, 135–142. [CrossRef]

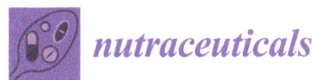

Article

Development of Quercetin-DHA Ester-Based Pectin Conjugates as New Functional Supplement: Effects on Cell Viability and Migration

Gabriele Carullo [1], Umile Gianfranco Spizzirri [2,*], Rocco Malivindi [2], Vittoria Rago [2], Marisa Francesca Motta [2], Danilo Lofaro [3], Donatella Restuccia [2,†] and Francesca Aiello [2,†]

[1] Department of Life Sciences, University of Siena, Via Aldo Moro 2, 53100 Siena, Italy
[2] Department of Pharmacy, Health and Nutritional Sciences, DoE 2018–2022, University of Calabria, Edificio Polifunzionale, 87036 Rende, Italy
[3] de-Health Laboratory, DIMEG, University of Calabria, 87100 Rende, Italy
* Correspondence: g.spizzirri@unical.it
† These authors contributed equally to this work.

Abstract: A quercetin derivative with remarkable biological performance was successfully synthesized by chemical modification of the flavonoid with docosahexaenoic acid to synthesize 2-(2,2-diphenylbenzo[*d*][1,3]dioxol-5-yl)-5,7-dihydroxy-4-oxo-4*H*-chromen-3-yl-(4Z,7Z,10Z,13Z,16Z,19Z)-docosa-4,7,10,13,16,19-hexaenoate (**3**), deeply characterized by NMR spetroscopy. Modified quercetin and pectin were involved in a grafting process by an ecofriendly radical procedure able to preserve the biological features of the quercetin derivative. Antioxidant performances of the conjugate were evaluated both in term of total phenolic amount and scavenger activity in organic and aqueous environments. Additionally, in vitro acute oral toxicity was also tested against Caco-2 cells and 3T3 fibroblasts, confirming that pectin conjugate does not have any effect on cell viability at the dietary use concentrations. Finally, in vitro experiments highlighted the ability of the conjugate to counteract the migratory properties of Caco-2 and HepG2 cells, indicating its feature in the reduction of the migration of tumour cells. These data showed that the covalent binding of the quercetin derivative to the pectin chain represents a very interesting strategy to improve the bioavailability of the quercetin, representing an effective means of protecting and to transporting polyphenol molecules.

Keywords: quercetin; docosahexaenoic acid; pectin; polymeric conjugate; biological properties

Citation: Carullo, G.; Spizzirri, U.G.; Malivindi, R.; Rago, V.; Motta, M.F.; Lofaro, D.; Restuccia, D.; Aiello, F. Development of Quercetin-DHA Ester-Based Pectin Conjugates as New Functional Supplement: Effects on Cell Viability and Migration. *Nutraceuticals* **2022**, *2*, 278–288. https://doi.org/10.3390/nutraceuticals2040021

Academic Editor: Ivan Cruz-Chamorro

Received: 27 July 2022
Accepted: 30 September 2022
Published: 11 October 2022

Publisher's Note: MDPI stays neutral with regard to jurisdictional claims in published maps and institutional affiliations.

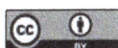

Copyright: © 2022 by the authors. Licensee MDPI, Basel, Switzerland. This article is an open access article distributed under the terms and conditions of the Creative Commons Attribution (CC BY) license (https://creativecommons.org/licenses/by/4.0/).

1. Introduction

Nowadays, to have a healthy human body, people are paying more attention to their foods, preferring minimally processed ones, consuming a large number of fruits and vegetables, and also taking nutraceuticals and dietary supplements [1–5]. Considering that the definition of "healthy food" can be ascribed to improved immune function, preventing specific diseases, and reducing side effects and health care costs, nutraceuticals comprise prebiotics, polyunsaturated fatty acids, probiotics, herbal products, and antioxidants, and consequently, the nutraceutical industry has encountered large consumer compliance so far [6]. Additionally, with both a growing population and the prevalence of chronic diseases as the population ages, future demands for eicosapentaenoic acid/docosahexaenoic acid (EPA/DHA) will further increase [7]. Recently, during the COVID-19 pandemic, scientific shreds of evidence confirmed that quercetin [8], astaxanthin, lactoferrin, glycyrrhizin, hesperidin, and curcumin have shown encouraging data in reverting long COVID-19 phenomena, suggesting their use in preventing and counteracting the symptoms of the infection [9,10]. In this work, we carried out the synthesis of a hybrid molecule, obtained by a Steglich coupling between quercetin and DHA, at position 3, and its grafting with pectin, to obtain a functional polymer, endowing better antioxidant performance of parent compounds and probably improving bioavailability. Quercetin is a flavonol characterized by the presence of an oxogroup at the 4 position and a 2,3-double bond on ring C, which allows conjugation between rings A and B and strongly affects the redox properties of this compound. They differ from the flavones for the presence of a nonphenolic hydroxyl group at the 3 position. Quercetin is the most powerful antioxidant flavonoid in nature, and it is present in many vegetal sources, particularly belonging to *Mangifera indica*, *Curcuma domestica valenton*, and others. In vitro experiments highlighted the anticancer, antidiabetic, antifungal, antibacterial, anti-inflammatory, antiobesity, antiviral, and neuroprotective properties of quercetin and its derivatives, as well as its feature to accelerate wound healing. These findings allowed for the employment of quercetin as an ingredient in the preparation of different nutraceuticals and cosmeceuticals [11]. The absorption of quercetin, broadly found in foods, is extremely variable relative to the type—and particularly the position—of sugar linked to the aglycone. The absorption of quercetin is strictly correlated to the food matrix, whilst plasma concentration of quercetin was found higher after onion intake than in red wine or tea. Some authors have demonstrated that absorption rate is not affected of the glucose position ($3'$ and $4'$) [12]. However, the main challenge related to the employment of the quercetin is its bioavailability, which appears particularly low (<10%). Poor water solubility, absorption profile, and chemical stability represent the main causes, and they could be overcome by encapsulating it in suitable macromolecular systems collected from food-grade ingredients. More effective nutraceuticals and functional foods can definitely be developed by improving the bioavailability of quercetin [13]. The nutraceutical effect of quercetin, assayed in vivo in two experiments, is measurable with the ability to work as an antioxidant and anti-inflammatory agent when the basal level of oxidative stress and inflammation is high. This scientific evidence confirms that quercetin supplementation is useful in people with diseases, but not in healthy ones. However, in chronic disorders, the safety of quercetin supplementation is still to be established [14]. In the last few years, there have been a lot of efforts to increase the bioavailability of active molecules, overcoming the problems often related to their poor solubility. Several systems have been developed to incorporate such compounds to improve stability, increase dispersion, and ensure maximum health benefits. There are many biopolymers already used for these purposes, and pectin displayed the best characteristics for the realization of macromolecular carriers for oral administration. Pectin is a linear heteropolysaccharide contained in the cell walls of plant tissues. More precisely, the name "pectin" refers to the compound extracted from fruit starting from the protopectin it contains. In particular, apples, apricots, and pears are rich in it (variable content from 1 to 1.5%), but also oranges (0.5–3.5%) and carrots (1.4%). Very high content of pectin is present in fruit peel; in that of oranges, the presence of the fibre in question is particularly high (about 30%) [15]. Alternative sources of pectin can be waste from the processing of sugar beet, mango, sunflowers, legumes, bananas, cabbage, carrots, and pomelo. In general, however, it would be more correct to speak of "pectins", because in nature there are different structures, the most common of which is composed of monomeric units of D-galacturonic acid joined together through α-(1→4) glycosidic bonds to form a long chain to which sugar functions such as rhamnose, arabinose, galactose, and xylose can bind, thus forming the side chains [15]. In this work, pectin was involved in an ecofriendly radical process, to synthesize polymeric conjugates with remarkable biological activities. Macromolecular compounds were deeply analysed in term of antioxidant activity and toxicity against Caco-2 and HepG2 cells, while their ability to counteract the migratory properties of cells was also investigated.

2. Materials and Methods
2.1. Chemistry

The synthesis of compound **3** was realized starting from **1**, which was previously protected as $3',4'$-diphenylmethylketal derivative by treating **1** with α,α-dichlorodiphenylmethane. The protected derivative **2** was then treated with docosahexaenoic acid in Steglich conditions to obtain the final compound, named **3**.

2.1.1. Synthesis of 2-(2,2-Diphenylbenzo[d][1,3]dioxol-5-yl)-3,5,7-trihydroxy-4H-chromen-4-one (2)

Compound **2** was synthesized according to our previous reported procedures (Scheme 1). Spectroscopic data are in line with those reported [16,17].

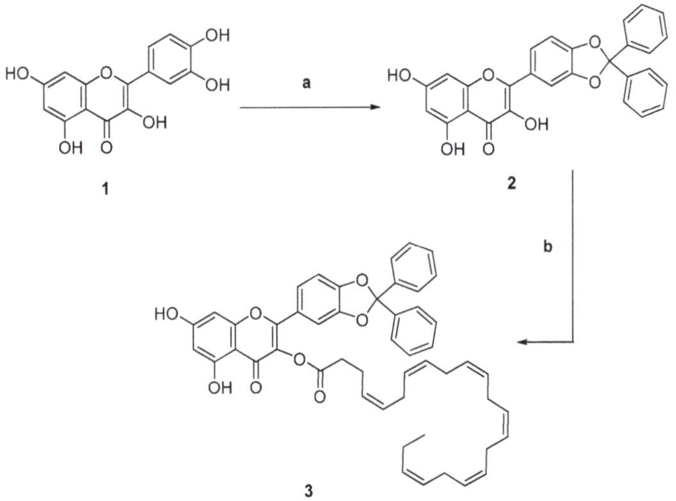

Scheme 1. Reagents and conditions: (**a**) α,α-dichlorodiphenylmethane, 180 °C, 10 min; (**b**) cervonic acid, N,N'-dicyclohexylcarbodiimmide, dry dichloromethane, 0 °C to RT, 24 h.

2.1.2. Synthesis of 2-(2,2-Diphenylbenzo[d][1,3]dioxol-5-yl)-5,7-dihydroxy-4-oxo-4H-chromen-3-yl (4Z,7Z,10Z,13Z,16Z,19Z)-Docosa-4,7,10,13,16,19-hexaenoate (3)

To a well-stirred solution of cervonic acid (128 µL, 0.386 mg) in dry DCM (2.0 mL) at 0 °C, N,N'-dicyclohexylcarbodiimmide (91.0 mg, 0.46 mmol) was added. The mixture was stirred for 1 h at 0 °C, after which **2** (180.0 mg, 0.39 mmol) was dropped and the resulting mixture warmed to RT and stirred for 23 h. The mixture was filtered on Celite® and treated with 5 mL of saturated $NaHCO_3$. The organic layer was dried, filtered, and evaporated under reduced pressure. The title compound **3** was purified through column chromatography (eluent n-hexanes/ethyl acetate 5:1 v/v) (Scheme 1). Yellow oil, 56% yield.
^{1}H NMR (300 MHz, DMSO-d_6) δ 11.5 (bs, 1H), 9.60 (bs, 1H), 7.7–7.3 (m, 11H), 7.25 (s, 1H), 7.10 (s, 1H), 6.90 (s, 1H), 6.20 (s, 1H), 5.5–5.0 (m, 12H), 4.1–3.8 (m, 9H), 2.9–2.6 (m, 2H), 2.4–2.2 (m, 2H), 2.0–1.9 (m, 2H), 1.3–1.0 (m, 2H). ^{13}C NMR (75 MHz, DMSO-d_6) δ 171.1, 170.1, 167.0, 159.8, 157.1, 154.0, 150.2, 143.0, 139.1, 133.3, 132.1, 131.9, 130.6, 129.1 (4C), 128.6, (3C), 128.3 (4C), 126.1 (3C), 126.0 (3C), 127.5 (2C), 122.0 (6C), 110.4, 98.8, 93.5, 39.10 (4C), 33.9, 25.6, 22.8, 20.5, 14.5. ESI-MS 775 [M-H]$^-$.

2.2. Disposable Phenolic Equivalents by Folin–Ciocalteu Procedure

Total phenolic groups were evaluated employing Folin–Ciocalteu procedure, according to the literature protocol with some changes [18]. In a volumetric flask 6.0 mL, of an aqueous solution of the active species was prepared, then 1.0 mL of the Folin–Ciocalteu reagent was added and mixed thoroughly. After 3 min, 3.0 mL of Na_2CO_3 (7.5% w/w) was added, and the mixture was intermittently shaken for 2 h. The absorbance was measured at 760 nm. Total phenolic equivalents were expressed as quercetin (Q) equivalent concentration (8.0, 16.0, 24.0, 32.0, and 40.0 µM). Least-squares method was employed to calculate a calibration curve, slope, correlation coefficient (R^2 = 0.9943), and intercept.

2.3. Total Antioxidant Activity

Total antioxidant activity of active species was investigated according to a literature protocol with some changes [19]. Briefly, 0.3 mL of an aqueous solution of the active species was mixed with 1.2 mL of reagent solution (28.0 M Na_3PO_4, 4.0 M $(NH_4)_2MoO_4$ and 0.6 M H_2SO_4,) and then incubated for 150 min at 95 °C. The solutions were analysed by a UV–Vis spectrophotometer (at 695 nm). The total antioxidant activities were expressed as catechin (CT) equivalent concentration, by recording a calibration curve at different antioxidants (8.0, 16.0, 24.0, 32.0, and 40.0 µM) and employing the method of least squares to calculate correlation coefficient (R^2), intercept, and slope of the regression equation.

2.4. Scavenging Activity against DPPH Radicals

Antioxidant species reacted with 2,2'-diphenyl-1-picrylhydrazyl radical (DPPH) free radicals to record their scavenging properties [20]. In each experiment, 12.5 mL of an aqueous solution of the active species was added to 12.5 mL of an ethanol solution of DPPH (200 µM) at 25 °C, and after 30 min, the absorbance was recorded (517 nm). The scavenging activity was expressed as percent inhibition of DPPH radicals, according to Equation (1):

$$\text{Inhibition (\%)} = (A_0 - A_1)/A_0 \times 100 \qquad (1)$$

where A_0 is the absorbance recorded in absence of active species, and A_1 is the absorbance recorded in presence of antioxidant compounds.

2.5. Scavenging Activity agaist ABTS Radical Cations

Scavenging properties of active species in the aqueous environment were evaluated against 2,2'-azino-bis(3-etylbenzotiazolin-6-sulphonic) radicals (ABTS) according to a literature protocol with some modifications [21,22]. An aqueous $ABTS^+$ solution able to guarantee an absorbance of 0.970 ± 0.020 at 734 nm was prepared. To evaluate the scavenging effect of the antioxidant compounds, 0.5 mL of each macromolecule solution was mixed with 2.0 mL of the ABTS radical solution and the mixture was incubated at 37 °C for 5 min. The antioxidant activity was expressed as a percentage of scavenging activity on the ABTS radical according to Equation (1).

2.6. Synthesis of Conjugates

Pectin conjugates were synthesized following a literature protocol with some modifications [23]. In a general procedure, 1.0 mL of H_2O_2 5.0 M (5.0 mmol) and 0.25 g of ascorbic acid (1.4 mmol) were added to 50.0 mL of pectin solution (10 mg mL^{-1}) at 25 °C. After 2 h, a suitable amount of extract corresponding to 0.150 mg of quercetin equivalent concentrations was added to the solution. After the reaction time, the mixture was dialysed by using dialysis membranes of 6–27/32" Medicell International LTD (MWCO: 10–12,000 Da). Purified pectin conjugates were checked to be free of unreacted low-molecular-weight molecules by liquid chromatography analysis (LC-DAD) of the washing medium. The purified solution was frozen and dried (Freeze drier Micro Modulyo, Edwards was employed) with a freeze drier to afford a vaporous solid. Additionally, blank pectin, exploited as a control, was prepared when the grafting process was carried out in absence of the antioxidant molecules.

2.7. Cell Culture

Balb/c 3T3 clone A31 cells were cultured in DMEM supplemented with 10% calf bovine serum and 1% penicillin-streptomycin. Caco-2 were maintained in MEM with fetal bovine serum (FBS) 20% (w/w), non-essential amino acids (1% w/w), L-glutamine (1% w/w) and penicillin–streptomycin (1% w/w), while HepG2 was cultured in MEM culture medium, supplemented with 10% FBS, non-essential amino acids (1% w/w), L-glutamine (1% w/w) and penicillin–streptomycin (1% w/w). The cells were grown in a 5% CO_2 atmosphere at 37 °C until 80% confluence, and subcultured twice a week. All cell lines were purchased from ATCC, Manassas, VA, USA.

2.8. Neutral Red Uptake (NRU)

The in vitro NRU test was described by the ISO 10993-5:2009 "Biological evaluation of medical devices-Part 5: Tests for in vitro cytotoxicity" on 3T3 cells. Cells with dimensions of 2.5×10^4 3T3 were treated with multiple concentrations of **PB**, **P_2**, and **P_3** overnight, in DMEM for 24 h at 37 °C and 5% CO_2 atmosphere. Cell viability was evaluated by neutral red uptake (NRU) assay, which included an incubation (3 h) with neutral red (50 µg/mL) followed by extraction with acetic acid, ethanol, and water (1:50:49 $v/v/v$) [24]. The absorbance was measured at 540 nm in a microplate reader Epoch (BioTek, Winooski, VT, USA). A percentage of viability was calculated as follows:

$$\%\text{Viability} = [\text{Abs}(540 \text{ nm})_{\text{test material}} - \text{Abs}(540 \text{ nm})_{\text{blank}}]/[\text{Abs}(540 \text{ nm})_{\text{control}} - \text{Abs}(540 \text{ nm})_{\text{blank}}] \quad (2)$$

2.9. Cell Viability Assay

Cell viability was measured by the 3-(4,5-dime-thylthiazol-2-yl)-2,5-diphenyltetrazolium (MTT) assay. The cells were seeded in 96-well plates at a density of 1×10^4 for Caco-2 and 2×10^4 for HepG2 and were synchronized in serum-free media (SFM) for 12 h. The cells were treated with increasing doses of **PB**, **P_2**, and **P_3**. After 24 h, 20 µL of MTT (5 mg mL^{-1}) was added to the cell media for 4 h. Finally, 200 µL of DMSO was added to each well, and the optical density was measured at 570 nm using a Beckman Coulter microplate reader [25]. Eight replicates were performed for each sample.

2.10. Wound-Healing Scratch Assay

Caco-2 and HepG2 cells were maintained in SFM for 12 h. The monolayers were scratched with a 100 µL pipet tip, as previously described [25]. After a wash with PBS, cells were treated with **PB**, **P_2**, and **P_3** for 24 h, and the resulting wound healing was photographed at 24 h at 4× magnifications using phase-contrast microscopy.

2.11. Statistical Analysis

Statistical analysis was performed by Student's t test using the GraphPad Prism 8.3.0 (GraphPad Software, Inc., San Diego, CA, USA). Antioxidant tests of the samples were assayed in triplicate. Data were expressed as means ± SD and analysed using the Wilcoxon test. A value of $p < 0.05$ was considered statistically significant. All analyses were conducted using GraphPad Prism 8.3.0 (GraphPad Software, Inc., San Diego, CA, USA).

3. Results

3.1. Antioxidant Performances

Antioxidant performances of **2** and **3** were deeply investigated in terms of total phenolic content, total antioxidant activity and scavenger activity against hydrophilic (ABTS) and lipophilic (DPPH) radical species, and the results are reported in Table 1.

Table 1. Antioxidant performances of **2** and **3**.

	Disposable Phenolic Groups (meq Q g^{-1})	Total Antioxidant Activity (meq CT g^{-1})	IC$_{50}$ (mg mL^{-1})	
			DPPH Radical	ABTS Radical
2	0.770 ± 0.011 [a]	0.866 ± 0.021 [a]	0.042 ± 0.005 [b]	0.153 ± 0.011 [b]
3	0.542 ± 0.010 [b]	0.580 ± 0.012 [b]	0.226 ± 0.015 [a]	0.530 ± 0.025 [a]

Q = quercetin; CT = catechin; DPPH = 2,2'-diphenyl-1-picrylhydrazyl radical; ABTS = 2,2'-azino-bis(3-etylbenzotiazolin-6-sulphonic). Different letters in the same column express significant differences ($p < 0.05$).

As expected, the chemical modification of **2** to **3** produced a significant reduction (29.6% lower) in phenolic content, and the total antioxidant capacity decreased by 33.0%. Additionally, the scavenging activities measured against DPPH and ABTS radical species displayed a substantial increase in IC_{50} values, which was more remarkable in the organic environment, concerning the aqueous medium. This loss of antioxidant performance can be attributed to the introduction of the docosahexaenoic acid in C_3, which is the disappearance of one of the reactive sites. At the same time, the spatial conformation of the hydrocarbon chain can hinder the interaction between the other hydroxylic groups and the radical species.

Widely used in the food industry, pectin is safe, passes through the gastrointestinal tract without any changes, and can be easily degraded by bacterial microflora in the colon. Among the many synthetic strategies proposed in the literature, for the synthesis of biopolymers coupled with antioxidant compounds, free-radical grafting is one of the most popular methods used due to its ability to avoid the generation of toxic by-products and perform chemical reactions at room temperature, thus preserving the molecules from degradation processes. Macromolecular conjugates were synthesized involving pectin as the polymeric structure, **2** and **3** as active molecules, and using the acid redox couple ascorbic acid/hydrogen peroxide, which constitutes a biocompatible and soluble radical initiation system [26]. The hydroxyl radical that starts the reaction is formed by the oxidation of ascorbic acid by hydrogen peroxide with the production of the ascorbate radical (Figure 1).

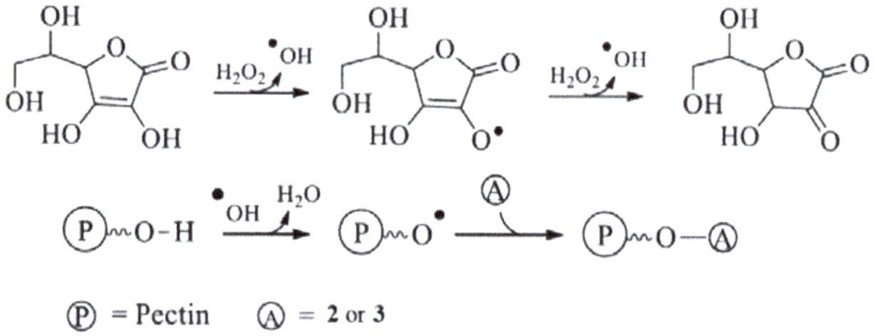

Figure 1. Schematic representation of the synthesis of the macromolecular conjugate.

The opportunity to graft antioxidant structures in a biomacromolecule by an ecofriendly procedure is an innovative strategy that significantly improves the performance of the natural compounds, opening new applications in the pharmaceutical field and in the food industry. The employment of the redox pair in the synthesis of the grafted biopolymer represents a synthetic strategy that allows for the preservation of antioxidant molecules from the damages related to the high temperatures. Additionally, these compounds avoid the production of toxic products, allowing for the employment of the final product in the food industry [27]. Finally the synthesis of polymeric antioxidants was a special deal able to guarantee a class of compounds having high stability and a slow degradation rate compared to the low-molecular-weight compounds [28].

The activation of the pectin toward radical reactions and the grafting of active species expects that the radical initiators preferably react with the macromolecule, avoiding self reactions. In Figure 1, a probable mechanism of interaction between active species and polysaccharide chains is proposed. Specifically, hydroxyl radicals attack the sensible residues in the side chains of the sugar, producing macroradical species in the sugar chain. The reaction of these radicals with the antioxidant molecules allows for the formation of a covalent bond between the antioxidant and the pectin. Literature data propose that ortho- and parapositions relative to the hydroxyl group are the main target of the free-radical macromolecule chains on the phenolic ring [29]. The heteroatom-centred radicals in the side chains of the pectin preferentially interact in some of the above-mentioned positions. This experimental strategy allowed for the synthesis of two pectin-based conjugates, labelled with the acronyms **P_2** and **P_3**. Additionally, a blank polymer (**PB**) was also synthesized, with pectin undergoing the same reaction but without any antioxidant molecules. Similarly, pectin–polyphenol conjugates were proposed by Karaki et al. that performed a grafting reaction via laccase catalysis methodology, employing ferulic acid as source on antioxidant moieties [30]. Ferulic acid was also involved in the synthesis of pectin conjugate by Wang et al., which activated reactive sites of ultrasound-treated pectins by vitamin C/hydrogen peroxide redox pair to obtain chain conformations more flexible than those of native sugar [31].

The antioxidant molecules' inclusion in the backbone of the polysaccharide was verified by measuring the antioxidant activity of the conjugates by the Folin–Ciocalteu test, total antioxidant capacity, and scavenger activity against DPPH and ABTS radicals, and the results are reported in Table 2.

Table 2. Antioxidant performances of pectin conjugates.

	Disposable Phenolic Groups (meq Q/g)	Total Antioxidant Activity (meq CT/g)	IC_{50} (mg mL^{-1})	
			DPPH Radical	**ABTS Radical**
P_2	0.243 ± 0.011 [a]	0.241 ± 0.008 [a]	0.480 ± 0.031 [a]	31.1% at 0.9 [a] mg mL^{-1}
P_3	0.051 ± 0.002 [b]	0.159 ± 0.009 [b]	44.1% at 1.3 [b] mg mL^{-1}	16.5% at 0.9 [b] mg mL^{-1}
PB	-	-	-	-

Q = quercetin; CT = catechin; DPPH = 2,2′-diphenyl-1- picrylhydrazyl radical; ABTS = 2,2′-azino-bis(3-etylbenzotiazolin-6-sulphonic). Different letters in the same column express significant differences ($p < 0.05$).

P_2 displayed the greatest antiradical activity: the polyphenolic content was significantly higher than **P_3**, which recorded a more than 30% increase in total antioxidant capacity. Disposable phenolic groups were in the same order of magnitude of the pectin–ferulic acid conjugates synthetized by employing ultrasound-treated pectins (0.335–0.386 meq of ferulic acid/g) that were able to ensure more flexible chains in respect to the native pectin [31]. Furthermore, between the two polymers, **P_2** was the only one able to reach the IC_{50}, while for **P_3** only 44.1% of inhibition was observed, at a concentration of 1.3 mg mL^{-1}. Wang et al. also recorded scavenging properties with IC_{50} values of about 0.5 mg mL^{-1}, while a reduced activity was recorded in the pectin conjugates synthesized by enzyme-catalysed grafting, due to the decrease in free hydroxyl groups that are involved in the covalent linkage. In the hydrophilic environment, against ABTS radicals, both polymers were poorly responsive; **P_2** reached an IC_{30} value, while **P_3** showed a 50% lower efficacy. This finding was confirmed by literature data that analysed the antioxidant activity of similar pectin conjugates [30,31]. Finally, **PB** did not show any activity.

3.2. Toxicity Evaluation

3.2.1. NRU Test

The effect of **PB**, **P_2**, and **P_3** on 3T3 cells was detected by in vitro NRU assay (Figure 2) The treatment with increasing doses of **PB**, **P_2**, and **P_3** did not alter cell viability versus control, in all treatments.

3.2.2. Cell Viability

As previously reported, quercetin has effects on the cell viability of tumour cell lines [32,33]. In this study, the cellular effects of **PB**, **P_2**, and **P_3** on cell motility were evaluated by MTT assay. This assay evaluates mitochondrial activity through the formation of the purple formazan in metabolically active cells, an NADP-dependent reaction catalysed by succinate dehydrogenase. This reaction was evaluated by measuring absorbance using a spectrophotometer [34]. Figure 3 shows the treatments with increasing concentrations of **PB**, **P_2**, and **P_3**. The results indicate a dose-dependent reduction in cell viability after treatment with **P_2** and **P_3**. On the contrary, the treatment with **PB** did not produce any effect.

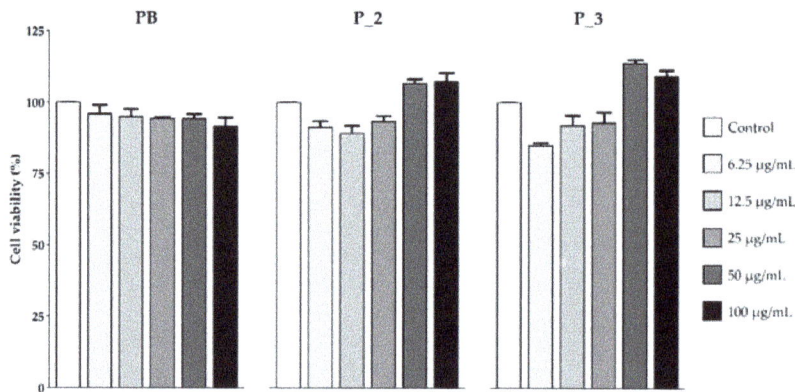

Figure 2. 3T3 cells' viability (%) after treatment with increased concentrations of **PB**, **P_2**, and **P_3** (µg mL^{-1}). Each column represents the mean + SD of 3 wells/group.

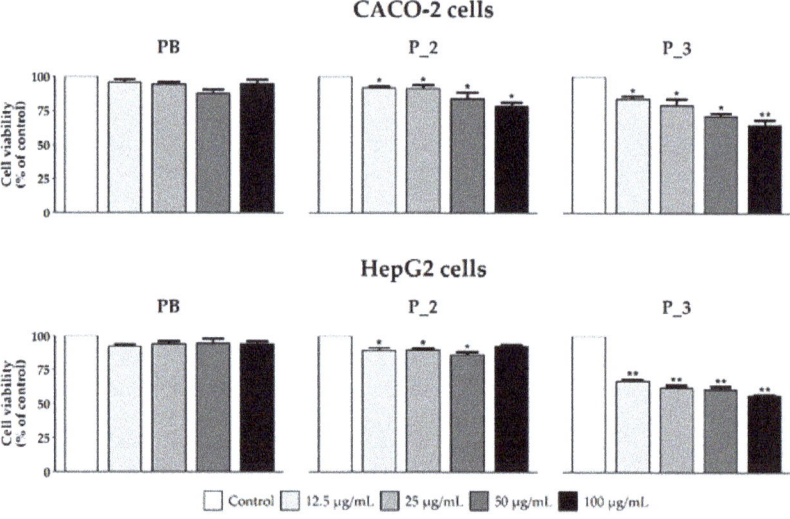

Figure 3. Effect of **PB**, **P_2**, and **P_3** on Caco-2 and HepG2 cells' viability. Each column represents the mean + SD of 3 wells/group. * $p < 0.01$; ** $p < 0.005$ treated vs. control.

3.2.3. Cells' Migratory Capability

Many studies report the effects of quercetin on cell motility in different intestinal cancer cell lines [32,33]. The capacity of **PB**, **P_2**, and **P_3** to oppose the migratory ability of Caco-2 and HepG2 cells is shown in Figure 4. The results obtained showed that **P_2** and **P_3** reduce the migration of tumour cells, while **PB** has no effect.

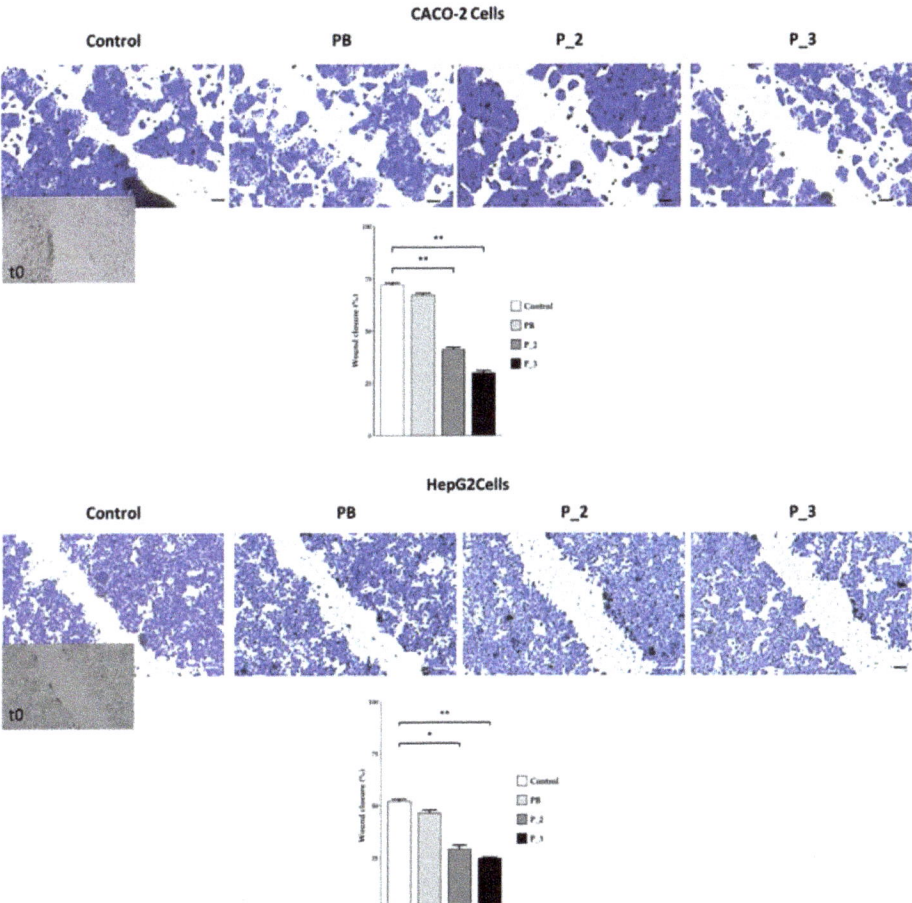

Figure 4. A wound-healing assay on Caco-2 and HepG2 cells after treatment with of **PB**, **P_2**, and **P_3** (50 μg mL^{-1}). The percentage of closure was quantified by ImageJ after 24 h. Scale bars: 100 μm, * $p < 0.01$; ** $p < 0.005$ treated vs. control.

4. Conclusions

Quercetin derivatives displayed a remarkable antioxidant performance, as well as scavenger activity both in organic and aqueous environments. The inclusion of the synthesized molecules into a polymeric matrix is a useful tool to improve their application in the pharmaceutical and nutraceutical fields. In this regard, pectin was chosen as the polymeric backbone due to its chemical and biological characteristics compatible with our purposes, and an ecofriendly strategy was selected to preserve the biological features of the quercetin derivative. In vitro tests performed on the synthesized polymers highlighted a reduction in the antioxidant activity that was retained. However, our results indicated that quercetin reduced cell viability and migration, as indicated in previous reports [35,36]. These data suggest that quercetin slowed the growth and migration of Caco-2 and Hepg-2 cell lines. These data appear very interesting because they provide a useful alternative aimed to improve the bioavailability of quercetin-derivatives through their covalent binding to the pectin chain, which becomes a very versatile and effective means to transport polyphenol compounds, both in terms of protection of the polyphenol itself and in terms of biological activity manifested in the matrices in which it will be used.

Author Contributions: Conceptualization, U.G.S., G.C., D.R. and F.A.; methodology, G.C., U.G.S. and R.M.; validation, U.G.S., F.A. and R.M.; formal analysis, U.G.S., G.C., V.R. and M.F.M.; investigation, U.G.S., G.C. and R.M.; resources, D.R. and F.A.; data curation, G.C., U.G.S., V.R. and D.L.; writing—original draft preparation, U.G.S., G.C., R.M. and F.A.; writing—review and editing, U.G.S., G.C., V.R., D.L., D.R. and F.A.; visualization, G.C. and V.R.; supervision, D.R. and F.A.; funding acquisition, D.R. and F.A. All authors have read and agreed to the published version of the manuscript.

Funding: This research received no external funding.

Institutional Review Board Statement: Not applicable.

Informed Consent Statement: Not applicable.

Data Availability Statement: Not applicable.

Conflicts of Interest: The authors declare no conflict of interest.

References

1. Carullo, G.; Ahmed, A.; Fusi, F.; Sciubba, F.; Di Cocco, M.E.; Restuccia, D.; Spizzirri, U.G.; Saponara, S.; Aiello, F. Vasorelaxant Effects Induced by Red Wine and Pomace Extracts of Magliocco Dolce cv. *Pharmaceuticals* **2020**, *13*, 87. [CrossRef]
2. Carullo, G.; Ahmed, A.; Trezza, A.; Spiga, O.; Brizzi, A.; Saponara, S.; Fusi, F.; Aiello, F. A multitarget semi-synthetic derivative of the flavonoid morin with improved in vitro vasorelaxant activity: Role of CaV1.2 and KCa1.1 channels. *Biochem. Pharmacol.* **2021**, *185*, 114429. [CrossRef] [PubMed]
3. Carullo, G.; Mazzotta, S.; Koch, A.; Hartmann, K.M.; Friedrich, O.; Gilbert, D.F.; Vega-Holm, M.; Schneider-Stock, R.; Aiello, F. New oleoyl hybrids of natural antioxidants: Synthesis and in vitro evaluation as inducers of apoptosis in colorectal cancer cells. *Antioxidants* **2020**, *9*, 1077. [CrossRef]
4. Mazzotta, S.; Governa, P.; Borgonetti, V.; Marcolongo, P.; Nanni, C.; Gamberucci, A.; Manetti, F.; Pessina, F.; Carullo, G.; Brizzi, A.; et al. Pinocembrin and its linolenoyl ester derivative induce wound healing activity in HaCaT cell line potentially involving a GPR120/FFA4 mediated pathway. *Bioorg. Chem.* **2021**, *108*, 104657. [CrossRef]
5. Carullo, G.; Ahmed, A.; Trezza, A.; Spiga, O.; Brizzi, A.; Saponara, S.; Fusi, F.; Aiello, F. Design, synthesis and pharmacological evaluation of ester-based quercetin derivatives as selective vascular KCa1.1 channel stimulators. *Bioorg. Chem.* **2020**, *105*, 104404. [CrossRef] [PubMed]
6. Hoti, G.; Matencio, A.; Pedrazzo, A.R.; Cecone, C.; Appleton, S.L.; Monfared, Y.K.; Caldera, F.; Trotta, F. Nutraceutical Concepts and Dextrin-Based Delivery Systems. *Int. J. Mol. Sci.* **2022**, *23*, 4102. [CrossRef] [PubMed]
7. Panchal, S.K.; Brown, L. Addressing the insufficient availability of epa and dha to meet current and future nutritional demands. *Nutrients* **2021**, *13*, 2855. [CrossRef] [PubMed]
8. Imran, M.; Thabet, H.K.; Alaqel, S.I.; Alzahrani, A.R.; Abida, A.; Alshammari, M.K.; Kamal, M.; Diwan, A.; Asdaq, S.M.B.; Alshehri, S. The Therapeutic and Prophylactic Potential of Quercetin against COVID-19: An Outlook on the Clinical Studies, Inventive Compositions, and Patent Literature. *Antioxidants* **2022**, *11*, 876. [CrossRef]
9. Alesci, A.; Aragona, M.; Cicero, N.; Lauriano, E.R. Can nutraceuticals assist treatment and improve COVID-19 symptoms? *Nat. Prod. Res.* **2022**, *36*, 2672–2691. [CrossRef] [PubMed]
10. Pastor, N.; Collado, M.C.; Manzoni, P. Phytonutrient and nutraceutical action against COVID-19: Current review of characteristics and benefits. *Nutrients* **2021**, *13*, 464. [CrossRef] [PubMed]
11. Azeem, M.; Hanif, M.; Mahmood, K.; Ameer, N.; Chughtai, F.R.S.; Abid, U. An insight into anticancer, antioxidant, antimicrobial, antidiabetic and anti-inflammatory effects of quercetin: A review. *Polym. Bull.* **2022**. [CrossRef] [PubMed]
12. Barreca, D.; Trombetta, D.; Smeriglio, A.; Mandalari, G.; Romeo, O.; Felice, M.R.; Gattuso, G.; Nabavi, S.M. Food flavonols: Nutraceuticals with complex health benefits and functionalities. *Trends Food Sci. Technol.* **2021**, *117*, 194–204. [CrossRef]
13. Kandemir, K.; Tomas, M.; McClements, D.J.; Capanoglu, E. Recent advances on the improvement of quercetin bioavailability. *Trends Food Sci. Technol.* **2022**, *119*, 192–200. [CrossRef]
14. Boots, A.W.; Haenen, G.R.M.M.; Bast, A. Health effects of quercetin: From antioxidant to nutraceutical. *Eur. J. Pharmacol.* **2008**, *585*, 325–337. [CrossRef] [PubMed]
15. Sriamornsak, P. Application of pectin in oral drug delivery. *Expert Opin. Drug Deliv.* **2011**, *8*, 1009–1023. [CrossRef] [PubMed]
16. Badolato, M.; Carullo, G.; Perri, M.; Cione, E.; Manetti, F.; Di Gioia, M.L.; Brizzi, A.; Caroleo, M.C.; Aiello, F. Quercetin/oleic acid-based G-protein-coupled receptor 40 ligands as new insulin secretion modulators. *Future Med. Chem.* **2017**, *9*, 1873–1885. [CrossRef]
17. Carullo, G.; Perri, M.; Manetti, F.; Aiello, F.; Caroleo, M.C.; Cione, E. Quercetin-3-oleoyl derivatives as new GPR40 agonists: Molecular docking studies and functional evaluation. *Bioorg. Med. Chem. Lett.* **2019**, *29*, 1761–1764. [CrossRef]
18. Spizzirri, U.G.; Abduvakhidov, A.; Caputo, P.; Crupi, P.; Muraglia, M.; Oliviero Rossi, C.; Clodoveo, M.L.; Aiello, F.; Restuccia, D. Kefir Enriched with Carob (*Ceratonia siliqua* L.) Leaves Extract as a New Ingredient during a Gluten-Free Bread-Making Process. *Fermentation* **2022**, *8*, 305. [CrossRef]

19. Restuccia, D.; Giorgi, G.; Gianfranco Spizzirri, U.; Sciubba, F.; Capuani, G.; Rago, V.; Carullo, G.; Aiello, F. Autochthonous white grape pomaces as bioactive source for functional jams. *Int. J. Food Sci. Technol.* **2019**, *54*, 1313–1320. [CrossRef]
20. Spizzirri, U.G.; Carullo, G.; De Cicco, L.; Crispini, A.; Scarpelli, F.; Restuccia, D.; Aiello, F. Synthesis and characterization of a (+)-catechin and L-(+)-ascorbic acid cocrystal as a new functional ingredient for tea drinks. *Heliyon* **2019**, *5*, e02291. [CrossRef]
21. Carullo, G.; Spizzirri, U.G.; Loizzo, M.R.; Leporini, M.; Sicari, V.; Aiello, F.; Restuccia, D. Valorization of red grape (Vitis vinifera cv. Sangiovese) pomace as functional food ingredient. *Ital. J. Food Sci.* **2020**, *32*, 367–385. [CrossRef]
22. Restuccia, D.; Sicari, V.; Pellicanò, T.M.; Spizzirri, U.G.; Loizzo, M.R. The impact of cultivar on polyphenol and biogenic amine profiles in Calabrian red grapes during winemaking. *Food Res. Int.* **2017**, *102*, 303–312. [CrossRef]
23. Carullo, G.; Scarpelli, F.; Belsito, E.L.; Caputo, P.; Oliviero Rossi, C.; Mincione, A.; Leggio, A.; Crispini, A.; Restuccia, D.; Spizzirri, U.G.; et al. Formulation of New Baking (+)-Catechin Based Leavening Agents: Effects on Rheology, Sensory and Antioxidant Features during Muffin Preparation. *Foods* **2020**, *9*, 1569. [CrossRef]
24. Stokes, W.S.; Casati, S.; Strickland, J.; Paris, M. Neutral Red Uptake Cytotoxicity Tests for Estimating Starting Doses for Acute Oral Toxicity Tests. *Curr. Protoc. Toxicol.* **2008**, *36*, 20–24. [CrossRef] [PubMed]
25. Bossio, S.; Perri, A.; Malivindi, R.; Giordano, F.; Rago, V.; Mirabelli, M.; Salatino, A.; Brunetti, A.; Greco, E.A.; Aversa, A. Oleuropein Counteracts Both the Proliferation and Migration of Intra- and Extragonadal Seminoma Cells. *Nutrients* **2022**, *14*, 2323. [CrossRef] [PubMed]
26. Spizzirri, U.G.; Carullo, G.; Aiello, F.; Paolino, D.; Restuccia, D. Valorisation of olive oil pomace extracts for a functional pear beverage formulation. *Int. J. Food Sci. Technol.* **2021**, *56*, 5497–5505. [CrossRef]
27. Mishra, A.; Clark, J.H.; Vij, A.; Daswal, S. Synthesis of graft copolymers of xyloglucan and acrylonitrile. *Polym. Adv. Technol.* **2008**, *19*, 99–104. [CrossRef]
28. Pan, J.-Q.; Liu, N.C.; Lau, W.W.Y. Preparation and properties of new antioxidants with higher MW. *Polym. Degrad. Stab.* **1998**, *62*, 165–170. [CrossRef]
29. Kitagawa, M.; Tokiwa, Y. Polymerization of vinyl sugar ester using ascorbic acid and hydrogen peroxide as a redox reagent. *Carbohydr. Polym.* **2006**, *64*, 218–223. [CrossRef]
30. Karaki, N.; Aljawish, A.; Muniglia, L.; Humeau, C.; Jasniewski, J. Physico-chemical characterization of pectin grafted with exogenous phenols. *Food Hydrocoll.* **2016**, *60*, 486–493. [CrossRef]
31. Wang, C.; Cai, W.-D.; Yao, J.; Wu, L.-X.; Li, L.; Zhu, J.; Yan, J.-K. Conjugation of ferulic acid onto pectinaffected the physicochemical, functionaland antioxidant properties. *J. Sci. Food Agric.* **2020**, *100*, 5352–5362. [CrossRef] [PubMed]
32. Han, M.; Song, Y.; Zhang, X. Quercetin suppresses the migration and invasion in human colon cancer caco-2 cells through regulating toll-like receptor 4/nuclear factor-kappa B pathway. *Pharmacogn. Mag.* **2016**, *12*, 237–244. [CrossRef]
33. Zhou, J.; Fang, L.; Liao, J.; Li, L.; Yao, W.; Xiong, Z.; Zhou, X. Investigation of the anti-cancer effect of quercetin on HepG2 cells in vivo. *PLoS ONE* **2017**, *12*, e0172838. [CrossRef] [PubMed]
34. Liu, Y.; Nair, M.G. An Efficient and Economical MTT Assay for Determining the Antioxidant Activity of Plant Natural Product Extracts and Pure Compounds. *J. Nat. Prod.* **2010**, *73*, 1193–1195. [CrossRef] [PubMed]
35. Fernández-Palanca, P.; Fondevila, F.; Méndez-Blanco, C.; Tuñón, M.J.; González-Gallego, J.; Mauriz, J.L. Antitumor effects of quercetin in hepatocarcinoma in vitro and in vivo models: A systematic review. *Nutrients* **2019**, *11*, 2875. [CrossRef] [PubMed]
36. Wu, L.; Li, J.; Liu, T.; Li, S.; Feng, J.; Yu, Q.; Zhang, J.; Chen, J.; Zhou, Y.; Ji, J.; et al. Quercetin shows anti-tumor effect in hepatocellular carcinoma LM3 cells by abrogating JAK2/STAT3 signaling pathway. *Cancer Med.* **2019**, *8*, 4806–4820. [CrossRef] [PubMed]

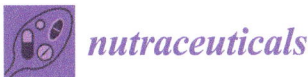

Article

Modulating the Gut Microbiota with Alginate Oligosaccharides In Vitro

Grégoire Bouillon [1,2,†], Olav Gåserød [2,‡], Łukasz Krych [1], Josué L. Castro-Mejía [1], Witold Kot [3], Markku T. Saarinen [4], Arthur C. Ouwehand [4,*], Dennis S. Nielsen [1] and Fergal P. Rattray [1,§]

[1] Department of Food Science, University of Copenhagen, Rolighedsvej 26, Frederiksberg C, DK-1958 Copenhagen, Denmark
[2] International Flavors and Fragrances, Industriveien 33, N-1337 Sandvika, Norway
[3] Department of Plant and Environmental Sciences, University of Copenhagen, Thorvaldsensvej 40, Frederiksberg C, DK-1871 Copenhagen, Denmark
[4] International Flavors and Fragrances, Sokeritehtaantie 20, 02460 Kantvik, Finland
[*] Correspondence: arthur.ouwehand@iff.com; Tel.: +358-40-5956-353
[†] Current address: Chr. Hansen A/S, Bøge Alle 10, 2970 Hørsholm, Denmark.
[‡] Current address: Gnosis by Lesaffre, Mustads vei 1, 0283 Oslo, Norway.
[§] Current address: Novozymes A/S, Biologensvej, 2, DK-2800 Lyngby, Denmark.

Abstract: Alginate oligosaccharides (AOS) are non-digestible carbohydrates from brown kelp. As such, they are dietary fibers and may have prebiotic potential. Therefore, we investigated the capacity of gut bacteria to utilize AOS with single-strain cultures and as a complex bacterial community. *Bifidobacterium adolescentis*, *Lacticaseibacillus casei* and *Lacticaseibacillus paracasei* showed weak growth (relative to unsupplemented medium; $p < 0.05$) in the presence of AOS and alginate, while strong growth ($p < 0.01$) was observed for *Bacteroides ovatus* when grown with alginate as carbohydrate source. *Enterococcus faecium* and *Enterococcus hirae* were for the first time reported to be able to grow on AOS. Further, AOS as substrate was investigated in a complex bacterial community with colonic fermentations in an in vitro gut model. The in vitro gut model indicated that AOS increased short-chain fatty acid (SCFA) levels in donors with a low endogenous SCFA production, but not to the same level as inulin. *Bacteroides* was found to dominate the bacteria community after in vitro gut simulation with alginate as substrate. Further, stimulation of *Bacteroides* was observed with AOS in the gut model for two out of three donors with the third donor being more resistant to change. Our results allowed the identification of AOS utilizers among common gut species. The results also demonstrated the capacity of AOS to elevate SCFA levels and positively modulate the gut microbiota during in vitro simulated colon fermentations, although some subjects appear to be resilient to perturbation via substrate changes.

Keywords: prebiotic; alginate; alginate oligosaccharides; intestinal microbiota; microbial metabolites; short-chain fatty acids; colon simulation

1. Introduction

In recent decades, development of functional foods has rapidly become a major focus of research [1]. The capacity of a food ingredient to selectively stimulate the growth of beneficial microbes is a key criterion for a prebiotic effect [2]. Numerous studies have been conducted to better understand the role and composition of the gut microbiota (GM) and its modulation by nutrition [3]. The composition of the GM has been reported to be highly variable even among people of the same region of the world [4]. Moreover, although a large number of oligosaccharides have been studied for prebiotic effects and are commonly incorporated into certain food preparations [5] their utilization by beneficial and nonbeneficial microbes is still open to different interpretations [6]. This underlines the need for a deeper understanding of the modulatory effect of a prebiotic food ingredient on the GM prior to its incorporation in a food product.

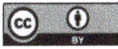

Alginate is an abundant polymer and represents up to 40% of the dry matter of brown seaweed, with about 30,000 metric tons produced industrially every year [7]. Alginate is a linear and naturally occurring copolymer of two main sugars: β-D-mannuronate (M) and α-L-guluronate (G) linked in 1,4-glycosidic bonds and organized in consecutive G residues (GGGGGG), M residues (MMMMMM), or alternating M and G residues (GMGMGM) [8]. Alginate is used in the food industry as a thickening agent with its viscosity directly correlated to its molecular weight and concentration. Moreover, alginate has the ability to form heat-stable gels through G-block-Ca^{2+} interactions described as the "egg-box model", where the calcium ions sit in the structural void of the polymer and form hydrogels by trapping water molecules [9]. Consequently, the gelling and thickening properties of alginate make it one of the most extensively used additives in the food industry [10,11].

The depolymerized form of alginate known as alginate oligosaccharide (AOS) has been investigated for diverse applications in the food and agriculture industries but also for human health applications [12]. Alginate is poorly digested in vivo, and the porcine microbiota has been reported to require a 39-day adaptation period prior to being able to degrade the oligomer [13]. After adaptation, the porcine microbiota was able to successfully utilize a broad range of AOS [14]. In rats, daily intake of AOS (2.5% of diet) over a two-week period increased fecal bifidobacteria and lactobacilli by 13-fold and 5-fold, respectively, while the abundance of *Enterobacteriaceae* and enterococci decreased [15]. However, in vitro fermentation of AOS using pig fecal samples or human fecal samples increased the abundance of *Bacteroides* and the production of short-chain fatty acids (SCFA), with no effect on the bifidobacteria or lactobacilli community [16,17]. *Bacteroides ovatus* was also established as the main gut bacterium able to degrade the 1,4-glycosidic bond of alginate [18]. While current literature indicates different effects of AOS on the gut microbiota, it also clearly demonstrates its potential as a gut microbiota modulatory agent.

In this study, a screening of several main representative bacteria of the GM was carried out in a single-strain approach to investigate their capacity to use AOS for growth. The modulation of the GM by the fermentation of AOS was further investigated using an in vitro colon model, CoMiniGut [19]. The dynamics of the simulated GM community was studied using Illumina-based NxtSeq-based 16S rRNA gene amplicon high throughput sequencing, and SCFA production was estimated using gas-chromatography analysis. To the best of our knowledge this study is the first to combine the single-strain approach of a broad range of gut bacteria with the use of an in vitro gut model, and will help to reach a better understanding of the prebiotic potential of AOS.

2. Materials and Methods

2.1. Substrates and Strains

Sodium alginate was extracted from the stem of the brown seaweed *Laminaria hyperborea* (supplied by IFF, Sandvika, Norway). The alginate was subsequently subjected to high-temperature acid hydrolysis, followed by neutralization with Na_2CO_3 before spray drying in order to produce the alginate oligosaccharide (AOS) with a purity of at least 90% [20]. Inulin was purchased from Sigma Aldrich (Søborg, Denmark). All bacteria used in the Bioscreen C study (Table 1) were collected from frozen stocks kept at both IFF facilities and the University of Copenhagen, or supplied from public collections. These strains were selected according to the following criteria: relevance for human gut microbiota and with published work with AOS, to investigate potential pre- and probiotic synergy, and availability in the culture collections.

Table 1. Growth after 24 h under anaerobic conditions of gut bacteria in basal medium supplemented with either glucose, AOS, alginate or inulin (n = 6).

Species	Source *	Strain Name	Glucose [a]	AOS [a]	Alginate [b]	Inulin [a]
Bifidobacterium breve	BCCM/LMG	LMG 13208	+++	-	-	-
Bifidobacterium longum	IFF	Bl-05	+++	-	-	-
Bifidobacterium lactis	IFF	Bl-04	+++	-	-	-
Bifidobacterium bifidum	IFF	Bb-06	+++	-	-	+++
Bifidobacterium adolescentis	DSMZ	DSM 20083	+++	+	+	+++
Bacteroides vulgatus	BCCM/LMG	LMG 17767	+++	-	-	-
Bacteroides acidifaciens	DSMZ	DSM 15896	+++	-	-	-
Bacteroides thetaiotaomicron	DSMZ	DSM 2079	+++	-	-	-
Bacteroides fragilis	DSMZ	DSM 2151	+++	-	-	-
Bacteroides ovatus	DSMZ	DSM 1896	+++	-	++	-
Escherichia coli	ATCC	ATCC 43888	+++	-	-	+++
Enterobacter cloacae	UCPH	NTCT 11572	+++	-	-	-
Klebsiella pneumoniae	UCPH	c132-98 WT	+++	-	-	-
Salmonella enterica Typhimurium	UCPH	SML 27C	+++	-	-	-
Cronobacter sakazakii	DSMZ	DSM 4485	+++	-	+	-
Lactobacillus acidophilus	BCCM/LMG	LMG 9433	+++	-	-	-
Lacticaseibacillus rhamnosus	DSMZ	DSM 20021	+++	-	-	-
Lacticaseibacillus casei	DSMZ	DSM 20011	+++	+	+	-
Lacticaseibacillus paracasei	NCIMB	NCFB 151	+++	+	+	+++
Enterococcus faecium	DSMZ	DSM 2146	+++	+	-	++
Enterococcus hirae	DSMZ	DSM 3320	+++	+	+	++
Clostridium clostridioforme	DSMZ	DSM 933	+++	-	-	-
Anaerostipes hardus	DSMZ	DSM 3319	+++	-	-	-

[a] added at 10 g L^{-1}; [b] added at 4 g L^{-1} (-) no growth; (+) weak growth; (++) moderate growth; (+++) strong growth.
* Source of bacteria strain: Belgium Coordinated Collection of Microorganism (BCCM/LMG); German Collection of Microorganism and Cell Culture (DSMZ); International Flavors & Fragrances (IFF); National Collection of Industrial, Food and Marine Bacteria (NCIMB); American Type Culture Collection (ATCC); University of Copenhagen (UCPH).

2.2. Basal Colon Media

Basal medium was prepared as described by Wiese et al. [19]. Briefly, the following reagents (all purchased from Merck, Darmstadt, Germany) were dissolved in one liter of ultrapure water (Milli-Q®, Merck, Darmstadt, Germany): 0.5 g bile salts, 2 g peptone, 2 g yeast extract, 0.1 g NaCl, 0.04 g K_2HPO_4, 0.04 g KH_2PO_4, 0.01 g $MgSO_4 \cdot 7H_2O$, 0.01 g $CaCl_2 \cdot 6H_2O$, 2 g $NaHCO_3$ and 2 mL Tween-80. After full dissolution, the pH of the medium was adjusted to 5.6 using 1M HCl and anaerobic conditions were generated using the Hungate boiling system prior to autoclaving at 121 °C for 20 min. Finally, 0.002 g hemin, 10 µL vitamin K1 and 0.5 g L-cysteine HCl were aseptically added under anaerobic conditions. The medium was further supplemented with 10 g L^{-1} of glucose, AOS or inulin, used as a reference prebiotic. A concentration of 4 g L^{-1} of alginate was used to avoid too high a level of viscosity. Once all ingredients were fully dissolved, the medium was filter-sterilized and kept anaerobically at 4 °C in the dark, prior to use in both in vitro screening method using Bioscreen C (Growth Curves Ltd., Helsinki, Finland) and in vitro fermentation within the CoMiniGut.

2.3. Single-Strain Growth Experiment

The single-strain growth experiment was performed as described by Mäkeläinen et al. [21]. Prior to each run, pre-cultures were prepared in fresh glucose containing medium to maximize the growth over 24 h. The cultures were centrifuged at 4000× g for 10 min at 4 °C. The pellet was resuspended in saline solution (0.9% NaCl) and diluted accordingly to obtain a 10^6 CFU mL^{-1} inoculum. Twenty µL of inoculum was anaerobically added to 180 µL of each medium into a 10 × 10-well honeycomb plate. All treatments and appropriate controls were tested in triplicate, and every experiment was performed in duplicate (n = 6). Incubation was carried out using a Bioscreen C. Anaerobic conditions (80% N_2, 10% H_2, and 10% CO_2) were maintained using a Concept 400 anaerobic chamber (Ruskin Technologies, Leeds, UK). The optical density (OD 600 nm) was measured every 30 min for 24 h. The area under the curve for each growth kinetic was computed after subtracting the blank values. Significant differences between data sets compared to the basal medium were determined by two-way ANOVA, and $p < 0.05$ was considered significant.

2.4. Faecal Sample Preparation

Fresh stool samples were collected from 3 healthy adults (18–65 years of age), healthy as self-reported and without antibiotics or probiotics intake 3 months prior to donation. The samples were donated anonymously and no further details were collected in accordance with the ethical approval (Ethical Committee of the Capital Region of Denmark, registration number H-20028549) were collected and homogenized in a 1:1 ratio with phosphate saline solution (per liter: 8 g NaCl, 0.2 g KCl, 1.44 g Na_2HPO_4 and 0.24 g K_2HPO_4) with 30% (v/v) glycerol in a stomacher bag for 120 s using a stomacher (Stomacher 400; Seward, Worthing, UK) at medium speed. Due to limitation in the collection process, fecal slurries with a final glycerol content of 15% (v/v) were aliquoted into cryotubes and stored at −60 °C prior to further use to minimize variation between fermentation. Faecal sample preparations were used separately and not pooled.

2.5. In Vitro Gut Model CoMiniGut

The in vitro gut fermentations were carried out using the CoMiniGut model as described by Wiese et al. [19]. In brief, the model consisted of a climate box with five parallel anaerobic reactor units. A circulating water bath connected to a heat-exchange plate and coupled with a ventilation system ensured a stable and evenly distributed heat throughout the experiment within the climate box. Each unit contained a 5 mL reaction vessel with a magnetic stirrer, an anaerogen bag (AN0020D; ThermoScientific, Waltham, MA, USA) and a resazurin indicator (Anaerobe Indicator Test; Sigma-Aldrich, St. Louis, MO, USA). The units were placed on a magnetic stirrer bench and pH probes were inserted into each reactor. The pH was monitored using a 6-channel pH meter and a data logger (Consort multi-parameter analyzer C3040) and connected to a laptop running Matlab scripts for pH control (ver. R2015a; The MathWorks, Inc., Natick, MA, USA). The pH was maintained at the desired level during the fermentation by addition of 0.5 M NaOH through a multi-channel syringe pump connected to the reactors using injection needles (Frisenette, Knebel, Østjylland, Denmark) and controlled by the Matlab script. The pH was set to incrementally increase from 5.7 to 6.1 over the first 8 h of fermentation to mimic the proximal colon, from 6.1 to 6.5 over the following 8 h to mimic the transverse colon and from 6.5 to 6.8 over the last 8 h to mimic the distal colon.

2.6. Fermentation Conditions

The five reactor units were assembled the day prior to the experiment to generate anaerobic conditions. Fecal glycerol stocks were thawed for 30 min at refrigerated temperatures prior to the experiment. One millilitre of fecal stock (1:1 ratio of fecal matter with PBS 15% glycerol) was diluted with 4 mL of 0.1 M PBS pH 5.6. CoMiniGut reaction vessels were aseptically filled with 4.5 mL of basal medium and further inoculated with 0.5 mL of fecal slurry to achieve a final inoculation at 1% original fecal matter. Using the control media or media supplemented with AOS, alginate or inulin, the fermentations were performed for each fecal sample in quadruplicate. After 24 h, the products of fermentation were aliquoted in cryotubes and kept at −60 °C until further analysis.

2.7. SCFA Analysis

The level of acetic, butyric, propionic, valeric, isobutyric, 2-methylbutyric, isovaleric and lactic acids were measured as previously described by Ouwehand et al. [22]. One hundred µL of internal standard (20 mM pivalic acid) was mixed with 300 µL of water, 250 µL of saturated oxalic acid solution and added to 100 µL of the simulator sample. After thorough mixing, the sample was kept at 4 °C for 60 min and subsequently centrifuged at $13,000 \times g$ for 5 min. Supernatant (1 mL) was analyzed by GC using a glass column packed with 80/120 Carbopack B-DA/4% on Carbowax 20M stationary phase (Supelco, Bellefonte, PA, USA) at 175 °C and with helium as the carrier gas at a flow rate of 24 mL min^{-1}. The temperature of the injector and the flame ionization detector were 200 and 250 °C, respectively. The concentration of acetic acid, propionic acid and butyric acid were determined using previously established standard curves. One-way ANOVA was performed (significance level $p < 0.05$) using the package "ggpubr" of the Rstudio platform.

2.8. DNA Extraction

One hundred µL from each gut reactor was used for genomic DNA extraction using the Bead-beat Micro AX Gravity kit (A&A Biotechnology, Gdynia, Poland) following the protocol of the manufacturer. The bead-beating step was performed in 3 cycles of 15 s each at a speed of 6.5 ms^{-1} in a FastPrep-24TM Homogenizer (MP) at room temperature. DNA quantity was measured using Qubit® (dsDNA HS assay; Invitrogen, Carlsbad, CA, USA).

2.9. Amplicon Sequencing

The bacterial community composition was determined using high throughput tag-encoded 16S rRNA gene amplicon NxtSeq-based sequencing (Illumina, San Diego, CA, USA). The V3 region of the 16S rRNA gene was amplified using primers compatible with the Nextera Index Kit (Illumina) NXt_338_F:50- 5′-TCGTCGGCAGCGTCAGATGT GTATAAGAGACAGACWCCTACGGGWGGCAGCAG-3′ and NXt_518_R: 5′-GTCTCGTG GGCTCGGAGATGTGTATAAGAGACAGATTACCGC GGCTGCTGG-3′ (Integrated DNA Technologies; Leuven, Belgium). The PCR reactions and library preparation were performed as described previously [23].

2.10. High Throughput Sequencing and Data Treatment

The raw data set containing pair-ended reads with corresponding quality scores were merged and trimmed using fastq_mergepairs and fastq_filter scripts implemented in the UPARSE pipeline. The minimum overlap length was set to 10 base pairs (bp). The minimum length of merged reads was 150 bp, the maximum expected error E was 2.0, and the first truncating position with quality score was $n \leq 4$. Purging the dataset from chimeric reads and constructing zero radius Operational Taxonomic Units (zOTU) were conducted using the UNOISE3 pipeline [24]. The Green Genes (13.8) 16S rRNA gene collection was used as a reference database [25]. Quantitative Insight Into Microbial Ecology 2 (QIIME2) open source software [26] (version 2019.4.0) was used for the subsequent analysis steps. Principal coordinate analysis (PCoA) plots were generated with the diversity core-metrics-phylogenetic workflow based on 10 UniFrac distance metrics calculated using 10 subsampled OTU tables. The number of sequences taken for each jack-knifed subset was set to 90% of the sequence number within the most indigent sample, hence 14,000 reads per sample. Analysis of similarities (ANOSIM) was used to evaluate group differences using weighted and unweighted [27] UniFrac distance metrics that were generated based on rarefied zOTU tables. The relative distribution of the genera registered was calculated for unified and summarized in genus level zOTU tables. Alpha diversity measures expressed as observed species values (sequence similarity 97%) were computed for rarefied zOTU tables. Differences in alpha diversity were determined using the alpha-group-significance workflow.

3. Results

3.1. Single-Strain Growth Analysis

A single-strain screening of selected bacteria was carried out in vitro (Table 1) to assess their potential for the utilization of AOS. Very little or no growth was observed for all the species inoculated into the basal medium (without carbohydrate), while the addition of glucose was sufficient to give satisfactory growth for all species tested after 24 h incubation. These initial results confirmed that the conditions were suitable for the growth of all tested bacteria in the presence of a carbon source. *Bif. adolescentis*, *L. casei*, *L. paracasei* and *E. hirae* showed a moderate yet significant growth ($p < 0.05$) in presence of both AOS and alginate relative to baseline. Strong growth ($p < 0.01$) was observed for *B. ovatus* using alginate as substrate, while *Bif. adolescentis*, *L. casei*, *L. paracasei* and *E. hirae* showed no growth in the presence of AOS. In comparison, significant growth ($p < 0.01$) was observed for *Bif. bifidum* Bb-06, *Bif. adolescentis*, *E. coli*, *L. paracasei*, *E. faecium*, and *E. hirae* in the presence of inulin.

3.2. SCFA Production during In Vitro Simulated Colon Passage

The production of SCFA was measured as an indication of the fermentation capacity by the simulated GM (Table 2). Although valeric, isobutyric, 2-methylbutyric, isovaleric and lactic acids were also measured, these acids were only present in trace amounts and under the certainty thresholds (results not shown). Interestingly, AOS and alginate mainly stimulated the production of acetic acid compared to the control from 14.4 ± 0.4 to 26.4 ± 0.5 and 25.9 ± 3.2 µmol mL^{-1}, respectively, for donor 1, and from 13.3 ± 3.9 to 29.2 ± 5.7 and 21.9 ± 4.2 µmol mL^{-1} for donor 3. Additionally, the level of propionic acid was increased for donor 3 in presence of both AOS and alginate from 2.0 ± 0.3 to 5.0 ± 1.7 and 2.8 ± 0.2 µmol mL^{-1}, respectively. These results indicate the capacity of AOS to stimulate acetic acid production in a donor-dependent manner. Inulin strongly increased the level of acetic acid for each donor, while butyric and propionic acid production was increased by inulin in a donor-dependent manner for donor 1 and donor 3, and no significant difference was observed for donor 2. Additionally, no significant increase in the level of any analyzed SCFAs was observed for donor 2 in the presence of both AOS and alginate. Inulin fermentation resulted in the highest activity and led to the largest amount of total SCFA with every donor.

Table 2. Concentration of SCFA after 24 h fermentation in the gut model *CoMiniGut* for each substrate ($n = 4$).

Donor	Substrate	Concentration of Fatty Acids (µmol mL^{-1})			
		Acetic Acid	Butyric Acid	Propionic Acid	Total
1	Control	14.4 ± 0.4	0.9 ± 0.0	1.6 ± 0.0	16.90
	AOS	26.4 ± 0.5 ***	0.6 ± 0.1 ***	1.6 ± 0.1	28.60 *
	Alginate	25.9 ± 3.2 **	1.0 ± 0.2	2.6 ± 0.6 *	29.50 *
	Inulin	60.5 ± 5.6 **	5.1 ± 1.8 *	17.9 ± 5.4 **	83.50 **
2	Control	23.4 ± 0.8	2.7 ± 0.3	2.0 ± 0.1	28.10
	AOS	28.3 ± 5.7	2.3 ± 0.2	2.6 ± 0.4	33.20
	Alginate	23.3 ± 6.2	1.0 ± 0.6 **	2.0 ± 0.5	26.30
	Inulin	44.5 ± 6.9 **	4.1 ± 7.7	1.8 ± 0.7	50.40 **
3	Control	13.3 ± 3.9	1.9 ± 0.5	2.0 ± 0.3	17.20
	AOS	29.2 ± 5.7 **	2.3 ± 0.6	5.0 ± 1.7 *	36.50 *
	Alginate	21.9 ± 4.2 *	1.0 ± 0.2 *	2.8 ± 0.2 **	25.70 *
	Inulin	30.7 ± 8.0 *	22.6 ± 4.2 **	4.7 ± 1.1 *	58.00 **

Significative differences compared to control are expressed as * (p-value ≤ 0.05); ** (≤ 0.01) and *** (≤ 0.001).

3.3. Changes in the Simulated GM Composition during Gut Model CoMiniGut

Alpha diversity analysis using Richness (observed species; Figure 1) and Shannon indices (Figure 2) revealed significant differences in bacterial diversity with all three tested carbohydrates. As expected, the highest diversity measured with both indexes was found in the control fermentation for all donors. The fermentation of AOS, alginate and inulin resulted in a similar index value for the overall analysis; however, some donor-dependent differences were also observed. A higher diversity of the bacteria community was found with AOS for donor 1 and donor 2 compared to inulin, while the opposite result was observed in donor 3.

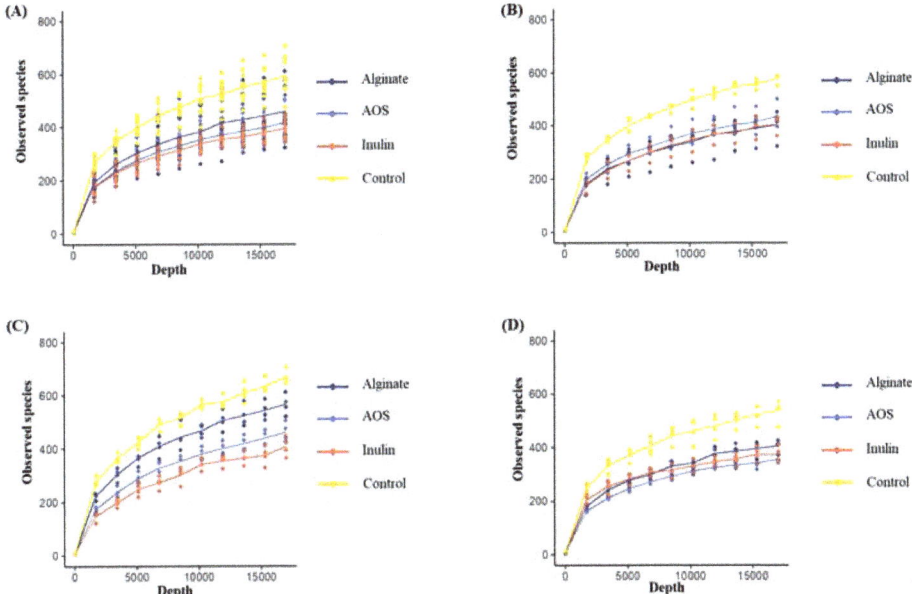

Figure 1. Richness rarefaction analysis. The Richness index (observed species per fermentation) was calculated for each treatment using the samples of combined donors (**A**), or for each individual donor: donor 1 (**B**), donor 2 (**C**) and donor 3 (**D**). The highest number of species observed were obtained in the control fermentation.

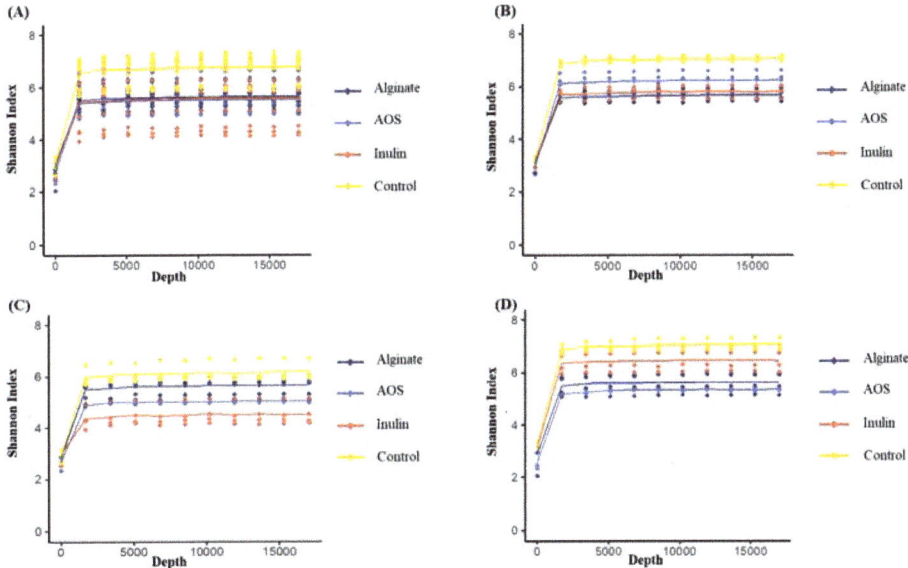

Figure 2. Shannon rarefaction analysis. The Shannon index was calculated for each treatment using the samples of combined donors (**A**), or for each individual donor: donor 1 (**B**), donor 2 (**C**) and donor 3 (**D**). Highest index value was observed in the control fermentation for each donor, while the effect of each substrate appeared to be donor dependent.

An analysis of composition of microbes (ANCOM) [28] test confirmed significant changes within microbial relative abundance and/or presence–absence due to substrate (Figure 3). Bacteria belonging to the genus *Bacteroides* overall had higher relative abundance in the fermentations with AOS and alginate. *B. ovatus* was found to be significantly represented among these fermentations compared to the control fermentation for each of the three donors. Furthermore, inulin strongly stimulated the *Bifidobacterium* community across all donors. Although similar features were noted among fermentations, the relative frequency of bacteria observed for each community was found to be strictly donor-dependent. Clear effects on the gut microbial composition within the AOS were also more specific for each donor. The relative abundance of *Bif. adolescentis* was slightly stimulated after fermentation with AOS compared to the control only for donor 1. The relative abundance of *Clostridiaceae* and *Enterobacteriaceae* markedly decreased after fermentation with AOS compared to the control for donor 2 and 3. All tested substrates caused a donor-dependent modulation of the simulated GM. However, the relative abundance of *Bacteroides* was significantly increased for all substrates.

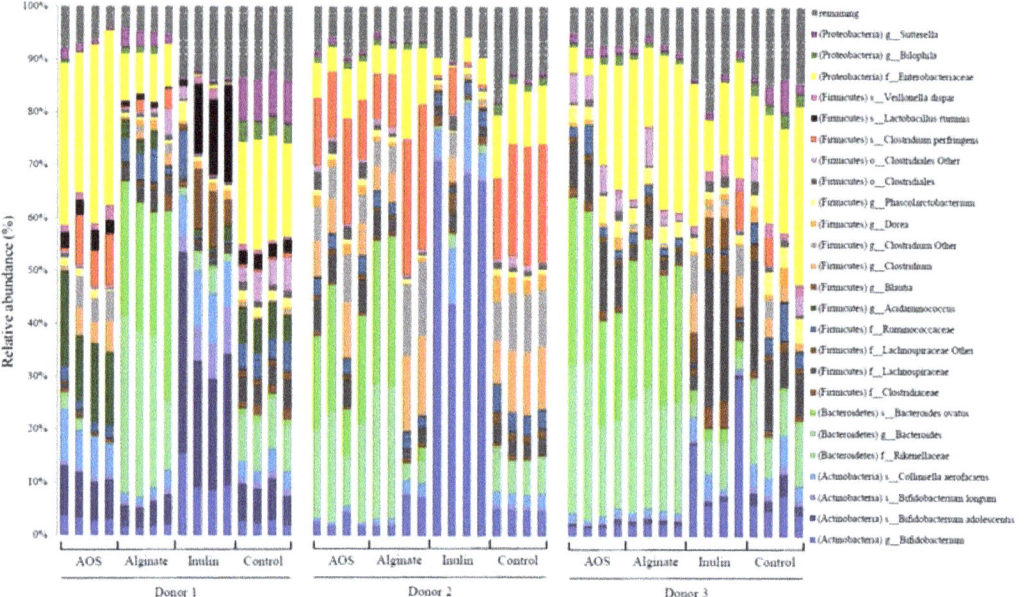

Figure 3. Relative abundance of bacterial community of the three donors in in vitro colon simulations performed in quadruplicate. The bar chart presents the bacterial relative distribution of 25 of the most abundant taxa determined by 16S rRNA gene amplicon sequencing (NxtSeq, Illumina). A clear increase in the bifidobacteria community was observed with inulin for each donor, while alginate oligosaccharide (AOS) and alginate stimulated *Bacteroides* abundance.

Beta-diversity analysis based on unweighted (qualitative) and weighted (quantitative) UniFrac distance matrices showed significant effects on gut microbial composition due to substrate (Figure 4A,B), and donor (Figure 4E,F). Although the donor effect was the strongest using unweighted UniFrac-based analysis, indicating the presence of donor-specific taxa, the proportions of the most abundant groups of bacteria were affected by the carbohydrate, resulting in the somewhat stronger effect of the carbohydrates (Figure 4B) than the donors (Figure 4F), observed with the weighted UniFrac-based analysis. Moreover, clear changes in the simulated GM were observed after 24 h for every donor in both abundance and diversity (Figure 4C,D).

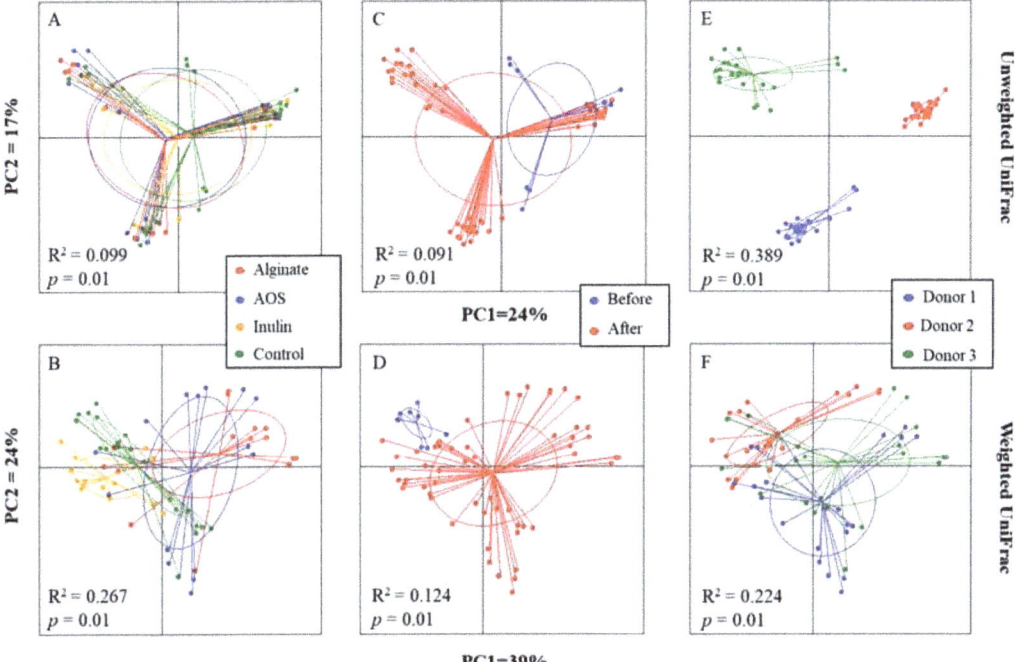

Figure 4. Beta-diversity analysis demonstrating differences in microbial composition of in vitro simulated colon fermentations. The Principal Coordinates Analysis (PCoA) plots are based on unweighted (**A,C,E**) and weighted (**B,D,F**) UniFrac distance matrices projecting similarities in microbial community between categories. AOS, alginate and inulin had little effect on the bacterial qualitative composition (**A**) and a pronounced effect on the bacterial relative abundance (**B**). The effect of fermentation on qualitative and quantitative characteristics of microbial community was weak yet significant (**C,D**). The donor effect was the strongest and clear on both unweighted (**E**) and weighted (**F**) UniFrac distance based on PCoA plots. The PERMANOVA results are given in each plot.

4. Discussion

An initial screening was carried out to gain insight into the capacity of AOS to influence bacterial growth. The growth of *Bif. adolescentis*, *L. casei* and *L. paracasei* was slightly stimulated in the presence of AOS, while no growth of the other tested bifidobacteria or lactobacilli was observed. Interestingly, previous studies reported that *Bif. longum*, *Bif. breve*, *Bif. bifidum*, *Bif. adolescentis*, *Bif. infantis* and *L. delbrueckii* subsp. *bulgaricus* were stimulated in the presence of AOS [15,29]. *Bacteroides ovatus* and *Bacteroides thetaiotaomicron* were also previously reported to be involved in the degradation of alginate and its derivatives [18]. *Bacteroides* spp. have been described as the main carbohydrate utilizers of the human microbiota, accounting for a large number of glycoside hydrolases (GH) and polysaccharide lyases (PL) genes per genome [30]. A significant amount of GH and PL genes were also found in the genome of certain bifidobacteria [30]. The capacity of these bacteria to grow in alginate and AOS-supplemented medium may be linked to their capacity to produce enzymes capable of degrading these substrates into smaller sugars. However, some of these studies evaluated the addition of enzymatically depolymerized alginate into skim-milk media or carbohydrate-free MRS [15,29]. In the present study, the use of colon basal medium aimed to recreate conditions similar to the colon model while enabling a better appreciation of the effect of AOS, as the basal medium is a less favorable growth environment compared to commonly used nutrient-rich media. Moreover, the AOS used here were obtained through acid hydrolysis of alginate. Thus, although similarities were found within the previous studies, differences indicated the capacity of certain bacteria to use AOS as substrate may be strain-dependent. It is also thought that this capacity is influenced by the chemical structure of AOS which is linked to the method used to produce these. Recent studies reported a relationship between the structure of the AOS and their biological properties [31,32]. Therefore, it is believed that further investigation of such structure–activity relationship for the prebiotic capacity of AOS should be considered.

The biological properties of SCFA, such as the acidification of the colon, reduced risk of pathogen colonization, modulation of water and salt retention, energy supply for colonocytes and peripheral tissues, as well as the stimulation of mucin production through modulation of the gene expression of epithelial cells, have driven the search for food ingredients that can stimulate the production of these metabolites [33]. In the present study, it was demonstrated that the level of acetic acid increased after 24 h fermentation in the presence of AOS compared to control conditions for donor 1 and donor 3, by 80% and 119%, respectively. For donor 3, the level of acetic acid was similar to that detected in the fermentation with inulin. A tendency to increase acetic acid was also noted in donor 2, although it was not statistically significant. These results indicated the capacity of AOS to stimulate SCFA production in a donor-dependent manner, although SCFA levels were often lower than those found in the fermentation with inulin. These results were in agreement with previous studies carried out in vitro using human GM inoculum [18], as well as some in vivo studies performed in weaned pigs and broiler chickens [34,35], which indicate that AOS may have prebiotic potential.

A UniFrac analysis confirmed the donor-specific aspect of each simulated GM profile, which was consistent with the current literature on the variability of GM composition among individuals. An elevated proportion of *Bacteroides*, especially *B. ovatus* was found for all donors after fermentation with AOS. Although these results are in agreement with earlier in vitro fermentation studies [17,18], they do not correlate entirely with the single-strain growth experiments, where we failed to observed growth of this species on AOS (Table 1). Along with an increased proportion of *Bacteroides*, a donor-dependent effect was observed for other bacterial taxa. A reduction in the relative abundance of *Clostridiaceae* and *Enterobacteriaceae* families was observed for donor 2 and 3 after the fermentation with AOS. This correlates with the single-strain growth experiments where *E. coli*, *E. cloacae*, *K. pneumoniae* and *S. enterica* Typhimurium failed to grow on AOS and thus were outcompeted by species that were able to utilise this substrate. *Bif. adolescentis* was mainly observed in donor 1 and to a lesser extent in donor 3. *Bif. adolescentis* showed growth with AOS and inulin in the single-strain culture tests. In the in vitro colon simulations, AOS only modestly increased the relative proportion of *Bif. adolescentis* in donor 1 while no effect was observed on *Bif. adolescentis* in donor 3. Moreover, inulin substantially increased the relative abundance of *Bif. aolescentis* only in donor 1, which was in line with the single-strain growth experiments. However, inulin showed stimulation of the growth of genus *Bifidobacterium* in all three donors, in agreement with the single-strain screening. Although several lactobacilli and enterococci species were observed to grow on AOS in the single-strain testing, their numbers were too low to be observed in the community analyses.

Although only three donors were included in the present study, it is clear that there is a donor-dependent ability to utilise AOS and alginate. The influence of the host microbiota composition on its ability to utilise alginates has recently been reported [36] and is also influenced by cross-feeding between members of the intestinal microbiota [37]. The absence of cross-feeding in the single-strain growth experiments may be one of the explanations why the results do not fully correlate with the in vitro colon simulations.

Therefore, it can be suggested that although the single-strain approach led to a better understanding of the capacity of certain species of bacteria to use AOS for their growth, the presence of a complex bacteria community such as in the colon is necessary to further investigate the impact of AOS onto the simulated GM. Although AOS led to limited growth improvement in single-strain culture, important changes in the gut microbiota profile were noted after fermentation in the colon-model approach. As previously mentioned, AOS and alginate stimulated the growth of only a few specific bacterial taxa. Accordingly, the lower value obtained by the Richness and Shannon indices of the gut model carried out with the substrates was explained by the stimulation of these specific bacteria and therefore their preferential growth among the simulated GM community compared to the control. Overall, AOS possesses the capacity to shape the GM in vitro, although this effect differs by its selectiveness and its intensity from the effect of inulin. The use of the combined approach led to a better understanding of the results of each experiment.

5. Conclusions

This study aimed to provide a better insight into the prebiotic capacity of AOS. For the first time using an in vitro approach, the effect of AOS on both bifidobacteria and *Bacteroides* communities was observed and explained by donor-dependent variations, while the capacity of certain gut bacteria to utilize AOS was validated through the single-strain method. Although of a lesser intensity compared to inulin, the production of acetic acid was increased by AOS in a gut-model fermentation. AOS effectively stimulated the growth of *Bacteroides* in all fecal samples tested, while they also increased the abundance of *Bif. adolescentis* and decreased the abundance of *Clostridiaceae* and *Enterobacteriaceae* families in a donor-dependent manner. These results were in agreement with previous findings and confirmed the potential of AOS to be used as a prebiotic ingredient, although more studies are needed to further evaluate the prebiotic capacity and the link with the chemical structure of AOS.

Author Contributions: Conceptualization, G.B., O.G., Ł.K., D.S.N. and F.P.R.; methodology, G.B., J.L.C.-M., W.K., M.T.S., Ł.K., D.S.N. and F.P.R.; formal analysis, G.B. and M.T.S.; resources, Ł.K., A.C.O., D.S.N. and F.P.R.; data curation, W.K., G.B. and M.T.S.; writing—original draft preparation, G.B.; writing—review and editing, all authors; visualization, G.B.; supervision, O.G., A.C.O., D.S.N. and F.P.R.; project administration, O.G., A.C.O., D.S.N. and F.P.R.; funding acquisition, O.G. and F.P.R. All authors have read and agreed to the published version of the manuscript.

Funding: This research was funded by the Innovation Fund Denmark (5189-00028A) in collaboration with DuPont Nutrition and Biosciences and the University of Copenhagen. We would like to express our sincere gratitude to Kirsi Stenström and Nicolas Yeung at DuPont Nutrition and Biosciences, and Bashir Aideh and Denitsa Stefanova at the University of Copenhagen for their precious and skillful help.

Institutional Review Board Statement: The study was conducted in accordance with the Declaration of Helsinki, and approved by the Ethical Committee of the Capital Region of Denmark registration number H-20028549 (25 June 2020).

Informed Consent Statement: Not applicable.

Data Availability Statement: For the genome data, a SRA submission was done (PRJNA646360).

Conflicts of Interest: At the time of the study GB, OG, MS and ACO were employees of DuPont Nutrition and Biosciences (now International Flavors & Fragrances) which manufactures and markets alginates and probiotics. The other authors—GB, LK, JLC-M, WK, DSN and FPR—declare no conflict of interest.

References

1. Topolska, K.; Florkiewicz, A.; Filipiak-Florkiewicz, A. Functional Food-Consumer Motivations and Expectations. *Int. J. Environ. Res. Public Health* **2021**, *18*, 5327. [CrossRef] [PubMed]
2. Gibson, G.R.; Hutkins, R.; Sanders, M.E.; Prescott, S.L.; Reimer, R.A.; Salminen, S.J.; Scott, K.; Stanton, C.; Swanson, K.S.; Cani, P.D.; et al. Expert consensus document: The International Scientific Association for Probiotics and Prebiotics (ISAPP) consensus statement on the definition and scope of prebiotics. *Nat. Rev. Gastroenterol. Hepatol.* **2017**, *14*, 491–502. [CrossRef] [PubMed]
3. Attaye, I.; Warmbrunn, M.V.; Boot, A.; van der Wolk, S.C.; Hutten, B.A.; Daams, J.G.; Herrema, H.; Nieuwdorp, M. A Systematic Review and Meta-analysis of Dietary Interventions Modulating Gut Microbiota and Cardiometabolic Diseases-Striving for New Standards in Microbiome Studies. *Gastroenterology* **2022**, *162*, 1911–1932. [CrossRef] [PubMed]

4. Deschasaux, M.; Bouter, K.E.; Prodan, A.; Levin, E.; Groen, A.K.; Herrema, H.; Tremaroli, V.; Bakker, G.J.; Attaye, I.; Pinto-Sietsma, S.J.; et al. Depicting the composition of gut microbiota in a population with varied ethnic origins but shared geography. *Nat. Med.* **2018**, *24*, 1526–1531. [CrossRef]
5. Neri-Numa, I.A.; Pastore, G.M. Novel insights into prebiotic properties on human health: A review. *Food Res. Int* **2020**, *131*, 108973. [CrossRef]
6. Wang, Z.; Tauzin, A.S.; Laville, E.; Tedesco, P.; Letisse, F.; Terrapon, N.; Lepercq, P.; Mercade, M.; Potocki-Veronese, G. Harvesting of Prebiotic Fructooligosaccharides by Nonbeneficial Human Gut Bacteria. *mSphere* **2020**, *5*, e00771-19. [CrossRef]
7. Stephen, A.M.; Phillips, G.O. *Food Polysaccharides and Their Applications*; CRC Press: Boca Raton, FL, USA, 2006.
8. Lee, K.Y.; Mooney, D.J. Alginate: Properties and biomedical applications. *Prog. Polym. Sci.* **2012**, *37*, 106–126. [CrossRef]
9. August, A.D.; Kong, H.J.; Mooney, D.J. Alginate hydrogels as biomaterials. *Macromol. Biosci.* **2006**, *6*, 623–633. [CrossRef]
10. Brownlee, I.A.; Allen, A.; Pearson, J.P.; Dettmar, P.W.; Havler, M.E.; Atherton, M.R.; Onsoyen, E. Alginate as a source of dietary fiber. *Crit. Rev. Food Sci. Nutr.* **2005**, *45*, 497–510. [CrossRef]
11. Qin, Y.; Jiang, J.; Zhao, L.; Zhang, J.; Wang, F. Applications of Alginate as a Functional Food Ingredient. In *Biopolymers for Food Design; Handbook of Food Bioengineering*; Grumezescu, A.M., Holban, A.M., Eds.; Academic Press: London, UK, 2018; pp. 409–429.
12. Liu, J.; Yang, S.; Li, X.; Yan, Q.; Reaney, M.J.T.; Jiang, Z. Alginate Oligosaccharides: Production, Biological Activities, and Potential Applications. *Compr. Rev. Food Sci Food Saf.* **2019**, *18*, 1859–1881. [CrossRef]
13. Jonathan, M.; Souza da Silva, C.; Bosch, G.; Schols, H.; Gruppen, H. In vivo degradation of alginate in the presence and in the absence of resistant starch. *Food Chem.* **2015**, *172*, 117–120. [CrossRef] [PubMed]
14. Jonathan, M.C.; Bosch, G.; Schols, H.A.; Gruppen, H. Separation and identification of individual alginate oligosaccharides in the feces of alginate-fed pigs. *J. Agric. Food Chem.* **2013**, *61*, 553–560. [CrossRef] [PubMed]
15. Wang, Y.; Han, F.; Hu, B.; Li, J.; Yu, W. In vivo prebiotic properties of alginate oligosaccharides prepared through enzymatic hydrolysis of alginate. *Nutr. Res.* **2006**, *26*, 597–603. [CrossRef]
16. Ramnani, P.; Chitarrari, R.; Tuohy, K.; Grant, J.; Hotchkiss, S.; Philp, K.; Campbell, R.; Gill, C.; Rowland, I. In vitro fermentation and prebiotic potential of novel low molecular weight polysaccharides derived from agar and alginate seaweeds. *Anaerobe* **2012**, *18*, 1–6. [CrossRef] [PubMed]
17. Han, Z.L.; Yang, M.; Fu, X.D.; Chen, M.; Su, Q.; Zhao, Y.H.; Mou, H.J. Evaluation of Prebiotic Potential of Three Marine Algae Oligosaccharides from Enzymatic Hydrolysis. *Mar. Drugs* **2019**, *17*, 173. [CrossRef]
18. Li, M.; Li, G.; Shang, Q.; Chen, X.; Liu, W.; Pi, X.; Zhu, L.; Yin, Y.; Yu, G.; Wang, X. In vitro fermentation of alginate and its derivatives by human gut microbiota. *Anaerobe* **2016**, *39*, 19–25. [CrossRef]
19. Wiese, M.; Khakimov, B.; Nielsen, S.; Sorensen, H.; van den Berg, F.; Nielsen, D.S. CoMiniGut-a small volume in vitro colon model for the screening of gut microbial fermentation processes. *PeerJ* **2018**, *6*, e4268. [CrossRef]
20. Bouillon, G.A.; Gåserod, O.; Rattay, F.P. Evaluation of the inhibitory effect of alginate oligosaccharide on yeast and mould in yoghurt. *Int. Dairy J.* **2019**, *99*, 104544. [CrossRef]
21. Mäkeläinen, H.; Saarinen, M.; Stowell, J.; Rautonen, N.; Ouwehand, A.C. Xylo-oligosaccharides and lactitol promote the growth of *Bifidobacterium lactis* and *Lactobacillus* species in pure cultures. *Benef. Microbes* **2010**, *1*, 139–148. [CrossRef]
22. Ouwehand, A.C.; Tiihonen, K.; Saarinen, M.; Putaala, H.; Rautonen, N. Influence of a combination of *Lactobacillus acidophilus* NCFM and lactitol on healthy elderly: Intestinal and immune parameters. *Br. J. Nutr.* **2009**, *101*, 367–375. [CrossRef]
23. Krych, L.; Kot, W.; Bendtsen, K.M.B.; Hansen, A.K.; Vogensen, F.K.; Nielsen, D.S. Have you tried spermine? A rapid and cost-effective method to eliminate dextran sodium sulfate inhibition of PCR and RT-PCR. *J. Microbiol. Methods* **2018**, *144*, 1–7. [CrossRef] [PubMed]
24. Edgar, R.C. UNOISE2: Improved error-correction for Illumina 16S and ITS amplicon sequencing. *bioRxiv* **2016**. [CrossRef]
25. McDonald, D.; Price, M.N.; Goodrich, J.; Nawrocki, E.P.; DeSantis, T.Z.; Probst, A.; Andersen, G.L.; Knight, R.; Hugenholtz, P. An improved Greengenes taxonomy with explicit ranks for ecological and evolutionary analyses of bacteria and archaea. *ISME J.* **2012**, *6*, 610–618. [CrossRef] [PubMed]
26. Caporaso, J.G.; Kuczynski, J.; Stombaugh, J.; Bittinger, K.; Bushman, F.D.; Costello, E.K.; Fierer, N.; Pena, A.G.; Goodrich, J.K.; Gordon, J.I.; et al. QIIME allows analysis of high-throughput community sequencing data. *Nat. Meth.* **2010**, *7*, 335–336. [CrossRef] [PubMed]
27. Lozupone, C.; Knight, R. UniFrac: A new phylogenetic method for comparing microbial communities. *Appl. Environ. Microbiol.* **2005**, *71*, 8228–8235. [CrossRef] [PubMed]
28. Mandal, S.; Van Treuren, W.; White, R.A.; Eggesbo, M.; Knight, R.; Peddada, S.D. Analysis of composition of microbiomes: A novel method for studying microbial composition. *Microb. Ecol. Health Dis.* **2015**, *26*, 27663. [CrossRef] [PubMed]
29. Akiyama, H.; Endo, T.; Nakakita, R.; Murata, K.; Yonemoto, Y.; Okayama, K. Effect of depolymerized alginates on the growth of bifidobacteria. *Biosci. Biotechnol. Biochem.* **1992**, *56*, 355–356. [CrossRef] [PubMed]
30. El Kaoutari, A.; Armougom, F.; Gordon, J.I.; Raoult, D.; Henrissat, B. The abundance and variety of carbohydrate-active enzymes in the human gut microbiota. *Nat. Rev. Microbiol.* **2013**, *11*, 497–504. [CrossRef]
31. Xu, X.; Iwamoto, Y.; Kitamura, Y.; Oda, T.; Muramatsu, T. Root growth-promoting activity of unsaturated oligomeric uronates from alginate on carrot and rice plants. *Biosci. Biotechnol. Biochem.* **2003**, *67*, 2022–2025. [CrossRef]
32. Yamasaki, Y.; Yokose, T.; Nishikawa, T.; Kim, D.; Jiang, Z.; Yamaguchi, K.; Oda, T. Effects of alginate oligosaccharide mixtures on the growth and fatty acid composition of the green *alga Chlamydomonas reinhardtii*. *J. Biosci. Bioeng.* **2012**, *113*, 112–116. [CrossRef]

33. Roy, C.C.; Kien, C.L.; Bouthillier, L.; Levy, E. Short-chain fatty acids: Ready for prime time? *Nutr. Clin. Pract.* **2006**, *21*, 351–366. [CrossRef] [PubMed]
34. Zhu, W.; Li, D.; Wang, J.; Wu, H.; Xia, X.; Bi, W.; Guan, H.; Zhang, L. Effects of polymannuronate on performance, antioxidant capacity, immune status, cecal microflora, and volatile fatty acids in broiler chickens. *Poult. Sci.* **2015**, *94*, 345–352. [CrossRef] [PubMed]
35. Zhu, W.; Li, D.; Wu, H.; Li, J.; Chen, Y.; Guan, H.; Zhang, L. Effects of purified polymannuronate on the performance, immune status, antioxidant capacity, intestinal microbial populations and volatile fatty acid concentrations of weaned piglets. *Anim. Feed Sci. Technol.* **2016**, *216*, 161–168. [CrossRef]
36. Fu, T.; Zhou, L.; Fu, Z.; Zhang, B.; Li, Q.; Pan, L.; Zhou, C.; Zhao, Q.; Shang, Q.; Yu, G. Enterotype-Specific Effect of Human Gut Microbiota on the Fermentation of Marine Algae Oligosaccharides: A Preliminary Proof-of-Concept In Vitro Study. *Polymers* **2022**, *14*, 770. [CrossRef] [PubMed]
37. Murakami, R.; Hashikura, N.; Yoshida, K.; Xiao, J.Z.; Odamaki, T. Growth-promoting effect of alginate on *Faecalibacterium prausnitzii* through cross-feeding with Bacteroides. *Food Res. Int.* **2021**, *144*, 110326. [CrossRef] [PubMed]

Disclaimer/Publisher's Note: The statements, opinions and data contained in all publications are solely those of the individual author(s) and contributor(s) and not of MDPI and/or the editor(s). MDPI and/or the editor(s) disclaim responsibility for any injury to people or property resulting from any ideas, methods, instructions or products referred to in the content.

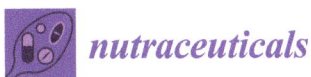

Article

Apple Puree as a Natural Fructose Source Provides an Effective Alternative to Artificial Fructose Sources for Fuelling Endurance Cycling Performance in Males

Kirsty M. Reynolds [1], Loris A. Juett [1], James Cobb [1], Carl J. Hulston [2], Stephen A. Mears [1] and Lewis J. James [1,*]

[1] National Centre for Sport and Exercise Medicine, School of Sport, Exercise and Health Sciences, Loughborough University, Loughborough LE11 3TU, UK
[2] Population Health Sciences Institute, Newcastle University, Newcastle upon Tyne NE1 7RU, UK
* Correspondence: l.james@lboro.ac.uk; Tel.: +44-1509-226305

Abstract: Carbohydrate consumption during exercise enhances endurance performance. A food-focused approach may offer an alternative, 'healthier' approach given the potential health concerns associated with artificial fructose sources, but food-based carbohydrate sources may increase gastrointestinal (GI) symptoms. This study compared the cycling performance and GI comfort of two different fructose sources (fruit and artificial) ingested during exercise. Nine trained male cyclists (age 24 ± 7 years; VO_{2peak} 65 ± 6 mL/kg/min) completed a familiarisation and two experimental trials (60 g/h carbohydrate, 120 min at 55% W_{max} and ~15 min time trial). In the two experimental trials, carbohydrate was ingested in a 2:1 glucose-to-fructose ratio, with fructose provided as artificial crystalline fructose (GLU/FRU) or natural apple puree (APPLE PUREE) and maltodextrin added to provide sufficient glucose. Time trial (TT) performance was not different between trials (GLU/FRU 792 ± 68 s, APPLE PUREE 800 ± 65 s; $p = 0.313$). No GI symptoms were significantly different between trials ($p \geq 0.085$). Heart rate, blood glucose/lactate concentrations, and RPE were not different between trials, but all, excluding blood glucose concentration, increased from rest to exercise and further increased post-TT. Apple puree as a natural fructose source provides an alternative to artificial fructose sources without influencing cycling performance or GI symptoms.

Keywords: fruit; food; health; sugar; athlete; comfort

1. Introduction

Carbohydrate is an important macronutrient for daily living and is the preferred exogenous fuel source during endurance exercise [1], as it has been demonstrated to benefit performance by maintaining blood glucose concentrations and delaying fatigue with exercise for >60 min. Carbohydrate is deemed to be a more efficient fuel source than fat during high-intensity or prolonged endurance exercise due to its ability to provide more adenosine triphosphate (ATP) for a given amount of oxygen [2]. Furthermore, ATP can be produced from carbohydrate in the absence of oxygen using glycolytic pathways [2]. Carbohydrate is stored in the body in the form of muscle and liver glycogen [2]; however, these stores are limited. Therefore, the provision of exogenous carbohydrate before and during exercise helps to preserve glycogen stores and is fundamental for optimal endurance performance. Current guidelines [3,4] suggest that during prolonged endurance exercise of >2 h, the intake of 60–90 g/h from mixed carbohydrate sources (i.e., glucose and fructose) is recommended, which should not cause acute gastrointestinal (GI) upset in the majority of athletes [5].

Whilst the current carbohydrate guidelines provide useful information on carbohydrate dosage and sugar type, they fail to offer suggestions and evidence on the source or form of the carbohydrate. Common sources of fructose used in commercial carbohydrate supplements are high-fructose corn syrup, isolated (crystalline) fructose, and sucrose.

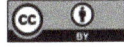

However, for some individuals, there may be potential long-term negative implications of high-fructose corn syrup and crystalline fructose ingestion [6,7]. These artificial fructose sources have been associated with increased levels of obesity and metabolic disease [6,7], possibly making them less attractive to some exercisers. Additionally, the consumption of high fructose drinks during and after exercise may exacerbate markers of acute kidney injury (AKI) [8].

However, natural sources of fructose, such as those in fruit, may not have the same potential negative health consequences and thus may provide 'healthier' options to the athlete/exerciser [9]. For example, apples naturally contain fructose (~60%) [10], and apple consumption has been related to a reduced risk of cancer [11,12] and cardiovascular disease [13]. The suggested mechanisms link back to the presence of phytochemicals and antioxidants contained within apples reducing oxidative damage. Thus, carbohydrate in the form of apple puree has the potential to provide health benefits, as well as energy intake during endurance exercise. There is a move towards more natural products, and our recent systematic review [14] concluded that whilst performance does not appear to be positively or negatively affected by carbohydrate sources (food vs. supplement), food carbohydrate sources might increase GI symptoms. Eight studies included in the systematic review assessed GI symptoms, and six of those studies reported increased negative symptoms in the food-based trial [15–20].

The increased GI symptoms experienced could occur due to the additional plant components and/or the greater volume of food that must be consumed to meet carbohydrate requirements for prolonged exercise. For example, many food sources of carbohydrate, particularly natural foods, such as fruits or vegetables, have a lower carbohydrate density, so a larger volume of food must be consumed to meet recommended intakes during prolonged exercise, e.g., [20]. This is an important consideration given the high prevalence of GI symptoms in endurance athletes when consuming high doses of carbohydrate [5,21]. Indeed, GI symptoms might impair performance or even lead to the failure to complete races [5]. Whole-food sources typically contain additional nutrients to carbohydrate (i.e., dietary fibre, fat, protein, vitamins, minerals, etc.). Whilst many of these nutrients might confer health benefits, some of them may also affect carbohydrate delivery to the working muscles or trigger negative effects on the GI system. However, nutrition in the form of a fruit puree may offer the carbohydrate delivery profile of a gel whilst minimising additional plant components that could upset the GI system, offering a natural and 'healthier' fructose source.

Research has tended to focus on the direct comparison between total carbohydrate sources from food or supplements and has not yet focused specifically on the sources of sugars, such as fructose (i.e., natural versus artificial sources), and whether they achieve the same endurance performance benefits without inducing adverse GI effects that may limit sporting outcomes [5]. Investigating natural versus artificial sugar sources is the novel aspect of our study, as it remains unknown whether such carbohydrate sources will have a negative impact on physiological function and performance. Therefore, the aim of this study was to examine endurance performance, GI comfort, and markers of renal injury associated with two different fructose sources (fruit and artificial) ingested during prolonged cycling exercise.

2. Materials and Methods

Participants. The study inclusion criteria included being a cyclist/triathlete (male or female, although no females volunteered), age 18–45 years, having ≥1 year of cycling experience, completing a minimum of 3 h cycling training per week, having previous experience ingesting carbohydrate during exercise. Individuals were not eligible if they had any conditions that could influence carbohydrate metabolism. Participants were healthy and free from injury. Nine trained male cyclists/triathletes completed the study, with an age (mean ± standard deviation) of 24 ± 7 years, a height of 179 ± 9 cm, a mass of 72.7 ± 6.5 kg (Adam CFW-150, Milton Keynes, UK), a VO_{2peak} of 65 ± 6 mL/kg/min, and a W_{max} of 373 ± 49 W. Initially, five additional participants (all male) started the study; four completed visit one, and one completed visits one and two. A National Lockdown in response to the COVID-19 pandemic meant that these participants were no longer able to participate in the study and limited some of the intended measures for the study. The study gained institutional ethical approval from the Loughborough University Ethics Approvals (Human Participants) Sub-Committee, and participants gave written informed consent and completed a medical screening questionnaire prior to testing.

Experimental Design

VO_{2peak} *test and familiarisation.* During the first visit, the participants completed a peak oxygen uptake (VO_{2peak}) test, and after a short break, they practised the time trial (TT). The VO_{2peak} test was completed on a cycle ergometer (Lode Excalibur Sport, Groningen, The Netherlands) starting at 95 W and increasing by 35 W every 3 min until volitional exhaustion. An expired breath sample was taken in the final 60 s to determine VO_{2peak}. The second visit consisted of a full familiarisation trial, which was identical to the experimental trials (detailed below). Carbohydrate was provided as 60 g/h of maltodextrin (MyProtein, Northwich, UK) only. Bike set-up was determined during the initial visit and then replicated for all trials.

Pre-trial Standardisation. Participants were required to complete an activity and food diary in the 24 h before the familiarisation trial, which was replicated before each subsequent trial. They were asked to abstain from alcohol and strenuous exercise for 24 h prior to each trial. Participants were instructed to consume at least 40 mL/kg body mass from beverages the day before the trials. A standardised breakfast providing 1.5 g carbohydrate/kg body mass and 8 mL water/kg body mass was consumed 2 h prior to arrival at the laboratory (consisting of cereal bars (Nutrigrain, Kellogg's, Salford, UK), orange juice (Tesco, Welwyn Garden City, UK), and water). Compliance with the pre-trial breakfast was assessed by photographic record, whilst compliance with other pre-trial standardisation procedures was verbally confirmed by participants on arrival. Trials started between 09:00 and 10:00, with each participant starting all trials at the same time to control for circadian rhythm and diurnal variation in performance [22].

Protocol. The study utilised a repeated-measures design. Participants completed the two experimental trials in a randomised order, separated by at least seven days. The exercise protocol consisted of 2 h at ~55% W_{max} (preload), followed by a TT designed to last ~15 min. A fan was provided in front of the participants providing a windspeed of ~4.7 m/s. For both trials, carbohydrate was provided at 60 g/h, (15 g at 0 and then every 15 min; ~22% carbohydrate solution) via a 50 mL syringe in a glucose-to-fructose ratio of 2:1, but the sources of fructose differed. No specific information was given to the participants about what the carbohydrate sources were. In the APPLE PUREE trial, the carbohydrate source was apple puree (BIONA ORGANIC; Surrey, UK), which provided natural sources of fructose and glucose (per 100 g of puree: 237 kcal, glucose 3.28 g, fructose 7.08 g, sucrose 2.15 g, dietary fibre 1.3 g, fat 0.1 g, protein 0.2 g). The puree was analysed for full nutritional breakdown by Campden BRI (Campden, UK). Maltodextrin was added to the apple puree (7.3 g maltodextrin and 61.3 g apple puree; total 68.6 g per 15 g carbohydrate serving) to achieve the 2:1 glucose:fructose ratio. In the GLU/FRU trial, the carbohydrate sources and water content were matched to the APPLE PUREE (67.9 g per 15 g carbohydrate serving) and consisted of maltodextrin (MyProtein, Northwich, UK) and crystalline fructose (Bulk Powders, Colchester, UK), providing an artificial source of fructose. Apple flavouring (MyProtein, Northwich, UK) was added to both carbohydrate sources. Tap water was provided *ad libitum* at room temperature during the preload and before the TT, but no fluid was ingested during the TT.

Each participant completed a workload-directed TT based on delivering $0.75 \times W_{peak} \times 900$, meaning it would take ~15 min to complete the target amount of work (kJ) if the participant cycled at ~75% W_{peak}. The cycle ergometer was in linear mode, whereby the participants' preferred cadence would generate ~75% W_{peak} [23]. Participants were blinded to all visual feedback during the TT, except target workload and work completed. On completion of each 25% of the target workload, participants were verbally informed using set wording, but there was no further interaction with the investigators, who stood behind the participant to reduce peripheral distractions.

Study Blinding. Participants were informed that the purpose of the study was to investigate the effect of different types of carbohydrate, both providing an optimal dosage, and that they would be debriefed on the specific carbohydrate supplements at the end of the study.

Measures. At rest, every 30 min during the preload, and at the end of the TT, ambient temperature and humidity (Kestrel 4400; Nielsen-Kellerman) were recorded. On arrival, participants provided a total void urine sample, and baseline nude body mass was measured, with additional total void urine samples provided and nude body mass measures made post-preload and post-TT. Participants completed 5 min rest on the cycle ergometer before baseline measures were recorded. Heart Rate (HR) was measured using a chest strap (worn at position T9; Polar M400; Polar Electro Oy, Kempele, Finland) at rest every 30 min during the preload and after each 25% of the TT. Rating of perceived exertion (RPE; 6–20 scale; [24]), thermal sensation (TS; −10 to +10 Scale; [25]), and GI scales (all 11-point Likert scales assessing hunger, thirst, stomach fullness, stomach bloatedness, stomach cramps, urge to vomit, urge to urinate, and urge to defecate [26]) were recorded at rest, every 30 min during the preload, and immediately post-TT. *Ad libitum* water intake was recorded for each hour of the preload. The time to complete each 25% interval during the TT was recorded. A fingertip capillary blood sample was collected pre-exercise (~320 µL), with additional fingertip capillary blood samples (20 µL) collected every 30 min during the preload and post-TT.

Unfortunately, due to the COVID-19 pandemic, we were unable to collect gas samples to determine VO_2 or substrate use during exercise.

Sample Processing and Analysis. For each urine sample, the volume was determined and urine specific gravity was measured using a hand-held analyser (Ceti, Refractometer) before the sample was stored at −80 °C until analysis for biomarkers of kidney damage, KIM-1 (kidney injury molecule-1), and NGAL (neutrophil gelatinase-associated lipocalin), by enzyme-linked immunosorbent assay (ELISA) (Human, NGAL ELISA kit, Bioporto, Hellerup, Denmark; Human KIM-1, ELISA kit ADI-900-226-001, Enzo Life Sciences, Lausen, Switzerland) in the pre- and post-preload urine samples only. Samples from the familiarisation trial (maltodextrin only) were included in this analysis to provide a fructose-free comparison.

From the pre-exercise blood sample, 300 µL was collected in a tube containing a clotting catalyst (Sarstedt 100 microvette, Sarstedt AG & Co., Nümbrecht, Germany). This tube was centrifuged at $2500 \times g$, 4 °C for 20 min before serum was aliquoted and stored at −80 °C until analysis for osmolality by freezing point depression (Gonotec Osmomat 030, Cryoscopic Osmometer; Gonotec). At each blood sampling time point, blood was collected in a 20 µL capillary tube before being mixed with 1 mL of haemolysing solution (EKF Diagnostics, Cardiff, UK) and analysed for lactate and glucose concentrations (Biosen C-Line; EKF Diagnostics, Cardiff, UK).

Statistical Analysis Statistical analyses were completed using Statistical Package for Social Sciences (SPSS) for Windows version 25 SPSS; Chicago, IL, USA). Statistical significance was set at $p \leq 0.05$, and results are presented as mean ± SD, except for GI scale responses and renal injury biomarkers, which are presented as medians (IQR). The normality of data was assessed using Shapiro–Wilk tests. Two-way repeated measures ANOVA was used to analyse data containing two factors (trial × time), whilst paired t-tests or Wilcoxon signed rank tests were used, as appropriate, to analyse data containing one factor. To correct for violation of sphericity, the degrees of freedom were corrected using Greenhouse–Geisser ($\varepsilon > 0.75$) or Huynh–Felt ($\varepsilon < 0.75$) [27].

3. Results

3.1. Pre-Trial Measures

There were no differences between trials for pre-trial body mass (Table 1; $p = 0.526$), urine specific gravity (Table 1; $p = 0.195$), serum osmolality (GLU/FRU 288 ± 2 mosmol/kg; APPLE PUREE 288 ± 2 mosmol/kg; $p = 0.864$), heart rate (Figure 1; $p = 0.483$) or any subjective variable (Figure 2; $p \geq 0.447$), indicating that participants started trials in a similar state.

Table 1. Urine specific gravity; body mass (kg) at rest, after 120 min preload, and post time trial (TT). Sweat loss (L) and dehydration (%) accrued after 120 min preload and post time trial (TT). Data presented as mean ± SD. * denotes a significant difference between carbohydrate supplements ($p > 0.05$).

	0	120	Post-TT
Urine Specific Gravity			
GLU/FRU	1.008 ± 0.01	1.009 ± 0.00	1.010 ± 0.01
APPLE PUREE	1.010 ± 0.01	1.012 ± 0.00	1.014 ± 0.01 *
Body Mass (kg)			
GLU/FRU	72.69 ± 6.50	72.36 ± 6.60	71.71 ± 6.63
APPLE PUREE	72.58 ± 6.66	72.27 ± 6.76	71.78 ± 6.73
Total Cumulative Sweat Loss (L)			
GLU/FRU		1.68 ± 0.35	2.13 ± 0.50
APPLE PUREE		1.68 ± 0.30	2.09 ± 0.38
Dehydration (%)			
GLU/FRU		−0.47 ± 0.56	−1.28 ± 0.56
APPLE PUREE		−0.43 ± 0.35	−1.12 ± 0.38

3.2. Heart Rate, RPE, TS, Blood Glucose/Lactate Responses, and Environmental Conditions

Laboratory conditions were not different between trials (GLU/FRU 21.8 ± 2.1 °C; APPLE PUREE 21.7 ± 1.7 °C; $p = 0.556$), relative humidity (GLU/FRU 35.4 ± 11.9%; APPLE PUREE 37.5 ± 14.4%; $p = 0.272$), or barometric pressure (GLU/FRU 751 ± 12 mmHg and APPLE PUREE 758 ± 8 mmHg; $p = 0.128$).

Heart rate (trial effect $p = 0.670$; interaction effect $p = 0.325$), blood glucose concentration (trial effect $p = 0.837$; interaction effect $p = 0.622$), blood lactate concentration (trial effect $p = 0.228$; interaction effect $p = 0.510$), RPE (trial effect $p = 0.468$; interaction effect $p = 0.613$), and TS (trial effect $p > 0.999$; interaction effect $p = 0.240$) were not different between trials (Figure 1). There were, however, main effects of time for heart rate, blood lactate concentration, RPE, and TS ($p \leq 0.001$), with an increase from rest to exercise and a further increase post-TT.

3.3. Gastrointestinal Scale Responses

GI scales for all symptoms were not significantly different between trials (trial effect $p \geq 0.052$ interaction effect $p \geq 0.085$; Figure 2). On average, no symptoms were classed as severe (≥ 5 out of 10), although some individual participants did report symptoms ≥ 5, including hunger (GLU/FRU 4 participants; APPLE PUREE 4 participants), thirst (GLU/FRU 6 participants; APPLE PUREE 4 participants), stomach fullness (GLU/FRU 3 participants; APPLE PUREE 4 participants), stomach cramps (GLU/FRU 1 participant; APPLE PUREE 0 participants), bloatedness (GLU/FRU 0 participants; APPLE PUREE 1 participant), urge to vomit (GLU/FRU 1 participant; APPLE PUREE 3 participants), and urge to urinate (GLU/FRU 3 participants; APPLE PUREE 1 participants). Thirst also increased over time ($p = 0.007$).

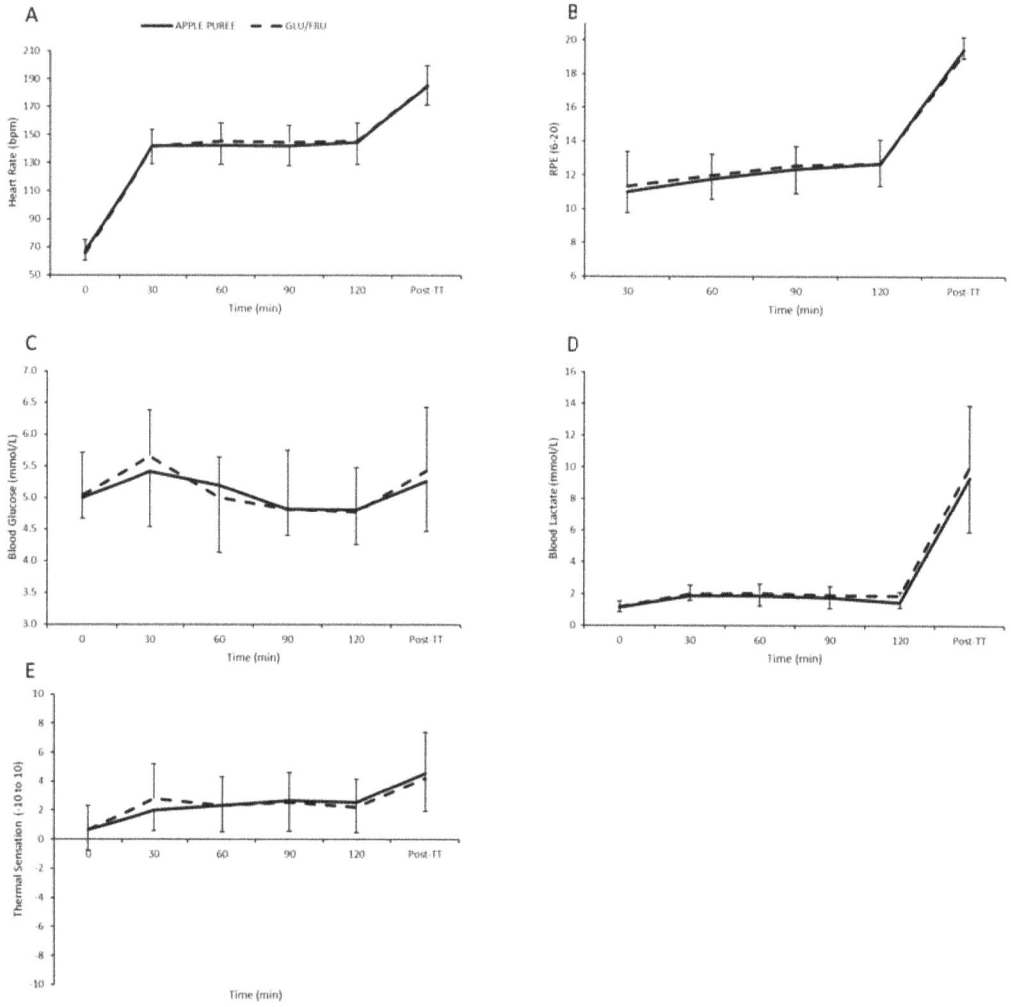

Figure 1. Heart rate (beat/min), (**A**); rating of perceived exertion (RPE) (6–20), (**B**); blood glucose (mmol/L), (**C**); blood lactate (mmol/L), (**D**); and thermal sensation (−10–10), (**E**) over the 2 h preload and post time trial (TT) for both carbohydrate supplements. Data presented as mean ± SD.

3.4. Fluid Balance Measures

There was no difference in ad libitum water intake (GLU/FRU 977 ± 464 g; APPLE PUREE 1018 ± 426 g; p = 0.722; Table 1), total fluid intake (GLU/FRU 1453 ± 464 g; APPLE PUREE 1493 ± 426 mL; p = 0.685), or sweat rate (p = 0.576; Table 1) between trials or in the dehydration accrued in trials (p = 0.555; Table 1). There was a significant trial effect for USG (p = 0.010) but no significant interaction (p = 0.968). Whilst USG was not different between trials upon arrival to the laboratory and after the 2 h preload, after the TT, USG values were slightly but significantly higher in the APPLE PUREE condition (p = 0.010; Table 1).

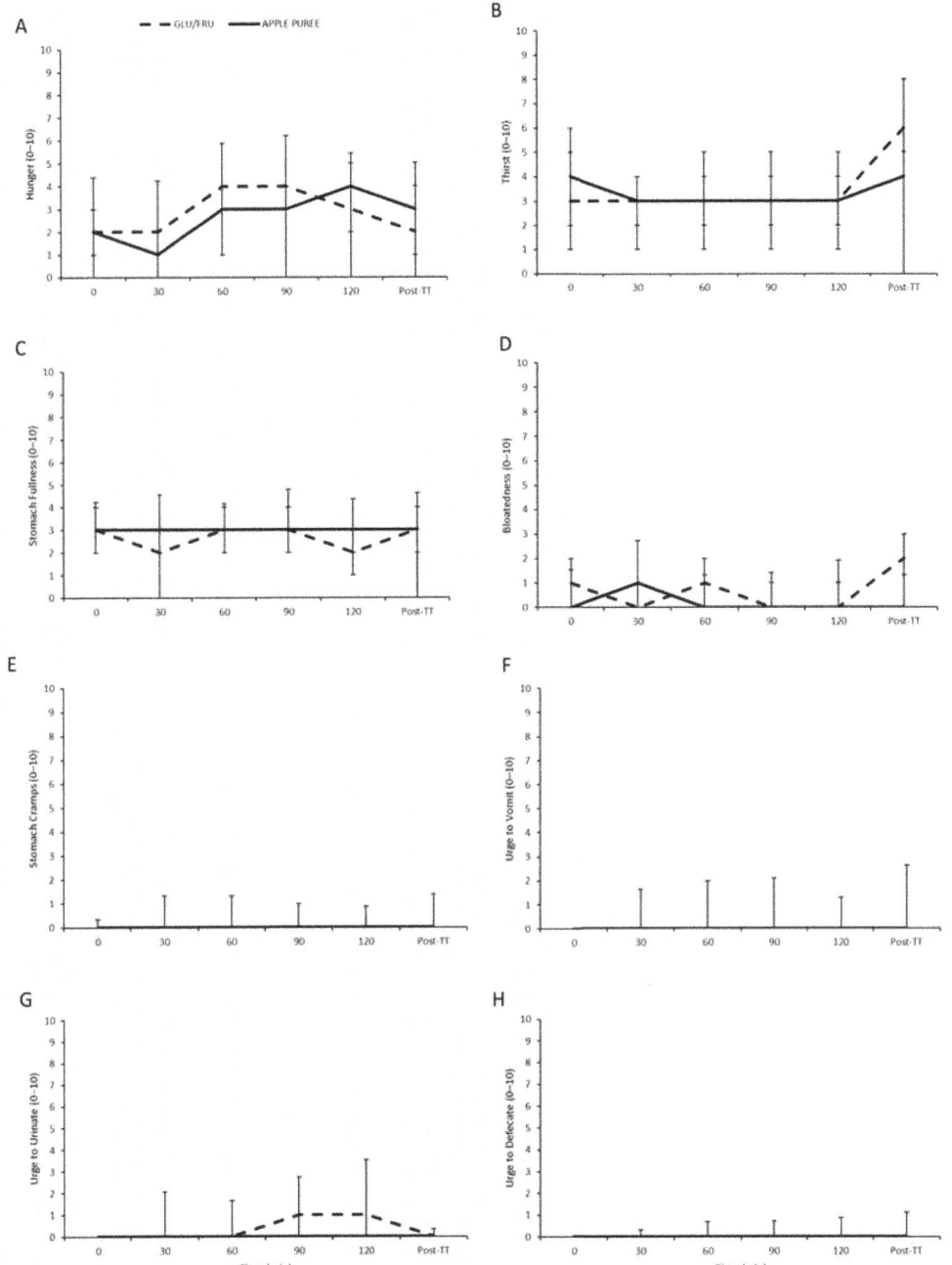

Figure 2. Gastrointestinal symptoms (hunger, (**A**); thirst, (**B**); stomach fullness, (**C**); bloatedness, (**D**); stomach cramps, (**E**); urge to vomit, (**F**); urge to urinate, (**G**); and urge to defecate, (**H**)) over the 2 h preload and post time trial (TT) for both carbohydrate supplements. Data presented as median ± IQR.

3.5. Time Trial (TT) Performance

The total time to complete the TT was not significantly different between the two trials (GLU/FRU 792 ± 68 s, APPLE PUREE 800 ± 65 s; $p = 0.313$, Figure 3). There was no influence on pacing between the trials or across each 25% section (condition × trial interaction $p = 0.909$).

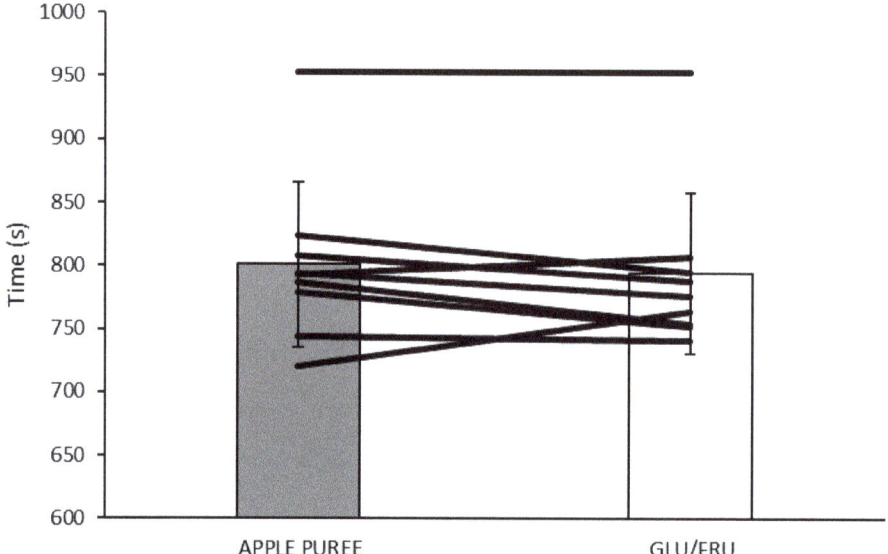

Figure 3. Time trial performance during GLU/FRU and APPLE PUREE. Bars are means ± SD. Lines are individual participant times.

3.6. Renal Injury Biomarkers

Only seven participants' data were included for the NGAL and KIM-1 analysis due to storage/analysis issues. Urine samples from familiarisation were also analysed, as they provided a fructose-free control. There were no significant differences for NGAL (trial effect $p = 0.538$; interaction effect $p = 0.974$) or KIM1 (trial effect $p = 0.591$; interaction effect $p = 0.440$) between trials (Figure 4) and no changes over time ($p \geq 0.069$).

3.7. Study Blinding and Trial Order Effects

No participant correctly identified both carbohydrate supplements or the aim of the study (i.e., to look at natural/fruit sources of fructose). Generally, participants thought the experiment was comparing the effects of different carbohydrate types on performance ($n = 7$) or different carbohydrate dosages ($n = 1$). One participant mentioned that he thought the study aim was something related to fructose but specified this to be in the breakfast content rather than in the carbohydrate provided during exercise. This suggests that the participants were successfully blinded to the study aims. Additionally, there was no trial order effect for any of the measured variables ($p \geq 0.055$), including the time to complete the time trial during the first and second visits (Trial 1, 788 ± 67 s, Trial 2, 804 ± 61 s), indicating that there was no learning effect over the trials.

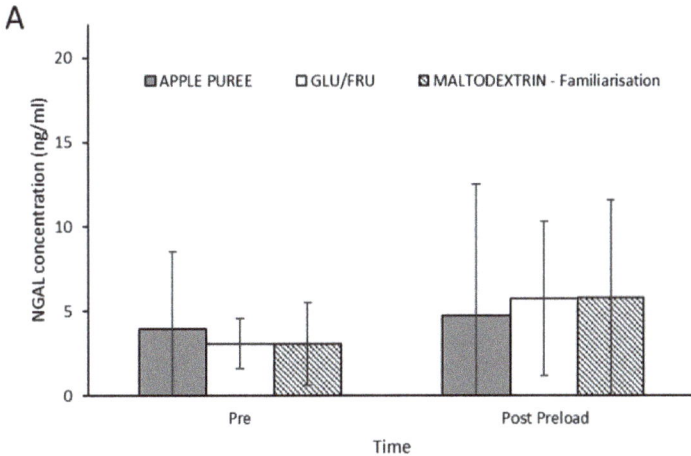
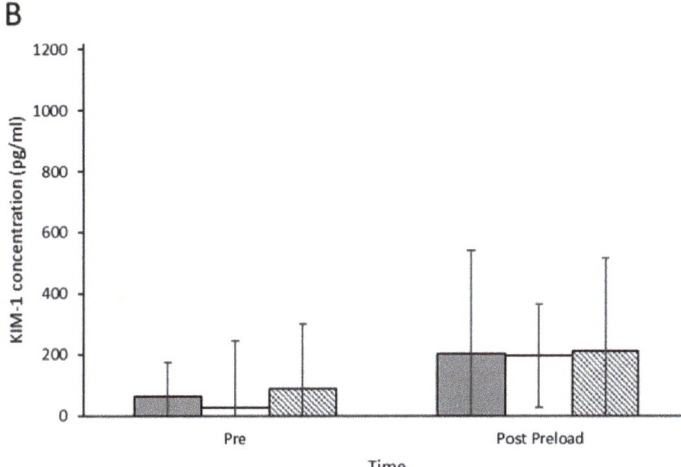

Figure 4. NGAL (ng/mL; (**A**)) and KIM-1 (pg/mL; (**B**)) urinary concentrations at rest and after the 2 h preload for both carbohydrate supplements and maltodextrin (fructose-free control). Data presented as median ± IQR. $n = 7$.

4. Discussion

The main findings of this study were that cycling TT performance and GI comfort were not different between fruit and artificial sources of fructose ingested during prolonged cycling. From a performance perspective, these results align with previous studies that have compared fruit or other whole-food sources with supplemental carbohydrate sources, including bananas [18,19], raisins [28–30], and pureed potato [20]. However, in contrast to many previous studies comparing supplemental and whole-food carbohydrate sources [15–20], there was no significant increase in GI disturbances with the consumption of apple puree. These results are of important practical relevance to the athlete/exerciser as they suggest that apple puree may be used to provide a more natural source of fructose in sports supplements without negatively impacting exercise performance or GI symptoms. Whole foods are more likely to delay taste and texture fatigue that can be associated with gels and drinks [31], and therefore, alternative carbohydrate sources may play an important role in encouraging athletes to meet fueling guidelines. Research suggests many endurance athletes do not meet the guidelines for carbohydrate intake during exercise, even in competition [5], meaning that widening the scope of appropriate sources through which athletes can obtain carbohydrate might be an important step in facilitating optimal carbohydrate intake during training/competition.

To meet the guidelines for carbohydrate dosage, the volume of whole foods needs to be considered, along with the potential for such volumes to cause GI upset. For example, when comparing potato consumption to a carbohydrate gel [20], 1028 g of potato puree was equitable to consuming 184 g of carbohydrate gel, which increased GI symptoms reported in the potato trial, likely due to the greater volume of food consumed. In the current study, the total amount consumed was similar between supplements (271.6 g/h in GLU/FRU vs. 274.4 g/h in APPLE PUREE), which may account for the lack of a difference in GI symptoms observed between trials, with all symptoms low, on average, in both trials. The current study provided carbohydrate at 60 g/h, whereas for longer durations, some athletes may consume carbohydrate at a higher intake rate (90g/h or more), and at higher dosages, there is the potential that GI symptoms may be increased. GI upset is often associated with increased exercise duration and intensity, and therefore, the finding that the high-intensity TT did not lead to any further exacerbation of GI symptoms in the apple puree trial is important.

The apple puree contained additional nutrients, including small amounts of fibre and protein. Whilst these additional components might be expected to slow gastric emptying [32,33], it seems the very small amounts (3.57 g fibre/h and 0.55 g protein/h) did not slow gastric emptying enough to induce any GI symptoms. This suggests that fruit puree, at least apple puree, might be an attractive option for a natural source of fructose in carbohydrate supplements. Research has suggested that the gut is a trainable organ [34,35], meaning that GI comfort could be improved with experience consuming carbohydrate foods and supplements during exercise with higher-volume feeding strategies. The participants in the current study all had previous experience consuming carbohydrate during exercise, which may have contributed to the low GI symptom scores compared with previous studies [15–20] as well as possibly the lack of a difference between trials.

The difference in carbohydrate supplement provided also did not affect other factors that might influence GI symptoms during exercise. High water intake during exercise can induce GI discomfort [36,37], and it is possible that the more viscous nature of the apple puree supplement could have induced increased drinking. However, neither *ad libitum* water intake throughout the preload nor subjective thirst were different between trials. These observations suggest that participants did not feel the need to drink more with the apple puree, which could have increased stomach volume and, consequently, GI symptoms. Indeed, hydration status was generally well maintained over the trial, with participants losing, on average, <0.5% body mass over the preload and <1.3% over the whole trial and no participant reaching >2% body mass loss during the preload when *ad libitum* drinking was permitted. Neither sweat rate nor dehydration accrued was different between trials, which was expected since the exercise intensity was the same. Hypohydration can impair endurance exercise performance [38,39], so this study suggests that *ad libitum* drinking is sufficient to prevent significant hypohydration from accruing during ~2 h of indoor cycling in a temperate environment.

Since it was not possible to measure carbohydrate oxidation, there is no definitive evidence of carbohydrate utilisation, but the performance and blood glucose data indicated no differences in carbohydrate availability or utilisation between trials. Therefore, the inclusion of the additional plant components and nutrients within the apple puree did not seem to hinder the bioavailability of carbohydrate during endurance exercise. However, the inclusion of fibre could explain the small but significant increase in USG in the apple puree trial (although there was no interaction effect). The presence of fibre in the gut has been linked to increased water retention in the lumen [40]. Although this increase was small and within a range considered euhydrated, it may be an important consideration for longer exercise durations or exercise in the heat, conditions in which there is a greater risk of dehydration [41]. Future studies should examine such conditions as well as measure changes in blood/plasma volume to ascertain the effects.

Urinary biomarkers of renal injury, KIM-1 and NGAL, have been shown to increase following various forms of exercise [42]. In the present study, urinary NGAL and KIM-1 concentrations only showed small, non-significant increases from rest to the end of the preload and were not significantly different between trials. It may be that hotter ambient temperatures and/or greater intensity/duration of exercise are required to increase renal injury, particularly with cycling (due to the lack of eccentric muscle contractions and thus muscle damage). Additionally, there is evidence to suggest that the consumption of high-fructose drinks during and after exercise heat stress increases biomarkers of renal injury [8], but that was not apparent in the present study. However, the fructose consumption was significantly greater in the Chapman study [8] (~234 g) compared with that in the present study (40 g). Whilst this may be a concern for individuals exercising for a prolonged duration in hot environments with high fructose intakes, most exercising recommendations suggest that intake rates for athletes have an upper fructose limit of ~30 g/h, which is less likely to produce negative effects.

As with all studies, the current study was not without limitations. The study was open to female participants, but none volunteered, which was very disappointing. Thus, these findings may not be transferable to females since females tend to have slower gastric emptying rates [43] and are more prone to experiencing GI symptoms during prolonged exercise [44].

5. Conclusions

Results from the current study indicate that apple puree as a fructose source may provide a suitable alternative to carbohydrate supplements when ingested during endurance cycling, with no difference in performance outcomes (GLU/FRU 792 ± 68 s, APPLE PUREE 800 ± 65 s; $p = 0.313$) or GI symptoms. Future research should examine running performance since runners are more prone to experience GI symptoms when exercising, and this could be exacerbated with natural carbohydrate sources. Additionally, further research on females is needed, as this group is poorly represented in studies and may be more prone to increased incidence of GI symptoms.

Author Contributions: The study was designed by K.M.R., C.J.H., S.A.M. and L.J.J.; K.M.R., J.C. and L.J.J. collected the data; K.M.R., L.A.J. and J.C. performed biochemical/data analysis; K.M.R. wrote the manuscript with assistance from L.A.J., J.C., C.J.H., S.A.M. and L.J.J. All authors have read and agreed to the published version of the manuscript.

Funding: K.M.R. is a doctoral researcher funded by Decathlon SA (Principal Investigator L.J.J.) and Loughborough University. Decathlon SA has read the final manuscript but played no role in the data collection, analysis, or writing of the manuscript.

Institutional Review Board Statement: The study was conducted in accordance with the Declaration of Helsinki, and approved by the Institutional Ethics Committee of Loughborough University (protocol code R2020-P008, approved February 2020).

Informed Consent Statement: Informed consent was obtained from all participants involved in the study.

Data Availability Statement: The data for this study is not publicly available.

Conflicts of Interest: L.J.J. is part of the National Institute for Health Research's Leicester Biomedical Research Centre, which is a partnership between the University Hospitals of Leicester NHS Trust, Loughborough University, and the University of Leicester. This report is independent research by the National Institute for Health Research. The views expressed in this publication are those of the authors and not necessarily those of the NHS, the National Institute for Health Research, or the Department of Health. L.J.J. has current/previous funding from Entrinsic Beverage Company LLP, Herbalife Europe Ltd., Bridge Farm Nurseries, Decathlon SA, PepsiCo Inc., and Volac International; has performed consultancy for PepsiCo Inc. and Lucozade, Ribena Suntory; and has received conference fees from PepsiCo Inc. and Danone Nutricia. In all cases, monies were paid to L.J.J.'s institution and not directly to L.J.J. SAM has current/previous funding from Entrinsic Beverage Company LLP and Decathlon SA. The authors declare no other conflict of interest.

References

1. Stellingwerf, T.; Cox, G.R. Systematic Review: Carbohydrate Supplementation on Exercise Performance or Capacity of Varying Duration. *Appl. Physiol. Nutr. Metab.* **2014**, *39*, 998–1011. [CrossRef] [PubMed]
2. Burke, L.M.; Castell, L.M.; Casa, D.J.; Close, G.L.; Costa, R.J.S.; Desbrow, B.; Halson, S.L.; Lis, D.M.; Melin, A.K.; Peeling, P.; et al. International Association of Athletics Federations Consensus Statement 2019: Nutrition for Athletes. *Int. J. Sport Nutr. Exerc. Metab.* **2019**, *29*, 73–84. [CrossRef] [PubMed]
3. Burke, L.M.; Hawley, J.A.; Wong, S.H.S.; Jeukendrup, A.E. Carbohydrate for Training and Competition. *J. Sports Sci.* **2011**, *29*, S17–S27. [CrossRef]
4. Jeukendrup, A. Nutrition for Endurance Sports: Marathon, Triathlon, and Road Cycling. *J. Sports Sci.* **2011**, *29* (Suppl. 1), S91–S99. [CrossRef] [PubMed]
5. Pfeiffer, B.; Stellingwerff, T.; Hodgson, A.B.; Randell, R.; Pöttgen, K.; Res, P.; Jeukendrup, A.E. Nutritional Intake and Gastrointestinal Problems during Competitive Endurance Events. *Med. Sci. Sports. Exerc.* **2012**, *44*, 344–351. [CrossRef]
6. Kelishadi, R.; Mansourian, M.; Heidari-Beni, M. Association of fructose consumption and components of metabolic syndrome in human studies: A systematic review and meta-analysis. *Nutrition* **2014**, *30*, 503–510. [CrossRef]
7. Liu, Q.; Ayoub-Charette, S.; Khan, T.A.; Au-Yeung, F.; Mejia, S.B.; De Souza, R.J.; Wolever, T.M.; Leiter, L.A.; Kendall, C.W.; Sievenpiper, J.L. Important food sources of fructose-containing sugars and incident hypertension: A systematic review and dose-response meta-analysis of prospective cohort studies. *J. Am. Heart Assoc.* **2019**, *8*, e010977. [CrossRef]
8. Chapman, C.L.; Johnson, B.D.; Sackett, J.R.; Parker, M.D.; Schlader, Z.J. Soft drink consumption during and following exercise in the heat elevates biomarkers of acute kidney injury. *Am. J. Physiol. Regul. Integr. Comp. Physiol.* **2019**, *316*, R189–R198. [CrossRef]
9. Hyson, D.A. A review and critical analysis of the scientific literature related to 100% fruit juice and human health. *Adv. Nutr.* **2015**, *6*, 37–51. [CrossRef]
10. Aprea, E.; Charles, M.; Endrizzi, I.; Corollaro, M.L.; Betta, E.; Biasioli, F.; Gasperi, F. Sweet taste in apple: The role of sorbitol, individual sugars, organic acids and volatile compounds. *Sci. Rep.* **2017**, *7*, 44950. [CrossRef]
11. Fabiani, R.; Minelli, L.; Rosignoli, P. Apple intake and cancer risk: A systematic review and meta-analysis of observational studies. *Public Health Nutr.* **2016**, *19*, 2603–2617. [CrossRef] [PubMed]
12. Hyson, D.A. A comprehensive review of apples and apple components and their relationship to human health. *Adv. Nutr.* **2011**, *2*, 408–420. [CrossRef] [PubMed]
13. Sandoval-Ramírez, B.A.; Catalán, Ú.; Calderón-Pérez, L.; Companys, J.; Pla-Pagà, L.; Ludwig, I.A.; Romero, M.P.; Solà, R. The effects and associations of whole-apple intake on diverse cardiovascular risk factors. A narrative review. *Crit. Rev. Food Sci. Nutr.* **2020**, *60*, 3862–3875. [CrossRef] [PubMed]
14. Reynolds, K.M.; Clifford, T.; Mears, S.A.; James, L.J. A Food First Approach to Carbohydrate Supplementation in Endurance Exercise: A Systematic Review. *Int. J. Sport Nutr. Exerc. Metab.* **2022**, *32*, 296–310. [CrossRef]
15. Guillochon, M.; Rowlands, D.S. Solid, Gel, and Liquid Carbohydrate Format Effects on Gut Comfort and Performance. *Int. J. Sport Nutr. Exerc. Metab.* **2011**, *27*, 247–254. [CrossRef]
16. Ishihara, K.; Taniguchi, H.; Akiyama, N.; Asami, Y. Easy to Swallow Rice Cake as a Carbohydrate Source during Endurance Exercise Suppressed Feelings of Thirst and Hunger without Changing Exercise Performance. *J. Nutr. Sci. Vitaminol.* **2020**, *66*, 128–135. [CrossRef] [PubMed]
17. Lee, J.K.W.; Maughan, R.J.; Shirreffs, S.M.; Watson, P. Effects of Milk Ingestion on Prolonged Exercise Capacity in Young, Healthy Men. *Nutrition* **2008**, *24*, 340–347. [CrossRef] [PubMed]
18. Nieman, D.C.; Gillitt, N.D.; Henson, D.A.; Sha, W.; Shanely, R.A.; Knab, A.M.; Cialdella-Kam, L.; Jin, F. Bananas as an Energy Source during Exercise: A Metabolomics Approach. *PLoS ONE* **2012**, *7*, E37479. [CrossRef]
19. Nieman, D.C.; Gillitt, N.D.; Sha, W.; Esposito, D.; Ramamoorthy, S. Metabolic Recovery from Heavy Exertion Following Banana Compared to Sugar Beverage or Water Only Ingestion: A Randomized, Crossover Trial. *PLoS ONE* **2018**, *13*, E0194843. [CrossRef]
20. Salvador, A.F.; Mckenna, C.F.; Alamilla, R.A.; Cloud, R.M.T.; Keeble, A.R.; Miltko, A.; Scaroni, S.E.; Beals, J.W.; Ulanov, A.V.; Dilger, R.N.; et al. Potato Ingestion Is as Effective as Carbohydrate Gels to Support Prolonged Cycling Performance. *J. Appl. Physiol.* **2019**, *127*, 1651–1659. [CrossRef]

21. Pugh, J.N.; Kirk, B.; Fearn, R.; Morton, J.P.; Close, G.L. Prevalence, Severity and Potential Nutritional Causes of Gastrointestinal Symptoms during a Marathon in Recreational Runners. *Nutrients* **2018**, *10*, 811. [CrossRef] [PubMed]
22. Drust, B.; Waterhouse, J.; Atkinson, G.; Edwards, B.; Reilly, T. Circadian rhythms in sports performance—An update. *Chronobiol. Int.* **2005**, *22*, 21–44. [CrossRef] [PubMed]
23. Jeukendrup, A.; Saris, W.H.; Brouns, F.J.P.H.; Kester, A.D. A new validated endurance performance test. *Med. Sci. Sports Exerc.* **1996**, *28*, 266–270. [CrossRef] [PubMed]
24. Borg, G.A. Psychophysical bases of perceived exertion. *Med. Sci. Sports Exerc.* **1982**, *14*, 377–381. [CrossRef] [PubMed]
25. Kenefick, R.W.; Cheuvront, S.N.; Palombo, L.J.; Ely, B.R.; Sawka, M.N. Skin temperature modifies the impact of hypohydration on aerobic performance. *J. Appl. Physiol.* **2010**, *109*, 79–86. [CrossRef]
26. Jeukendrup, A.E.; Vet-Joop, K.; Sturk, A.; Stegen, J.H.J.C.; Senden, J.; Saris, W.H.M.; Wagenmakers, A.J.M. Relationship between gastro-intestinal complaints and endotoxaemia, cytokine release and the acute-phase reaction during and after a long-distance triathlon in highly trained men. *Clin. Sci.* **2000**, *98*, 47–55. [CrossRef]
27. Field, A.P. *Discovering Statistics Using IBM SPSS: And Sex and Drugs and Rock'n'Roll*; SAGE: London, UK, 2013.
28. Rietschier, H.L.; Henagan, T.M.; Earnest, C.P.; Baker, B.L.; Cortez, C.C.; Stewart, L.K. Sun-Dried Raisins Are a Cost-Effective Alternative to Sports Jelly Beans in Prolonged Cycling. *J. Strength Cond. Res.* **2011**, *25*, 3150. [CrossRef]
29. Kern, M.; Heslin, C.J.; Rezende, R.S. Metabolic and Performance Effects of Raisins Versus Sports Gel as Pre-Exercise Feedings in Cyclists. *J. Strength Cond. Res.* **2007**, *21*, 1204–1207.
30. Too, B.W.; Cicai, S.; Hockett, K.R.; Applegate, E.; Davis, B.A.; Casazza, G.A. Natural Versus Commercial Carbohydrate Supplementation and Endurance Running Performance. *J. Int. Soc. Sports Nutr.* **2012**, *9*, 27. [CrossRef]
31. Tiller, N.B.; Roberts, J.D.; Beasley, L.; Chapman, S.; Pinto, J.M.; Smith, L.; Wiffin, M.; Russell, M.; Sparks, S.A.; Duckworth, L.; et al. International Society of Sports Nutrition Position Stand: Nutritional Considerations for Single-Stage Ultra-Marathon Training and Racing. *J. Int. Soc. Sports Nutr.* **2019**, *16*, 50. [CrossRef]
32. McIntyre, A.; Vincent, R.M.; Perkins, A.C.; Spiller, R.C. Effect of bran, ispaghula, and inert plastic particles on gastric emptying and small bowel transit in humans: The role of physical factors. *Gut* **1997**, *40*, 223–227. [CrossRef] [PubMed]
33. Babio, N.; Balanza, R.; Basulto, J.; Bulló, M.; Salas-Salvadó, J. Dietary fibre: Influence on body weight, glycemic control and plasma cholesterol profile. *Nutr. Hosp.* **2010**, *25*, 327–340. [PubMed]
34. Jeukendrup, A.E. Training the Gut for Athletes. *Sports Med.* **2017**, *47*, 101–110. [CrossRef] [PubMed]
35. Miall, A.; Khoo, A.; Rauch, C.; Snipe, R.M.J.; Camões-Costa, V.L.; Gibson, P.R.; Costa, R.J.S. Two Weeks of Repetitive Gut-Challenge Reduce Exercise-Associated Gastrointestinal Symptoms and Malabsorption. *Scand. J. Med. Sci. Sports* **2018**, *28*, 630–640. [CrossRef]
36. Robinson, T.A.; Hawley, J.A.; Palmer, G.S.; Wilson, G.R.; Gray, D.A.; Noakes, T.D.; Dennis, S.C. Water ingestion does not improve 1-h cycling performance in moderate ambient temperatures. *Eur. J. Appl. Physiol. Occup. Physiol.* **1995**, *71*, 153–160. [CrossRef]
37. Backx, K.; van Someren, K.A.; Palmer, G.S. One hour cycling performance is not affected by ingested fluid volume. *Int. J. Sport Nutr. Exerc. Metab.* **2003**, *13*, 333–342. [CrossRef]
38. Funnell, M.P.; Mears, S.A.; Bergin-Taylor, K.; James, L.J. Blinded and Unblinded Hypohydration Similarly Impair Cycling Time Trial Performance in the Heat in Trained Cyclists. *J. Appl. Physiol.* **2019**, *126*, 870–879. [CrossRef]
39. James, L.J.; Funnell, M.P.; James, R.M.; Mears, S.A. Does Hypohydration Really Impair Endurance Performance? Methodological Considerations for Interpreting Hydration Research. *Sports Med.* **2019**, *49*, 103–114. [CrossRef]
40. Eastwood, M.A.; Kay, R.M. An hypothesis for the action of dietary fiber along the gastrointestinal tract. *Am. J. Clin. Nutr.* **1979**, *32*, 364–367. [CrossRef]
41. Thomas, D.T.; Erdman, K.A.; Burke, L.M. American college of sports medicine joint position statement. nutrition and athletic performance. *Med. Sci. Sports Exerc.* **2016**, *48*, 543–568.
42. Juett, L.A.; James, L.J.; Mears, S.A. Effects of exercise on acute kidney injury biomarkers and the potential influence of fluid intake. *Ann. Nutr. Metab.* **2020**, *76*, 53–59. [CrossRef] [PubMed]
43. Datz, F.L.; Christian, P.E.; Moore, J. Gender-Related Differences in Gastric Emptying. *J. Nucl. Med.* **1987**, *28*, 1204–1207. [PubMed]
44. Ten Haaf, D.S.; van der Worp, M.P.; Groenewoud, H.M.; Leij-Halfwerk, S.; Nijhuis-van der Sanden, M.W.; Verbeek, A.L.; Staal, J.B. Nutritional Indicators for Gastrointestinal Symptoms in Female Runners: The 'Marikenloop Study'. *BMJ Open* **2014**, *4*, e005780. [CrossRef] [PubMed]

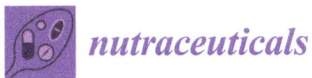

Article

Combined Therapy of Chitosan and Exercise Improves the Lipid Profile, Adipose Tissue and Hepatic Alterations in an In Vivo Model of Induced-Hyperlipidemia

João P. G. Passos [1], Carlisson R. Melo [1], Felipe M. A. Carvalho [1], Patricia Severino [1], Juliana C. Cardoso [1], John L. S. Cunha [2], Amanda Cano [3,4], Eliana B. Souto [3,5,6,*] and Ricardo L. C. de Albuquerque-Júnior [1,*]

[1] Institute of Technology and Research (ITP), University of Tiradentes, Aracaju 49010-390, Sergipe, Brazil; jp_gusmao@hotmail.com (J.P.G.P.); carlisson_melo@hotmail.com (C.R.M.); felipe_mendesdeandrade@hotmail.com (F.M.A.C.); patricia_severino@itp.org.br (P.S.); juliana_cordeiro@itp.org.br (J.C.C.)

[2] Post-Graduating Program in Stomatopathology, University of Campinas, Campinas 13083-970, São Paulo, Brazil; lennonrrr@gmail.com

[3] Department of Pharmacy, Pharmaceutical Technology and Physical Chemistry, Faculty of Pharmacy and Food Sciences, University of Barcelona, Av. Joan XXIII, 27-31, Campus Diagonal, 08028 Barcelona, Spain; acanofernandez@ub.edu

[4] Institute of Nanoscience and Nanotechnology (IN2UB), University of Barcelona, Av. Joan XXIII, 27-31, Campus Diagonal, 08028 Barcelona, Spain

[5] Department of Pharmaceutical Technology, Faculty of Pharmacy of University of Porto (FFUP), Rua Jorge de Viterbo Ferreira 228, 4050-313 Porto, Portugal

[6] REQUIMTE/UCIBIO, Faculty of Pharmacy, University of Porto (FFUP), Rua Jorge de Viterbo Ferreira 228, 4050-313 Porto, Portugal

* Correspondence: ebsouto@ff.up.pt (E.B.S.); ricardo_albuquerque@unit.br (R.L.C.d.A.-J.)

Citation: Passos, J.P.G.; Melo, C.R.; Carvalho, F.M.A.; Severino, P.; Cardoso, J.C.; Cunha, J.L.S.; Cano, A.; Souto, E.B.; de Albuquerque-Júnior, R.L.C. Combined Therapy of Chitosan and Exercise Improves the Lipid Profile, Adipose Tissue and Hepatic Alterations in an In Vivo Model of Induced-Hyperlipidemia. *Nutraceuticals* 2022, 2, 116–131. https://doi.org/10.3390/nutraceuticals2020009

Academic Editors: Ivan Cruz-Chamorro and Luisa Tesoriere

Received: 27 February 2022
Accepted: 7 June 2022
Published: 9 June 2022

Publisher's Note: MDPI stays neutral with regard to jurisdictional claims in published maps and institutional affiliations.

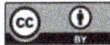

Copyright: © 2022 by the authors. Licensee MDPI, Basel, Switzerland. This article is an open access article distributed under the terms and conditions of the Creative Commons Attribution (CC BY) license (https://creativecommons.org/licenses/by/4.0/).

Abstract: Obesity is a prevalent public health concern in several countries, and is closely associated with several pathological disorders, including diabetes, hypertension, cardiovascular diseases, and increased dyslipidemia. Dyslipidemia is an asymptomatic condition characterized by high levels of low-density lipoproteins (LDL) and low levels of high-density lipoproteins (HDL), leading to the increased risk of ischemic heart disease. As lipid disorders are strongly associated with lifestyle and diet, in this work we have evaluated the effect of associating chitosan and exercise on the improvement of the lipid profile of high-fat diet-fed rats. Animals were submitted orally to hypercaloric diets based on liquid butter at 1 mL/100 g to induce a hyperlipidemic state for 8 weeks (as shown by body weight and measures of the Lee obesity index). After 8 weeks, the 40 rats were separated into five groups (n = 8) and adapted to different treatment strategies: physical exercise and/or treatment with chitosan (at a concentration of 2%). The hyperlipidemic group exhibited altered levels of glucose and hepatic enzymes, i.e., aspartate aminotransferase (AST) and alanine aminotransferase (ALT). The treatment with chitosan over 8 weeks significantly reduced the bodyweight of the animals, reaching values lower than the control group. Exercise reduced the Lee obesity index values of all the treated groups compared to non-treated rats. The concentration of total cholesterol, triglycerides, LDL, and VLDL was significantly reduced at the end of the study to healthy thresholds. The hepatic parenchyma of hyperlipidemic animals was recovered to show normal morphology when treated with chitosan; improved histological features (ca. 20–30% of parenchymal cells) could be achieved with physical exercise. In conclusion, oral administration of chitosan associated with physical exercise had a hypolipidemic effect in a model of dyslipidemia in rodents, showing decreased levels of total cholesterol, triglycerides, LDL-c, VLDL-c, glucose, and liver enzymes (AST and ALT). Our results are attributed to the synergism between the administration of chitosan and physical exercise that helps to reduce oxidative stress.

Keywords: chitosan; high-fat diet; hyperlipidemia; dyslipidemia; cardiovascular diseases; obesity

1. Introduction

Current lifestyle habits promote an unfavorable condition in the individual's overall health status with an increased risk of metabolic diseases [1,2]. The health–disease relationship is directly associated with the type and amount of fat contained in the diet and an inactive posture that characterizes a sedentary lifestyle, significantly contributing to the establishment of a positive energy imbalance [3,4]. More than 80% of adolescents aged between 11 and 17 years old do not follow the recommendations of the World Health Organization (WHO) about physical exercise for health improvement and, although the prevalence of physical inactivity varies greatly worldwide, about 80% of some adult populations [5] do not follow the recommendations.

A sedentary lifestyle and inadequate diet are environmental risk factors which, combined with individual factors (age, sex, education, genetic characteristics) [6–9], determine the onset of chronic diseases, including dyslipidemia [6]. Dyslipidemias are changes in serum levels of lipoproteins and present a significant public health concern due to their direct relationship with cardiovascular diseases [10,11]. These diseases are significant causes of mortality in both developed and developing countries, increasing the social and economic burden of health care systems [12–16].

The prevalence of dyslipidemia was found to be significantly higher in men than in women [17], but a higher prevalence of dyslipidemia components was reported for postmenopausal women [10]. Other studies demonstrate the trend of a higher lipid profile for men, which is associated with a higher risk of cardiovascular diseases when compared to women with the same lifestyle [18]. Food content directly influences plasma levels of triglycerides [19]. Guerra et al. (2007) [20] evaluated the effects of diet, serum lipids, and body weight in exercised rats. The authors observed that the intensity and time of physical exercise influenced high-density lipoprotein (HDL)-cholesterol (HDL-c) levels more acutely than the levels of triglycerides. Furthermore, a high-fat diet should follow a 14% change in lipid parameters and the use of the lipid substrate as a resource ergogenic.

The beneficial effects of healthy eating habits and physical exercise on dyslipidemia were demonstrated in the work by Mann et al. (2014) [21], in which serum levels of total cholesterol and low-density lipoprotein (LDL)-cholesterol (LDL-c) were reduced for individuals who performed physical exercise. On the other hand, total cholesterol, LDL-c, and weight had lower levels for the group submitted to physical exercise and to a specific diet, with an increase in HDL-c for this group as well. These results point out to the importance of the association between exercise and diet, optimizing changes in the lipoprotein profile.

The acute or chronic effect of aerobic exercise can improve the lipoprotein profile, stimulating a better functioning of the enzymatic processes involved in lipid metabolism, favoring the increase in HDL-c levels, and also modifying the chemical composition of LDL-c, making them the least atherogenic [21]. However, the association of diet and loss of body mass to aerobic exercise seems to be essential to obtaining an optimal lipid profile [22]. Hypocholesterolemic substances have been frequently used to decrease body mass and control hypercholesterolemia [23].

It is worth mentioning that cholesterol comes from two main sources, namely, from diet and from endogenous production [24]. Dietary cholesterol can be found free or esterified, while the latter needs to be de-esterified to be absorbed. For this absorption to occur, emulsification is necessary through the action of bile salts, fatty acids, and phospholipids, among others, forming the chylomicrons that will reach the bloodstream. The administration of substances capable of inhibiting the absorption of lipids has contributed to the control of serum cholesterol levels [25]. Although several studies report the effect of different treatment strategies with the use of lipid-lowering substances and different isolated diets [26–31], or just the practice of physical exercise on the plasma lipoprotein profile [9,32–35], the simultaneous approach to nutrition and physical exercise is important, as it encompasses a significant lifestyle change. A lifestyle change is also important in reducing the use of natural substances or lipid-lowering drugs needed to control dyslipidemia and, consequently, to prevent cardiovascular diseases [26].

In this process, polysaccharides can act by sequestering bile salts [24]. The viscosity and molecular weight of polysaccharides directly affect the aggregates formed in the intestinal lumen due to the ability to thicken and/or form gels enhanced by physical tangles, which, dependent on the monomeric units that make up the polysaccharide, benefit the non-internalization of cholesterol dietary [24]. Examples of polysaccharides are β-glucans, galactomannans, glucomannans, arabinoxylans, pectin, alginate, and chitosan. The latter is a linear polysaccharide composed of D-glucosamine and N-acetyl-D-glucosamine linked to positively charged β(1-4), which allows more efficient binding with bile salts that are negatively charged in the intestinal lumen [36–40].

It has already been reported that chitosan has hypocholesterolemic effects both in humans and in animals [41–45], behaving as an indigestible dietary fiber in the presence of mammalian enzymes from the gut [46]. The mechanism behind its beneficial effects for lipid metabolic disorders has however not been fully described. Tong et al. (2020) [47] demonstrated that *Ganoderma lucidum* polysaccharide and chitosan synergistically reduced hyperlipidemia in high-fat diet (HFD)-fed hamsters by lowering the contents of serum total triglycerides, total cholesterol, LDL-c, and aspartate aminotransferase (AST). The authors stressed that chitosan could even modify the composition of the gut microbiota with increased levels of beneficial bacteria, including those producing short-chain fatty acids.

Chiu et al. (2019) [46] compared the effect of chitosan of different molecular weights on cholesterol regulation in HFD-fed rats. This study confirmed chitosan of both high and low molecular weight could reduce hypercholesterolemia effectively by means of the activation of the hepatic AMPKα and PPARα cholesterol-modulators, inhibiting cholesterol-modulators in the intestine (ACAT2) and also modulating downstream LDLR and CYP7A1 signals. In this work, we evaluated the effect of a therapy combining chitosan and exercise on the lipid profile, adipose, and hepatic tissue, using an in vivo model of induced-hyperlipidemia.

2. Materials and Methods

2.1. Animals

Male rats of the Wistar lineage (45 days old, 220 ± 20 g) (n = 40) from the animal facility of Tiradentes University (Aracaju, Sergipe, Brazil) were used. The animals were kept under standardized conditions, with a 12 h light–dark cycle, treated with balanced feed and water *ad libitum*, with a temperature of 20 ± 4 °C and relative humidity of 70 ± 5%. The project was approved by the Research Ethics Committee of Tiradentes University under the embodied opinion number 060209-1.

2.2. Hyperlipidemia Induction

The liquid butter (bottle butter) used in the hyperlipidemia induction procedure was purchased at the Municipal Market of Aracaju, sold by one of the stores specializing in dairy products from family farms in the municipality of Glória (Sergipe, Brazil).

2.3. Chitosan

Low molecular weight chitosan (80 kDa) was purchased from the manufacturer Quimer Herbal (São Paulo, Brazil) as powdered crustacean fiber and distributed by Embrafarma *Produtos Químicos e Farmacêuticos* LTDA (São Paulo, Brazil), original batch: 029/3368.

2.4. Hyperlipidemia Induction Procedure

Of the 40 animals, 32 underwent an experimental process of induction of hyperlipidemia as described by Pan et al. (2016) [38]. These animals (45 days old) received the administration of liquid butter (1 mL/100 g of body weight) orally (gavage), to supplement the standard diet, developing a condition of hyperlipidemia for 8 weeks. This high-fat diet was administered from weaning onwards, continued for 8 weeks. The remaining

8 animals received a standard diet (NUVILAB® chow, Seoul, Korea) and distilled water orally (gavage) without the introduction of liquid butter (normolipidic diet) during the same period. NUVILAB® standard feed is composed of: calcium carbonate, corn, soybean, wheat bran, dicalcium phosphate, sodium chloride, mineral, amino acid premix, and an antioxidant additive. Confirmation of the hyperlipidemic state of the animals was performed by analyzing the serum lipid compositions (triglycerides, total cholesterol, high-density lipoproteins (HDL-c), low-density lipoproteins (LDL-c), and very low-density lipoprotein (VLDL-c)) and the blood glucose of the animals 8 weeks after induction.

2.5. Treatment Phase

Eight weeks after the hyperlipidemia induction phase, the 40 animals were separated into five groups (n = 8) and submitted to different treatment strategies: physical exercise, treatment with administration of chitosan, and the combination of both (Table 1).

Table 1. Distribution of experimental groups according to diet and recommended treatment.

Group (n = 8)	Systemic State	Oral Treatment	Physical Exercise
CTR	Normolipidemic	Distilled water	-
Hyp	Hyperlipidemic	Distilled water	-
Hyp–Ch	Hyperlipidemic	Chitosan	-
Hyp–Ex	Hyperlipidemic	Distilled water	Forced swimming
Hyp–ChEx	Hyperlipidemic	Chitosan	Forced swimming

2.5.1. Physical Training

The animals participated in aerobic physical exercises of light to moderate intensity, based on the adapted swimming training protocol as described by Dos Reis et al. (2018) [48]. The exercises were performed in tanks 100 cm deep by 60 cm wide and 80 cm long, with controlled temperatures between 28–32 °C. Initially, the animals were submitted to a period of adaptation to the liquid environment for one week, in which the time of sessions and the workload (caudal weight) were gradually increased until reaching that stipulated in the protocol. Work overload was up to 2% of body mass. The overload model was determined by using lead weights tied to the animal's tail with a pre-defined mass from the weekly measurement of the animals' body mass. The exercise took place in 45 min sessions with overload, 5 days a week, for 8 weeks.

2.5.2. Chitosan Treatment

For the use of chitosan, a solution in acetic acid 0.5 mol/L at a concentration of 2% was prepared, which was homogenized and made available for use. Gonçalves et al. (2017) [49] demonstrated that 2% chitosan in acetic acid has a high viscosity, as recommended for the oral sequestering of bile salts. The animals in the Hyp–Ch and Hyp–ChEx groups received 1 mL of the chitosan solution (corresponding to 20 mg of this product per animal) by oral gavage for 8 weeks. The other groups received 1.5 mL of water, replacing chitosan throughout the experiment, so that non-treated animals were subjected to similar stress procedures and conditions.

2.6. Assessment of Body Mass and Lee's Obesity Index

All animals were subjected to measurement of body mass at the beginning of the experiment, at the end of the induction phase, and at the end of the treatment phase, always at the same morning time, using a digital scale (Marte®, model AS2000C, São Paulo, Brazil). The gain in body mass at the end of the treatment phase was determined by the following equation:

$$BWG = \frac{W_i - W_f}{W_i} \times 100$$

where *BWG* is the body weight gain, W_i is the initial weight, and W_f is the final weight. The Lee's Obesity Index (*LOI*) was determined according to the following equation:

$$LOI = \frac{\sqrt[3]{BW}}{NaL}$$

where *LOI* is the Lee obesity index, *BW* is the body weight (g), and *NaL* is the nasoanal length (cm).

2.7. Determination of Lipid Percentage in Feces

Samples of 2 g of feces were collected using a spatula, weighed and submitted to extraction using petroleum ether in a Soxhlet type extractor. After 4 h of extraction, the solvent was recovered and the glass flask was weighed. The mass of lipids in the sample was calculated by the difference between the mass of the empty container and that obtained after the extraction and elimination of the solvent, with the results were expressed as the percentage.

2.8. Biochemical Analysis of Serum Lipid Concentrations

To obtain the serum, the animals were first anesthetized with 3% isofuran by inhalation, and blood samples were then collected by cardiac puncture using complete ether anesthesia and centrifuged at $3000 \times g$ for 10 min. Serum was stored in a freezer until the time of biochemical analysis. Triglycerides and cholesterol were measured with Trinder enzyme kits (Labtest, Belo Horizonte, MG, Brazil). This test is based on the hydrolysis of cholesteryl esters by cholesterol esterase to form free cholesterol and fatty acid. Subsequently, the cholesterol is oxidized to cholest-4-en-one and hydrogen peroxide which, in the presence of peroxidase and hydrogen peroxide, phenol, and 4-amino antipyrine, form antipyrylquinonimine that can be measured in a spectrophotometer at 500 nm. The color intensity is directly proportional to the cholesterol concentration in the sample. HDL-c was determined after precipitation of VLDL-c and LDL-c with phosphotungstic acid and magnesium chloride. VLDL-c and LDL-c concentrations were calculated using the Friedewald equation:

$$LDL = \text{Total Cholesterol} - (HDL + VLDL), \text{ where } VLDL = \frac{\text{Triglycerides}}{5}$$

2.9. Biochemical Analysis of Liver Enzyme and Glucose Dosages

Serum levels of liver enzymes (aspartate aminotransferase (AST) andalanine aminotransferase (ALT)) and glucose in serum samples were measured by the enzymatic method using commercial kits from Biorex Diagnostics (Antrim, UK) in a Roche Hitachi 911 Chemistry Analyzer (Ramsey, MN, USA).

2.10. Animal Euthanasia

After the eight weeks of treatment, the animals fasted overnight (12 h) and were then submitted to the procedure of euthanasia by anoxia in carbon dioxide chambers (model CGSCO2G, Beira-Mae, Aracaju, SE, Brazil), with 100% CO_2 (Bonther, Ribeirão Preto, São Paulo, Brazil, flow rate of 1–3 L/min) for 15 min. Lack of breathing and the fading of eye color were used to certify death. All animals were euthanized at the same time of day, after blood collection, following the same fasting period. The animal experiments were approved by the Research Ethics Committee of Universidade Tiradentes under the embodied opinion number 060209-1.

2.11. Assessment of Abdominal Adipose Tissue Weight

The assessment of abdominal adipose tissue Weight (AATW) was evaluated by weighing the subcutaneous and visceral adipose tissues. The weights of these two tissues were combined to form the ex vivo abdominal fat weight, which was expressed as the ratio of AATW and the bodyweight of each animal (wt/wt).

2.12. Histopathological Analysis of Liver Specimens

Immediately after euthanasia and ex vivo abdominal fat dissection, the animals' livers were removed and fixed in buffered formaldehyde (10%, pH 7.4) for 24 h. All livers were then dehydrated in increasing concentrations of ethanol (70 °gL, 80 °gL, 90 °gL, and 99.9 °gL), cleared in xylene, and embedded in paraffin for histological examination. Histological sections (5 µm thick) were obtained from specimens embedded in paraffin and stained with hematoxylin-eosin (HE), using a semi-automated rotary microtome HistoCore MULTICUT (Leica Geosystems, São Paulo, Brazil) [50]. Histological analysis was performed considering cytological and morphoarchitectural characteristics of the hepatic parenchymal and stromal components, as well as the presence of inflammatory infiltrate, necrosis, or degenerative changes.

2.13. Statistical Analysis

All data were subjected to normal distribution analysis using the Shapiro–Wilk test. Once the Gaussian (normal) distribution of the data was confirmed, the Student's t-test (comparison between two groups) and the ANOVA test were used, followed by the Tukey multiple comparisons test (comparison between three or more groups). All data are expressed as mean ± standard error of the mean (SEM). For all tests, a significance level of 5% was applied.

3. Results and Discussion

3.1. Hyperlipidemia Induction

As shown in Figure 1, both bodyweight and Lee obesity index (LOI) demonstrated that liquid butter at 1 mL/100 g of body weight induced a hyperlipidemic state in the animals after 8 weeks of feeding. Screening of the lipidic profile corroborated this. The total cholesterol, triglycerides, HDL-c, LDL-c, and VLDL-c concentrations were almost doubled in the hyperlipidemic group in comparison to the control group (Figure 2), showing statistically significant differences between both treated groups (Hyp and CTR) for both outputs (body weight and LOI). Moreover, the established threshold for the healthy condition was exceeded in all lipid measurements in the hyperlipidemic group.

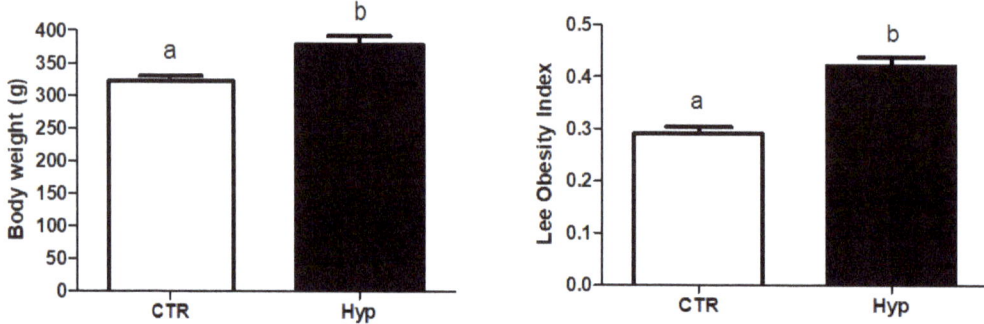

Figure 1. Assessment of body weight and Lee obesity index of the animals after the time-course of experimental induction of hyperlipidemia status (Hyp) using oral administration of liquid butter. Animals of the control group (CTR) were treated only with distilled water. Different letters (a,b) above the columns represent statistically different means (T Student test; $p < 0.05$).

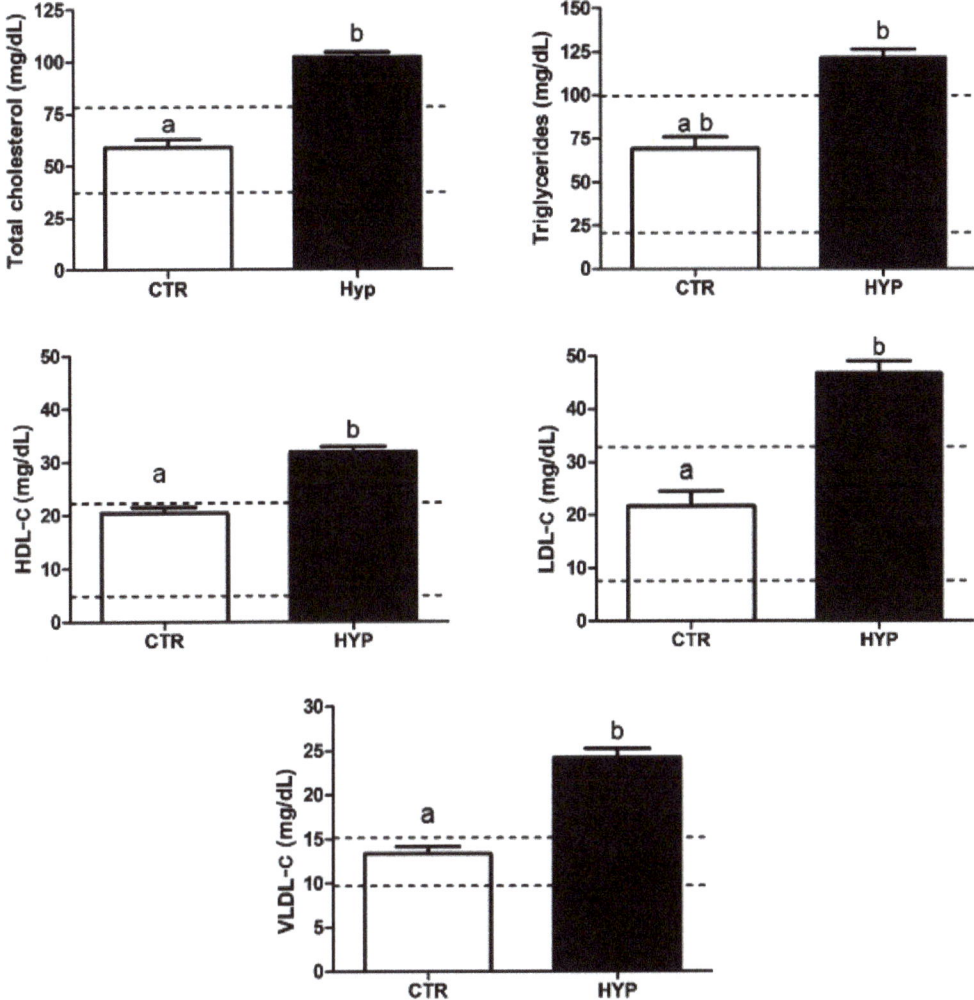

Figure 2. Assessment of lipidemic profile of the animals after the time-course of experimental induction of hyperlipidemia status (Hyp) using oral administration of liquid butter. Animals of the control group (CTR) were treated only with distilled water. Different letters (a,b) above the columns represent statistically different means (T Student test; $p < 0.05$). The normal range of the reference values is limited by the dashed lines.

Similarly, measurements of glucose and hepatic enzyme levels were also altered in the hyperlipidemic group. Whereas glucose levels of the control group were 104.1 ± 8.6 mg/dL, the hyperlipidemic group reached levels of 199.8 ± 3.8 mg/dL, surpassing the established threshold of healthy conditions (Figure 2, Total cholesterol). As for the hepatic enzymes, both AST and ALT were significantly increased (268.3 ± 25.8 UI/L and 109.4 ± 4.86 UI/L respectively) in the hyperlipidemic group ($p < 0.05$), and the established healthy threshold was exceeded too (Figure 3, AST) ($p < 0.05$).

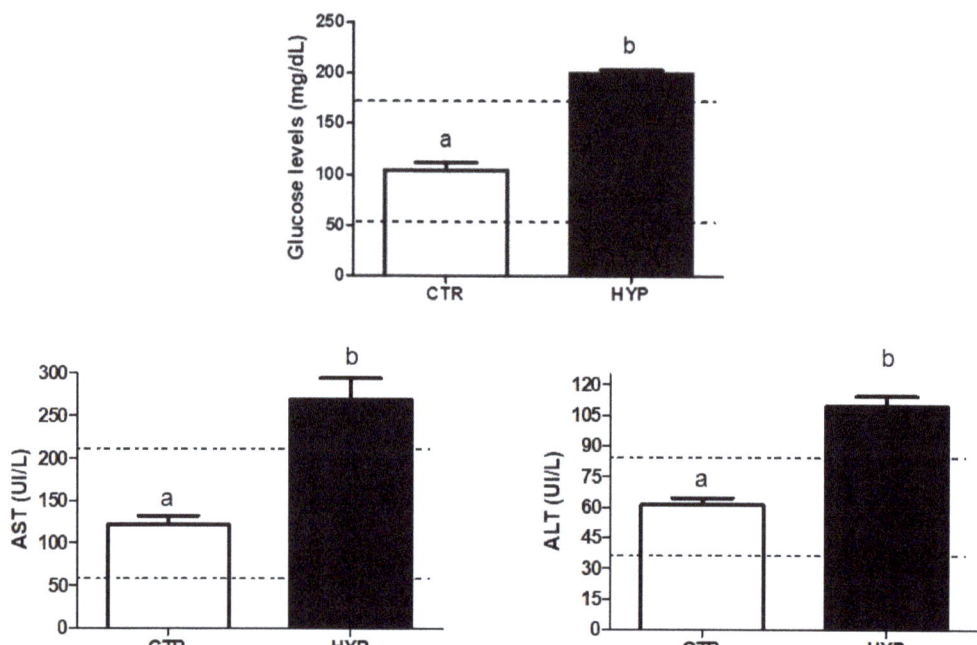

Figure 3. Assessment of the glucose and hepatic enzymes (Aspartate aminotransferase (AST) and alanine aminotransferase (ALT)) serum levels of the animals after the time-course of experimental induction of hyperlipidemia status (Hyp) using oral administration of liquid butter. Animals of the control group (CTR) were subjected to fake procedures using distilled water. Different letters (a,b) above the columns represent statistically different means (T Student test; $p < 0.05$). The normal range of the reference values is limited by the dashed lines.

3.2. Physical Training and Chitosan Treatment

After 8 weeks of treatment, hyperlipidemic rats exhibited a significant body gain weight compared to those littermates fed with the standard diet. However, those animals fed with liquid butter and simultaneously treated with chitosan significantly reduced their body weight ($p < 0.05$). When exercise was added to the treatment schedule, weight values were also significantly reduced ($p < 0.05$), reaching values even lower than the control group (Figure 4, body weight gain). Using Lee's obesity index, the same results were observed. Hyperlipidemic rats treated with chitosan and supplemented with physical exercise exhibited the lowest Lee obesity index values of all the treated groups compared to non-treated rats, reaching values close to similar to the standard diet-fed rats.

At the end of the study, the treatment of hyperlipidemic rats with chitosan was able to reduce total cholesterol, triglycerides, LDL-c, and VLDL-c concentrations compared to non-treated hyperlipidemic rats, but none of these molecules were reduced to the established healthy threshold (Figure 5). Total cholesterol and LDL-c were reduced to the established healthy threshold in those hyperlipidemic rats that underwent physical exercise only. Interestingly, the combination of chitosan treatment and physical exercise was able to significantly reduce the total cholesterol, triglycerides, LDL-c, and VLDL-c concentrations to the established healthy threshold ($p < 0.05$). Furthermore, in the case of LDL-c, this value was even lower than the control group. HDL-c results did not show any change in all the experimental groups compared to controls.

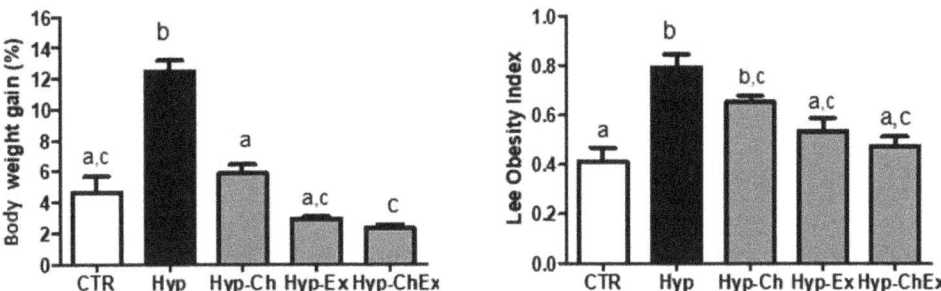

Figure 4. Assessment of body weight and Lee obesity index of the animals after the time-course of experimental induction of hyperlipidemia status (Hyp) using oral administration of liquid butter. Animals of the control group (CTR) were subjected to fake procedures using distilled water. Different letters (a,b,c) above the columns represent statistically different means (ANOVA and Tukey's test; $p < 0.05$).

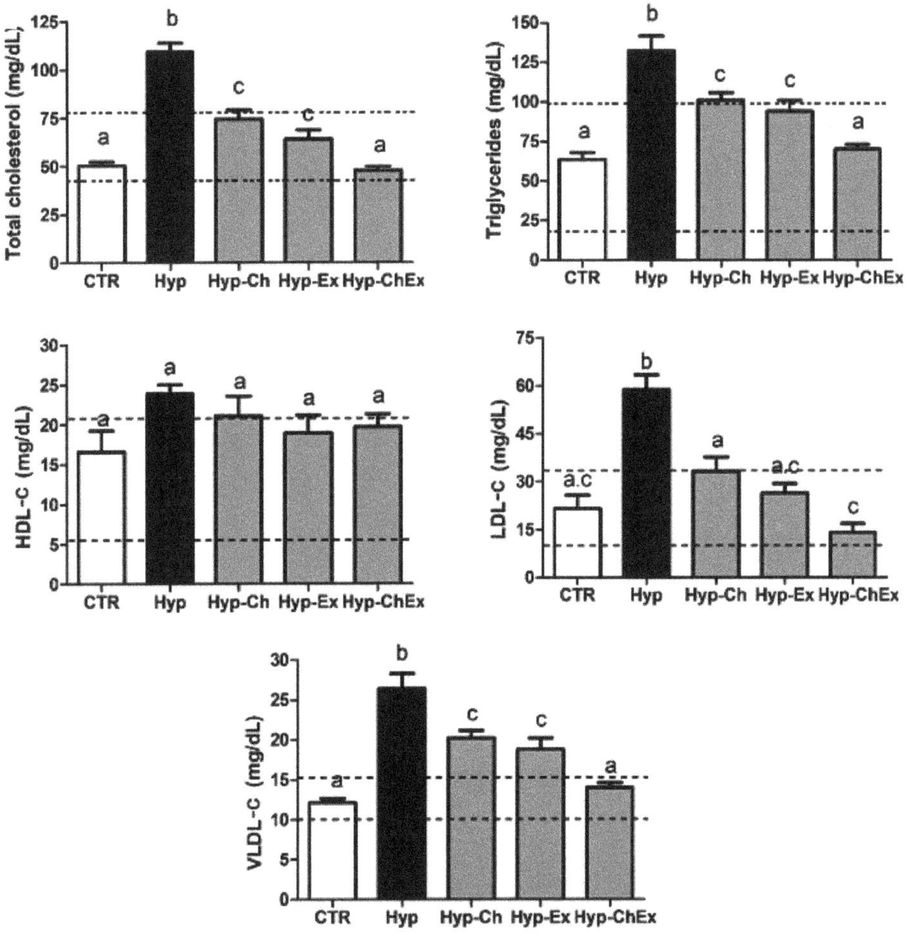

Figure 5. Assessment of lipidemic profile of the animals after treatment with oral administration of chitosan (Hyp–Ch), subjected to a standard protocol of physical exercises (Hyp–Ex) and combining

both treatments (Hyp–ChEx). The control group is represented as CTR and the untreated hyperlipidemic group as Hyp. All data are expressed as mean ± SEM. Different letters (a,b,c) above the columns represent statistically different values (ANOVA and Tukey's multiple comparisons tests; $p < 0.05$). The normal range of the reference values is limited by the dashed lines.

As observed with the lipid profile, the combination of chitosan and physical exercise exhibited the best results. Whereas chitosan's treatment only reduced the AST concentration in the hyperlipidemic rats, the supplementation of physical exercise significantly reduced glucose, AST, and ALT levels to the established healthy threshold (Figure 6) ($p < 0.05$). Moreover, in the case of AST, obtained values were even lower than in the control group.

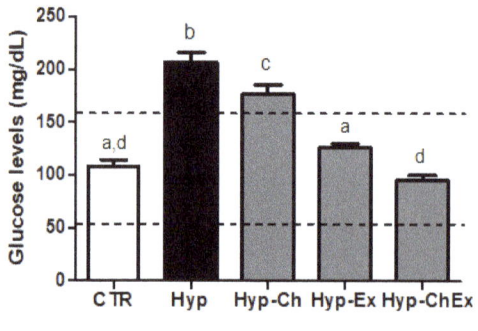

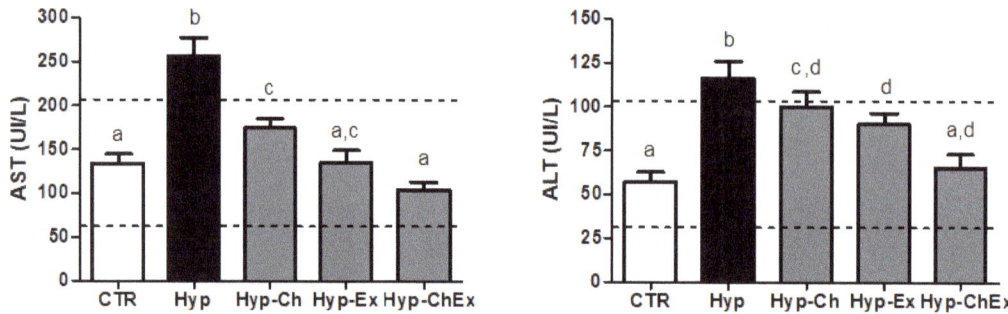

Figure 6. Assessment of the glucose and hepatic enzymes (Aspartate aminotransferase (AST) and alanine aminotransferase (ALT)) serum levels of the animals after treatment with oral administration of chitosan (Hyp–Ch), subject to a standard protocol of physical exercises (Hyp–Ex) and combining both treatments (Hyp–ChEx). The Control group is represented as CTR and the untreated hyperlipidemic group as Hyp. All data are expressed as mean ± SEM. Different letters (a,b,c,d) above the columns represent statistically different values (ANOVA and Tukey's multiple comparisons tests; $p < 0.05$). The normal range of the reference values is limited by the dashed lines.

Analysis of feces showed that the treatment with chitosan supplemented with physical exercise significantly reduces the lipid content of the feces compared to the non-treated hyperlipidemic littermates. Similar results were obtained in the hyperlipidemic rats that underwent physical exercise only (Figure 7, fecal lipid). Much higher differences were found in the abdominal fat assay. Once more, hyperlipidemic rats that received a combined treatment of chitosan and physical exercise exhibited the highest reduction of abdominal fat, reaching values close to the control group ($p < 0.05$). However, chitosan treatment and physical exercise separately were each also able to reduce abdominal fat in comparison to the non-treated hyperlipidemic group (Figure 6, AST).

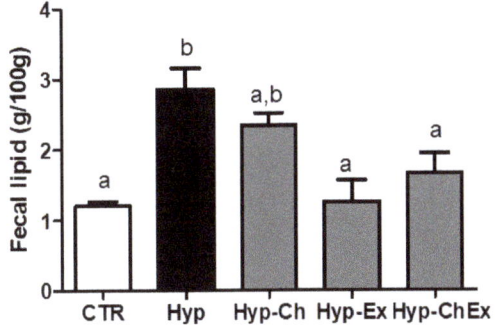
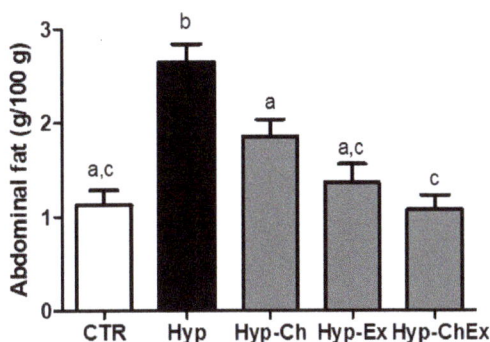

Figure 7. Assessment of fecal lipid and abdominal fat relative to the content of animals after treatment with oral administration of chitosan (Hyp–Ch), subjected to a standard protocol of physical exercises (Hyp–Ex), and the combination of both treatments (Hyp–ChEx). The control group is represented as CTR and the untreated hyperlipidemic group as Hyp. All data are expressed as mean ± SEM. Different letters (a,b,c) above the columns represent statistically different values (ANOVA and Tukey's multiple comparisons tests; $p < 0.05$). The normal range of the reference values is limited by the dashed lines.

Samples of the liver of the group CTR showed the usual morphological and architectural appearance of the hepatic parenchyma, characterized by a typical lobular structure and polygonal hepatocytes (over 50% of the liver parenchyma), with wide granular cytoplasm, bulky nuclei, and prominent nucleoli (Figure 8A,B). Non-treated hyperlipidemic animals (group Hyp), on the other hand, presented intense and diffusely distributed hepatocyte cytoplasmic vacuolization resulting from intracellular lipid accumulation (macrovesicular steatosis).

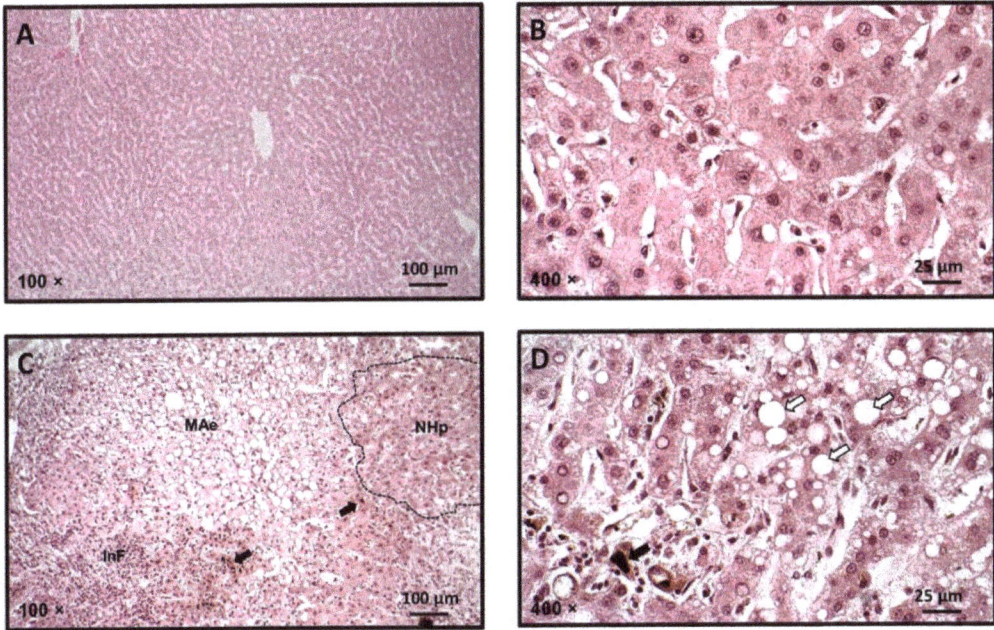

Figure 8. *Cont.*

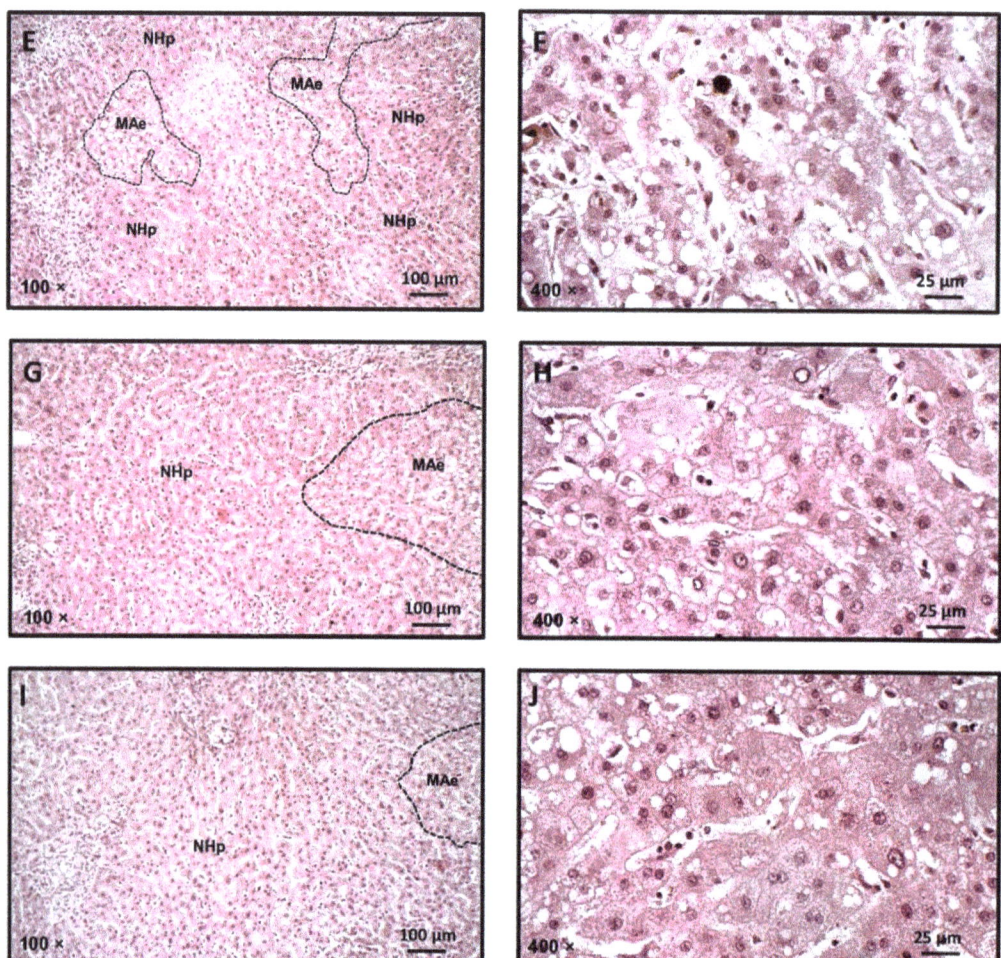

Figure 8. Histological sections of HE-stained samples of liver of the experimental groups. (**A,B**) Usual morphological and architectural appearance of the hepatic parenchyma is shown in CTR. (**C,D**) Hyperlipidemic animals showing intense and diffuse cytoplasmic round-shaped vacuolar changes of hepatocytes compatible with lipidic inclusions (macrovesicular steatosis); focal areas of chronic inflammatory infiltrate and droplets of brownish granular pigment compatible with bilirubin are also observed. In some focal areas, the reminiscent normal hepatic parenchyma can be observed. (**E,F**) Hyperlipidemic group treated with chitosan administration (Hyp–Ch) showing multiple and large foci of macrovesicular steatosis permeating the normal hepatic parenchyma. (**G,H**) Hyperlipidemic group treated with physical exercises (Hyp–Ex) showing large focal areas of reminiscent macrovesicular steatosis. (**I,J**) Hyperlipidemic group treated with combined chitosan administration and physical exercises (Hyp–ChEx) showing scant and less extensive foci of macrovesicular steatosis. NHp: Normal hepatic parenchyma; MAe: Macrovesicular steatosis; InF: chronic inflammatory infiltrate; black arrows: bilirubin pigment; white arrows: steatotic hepatocytes.

Focal areas of interlobular lymph-histiocytic inflammation, and both intracytoplasmic and intraductal accumulation of brown granular pigment compatible with bilirubin, were also observed (Figure 8C,D). All therapeutic approaches tested in the current work reduced the extent of the pathological changes observed in the liver tissues. However, the group treated only with oral administration of chitosan (Hyp–Ch) exhibited a persistence of multiple and large foci of macrovesicular steatosis (30–50% of the liver parenchyma) and intracellular/intraductal bilirubin accumulation (Figure 8E,F).

A better improvement of the histological features of the liver tissue occurred with the practice of physical exercises (20–30% of the parenchyma) (Figure 8G,H), but the reduction of the steatosis obtained from the combination of both treatments was remarkable, since less than 20% of the hepatocytes presented intracellular lipid inclusions, and no morphological signs of inflammation or cholestasis (reduction of the bile flow and consequent accumulation of bilirubin in the hepatic parenchyma) were observed (Figure 8I,J).

Studies of the effect of chitosan supplantation on the diet of overweight and obese patients have been published. The beneficial effects of this polysaccharide on hyperlipidemic individuals have been attributed to its role in the improvement of blood pressure and serum lipids status [51]. Trivedi et al. (2016) [52] conducted a randomized phase IV clinical study, which consisted of the administration of chitosan capsules (500 mg, five/day) and indistinguishable placebo capsules as daily supplements to 96 overweight and obese subjects over 90 days, resulting in a 10.91-fold reduction of the body mass index and loss of 3 kg [52]. Chitosan also reduced HbA1C levels (below 6%) in subjects who had initial higher values, but the lipid levels were not affected. Bahijri et al. (2017) [22] evaluated the effect of chitosan on markers of obesity and cardiometabolic risk in rats fed normal chow (NC) or a high-fat/high-cholesterol diet (HF/HCD) [20], concluding that chitosan improved lipid profile, insulin sensitivity, and oxidative stress caused by a high-cholesterol diet [38–40,53].

In our study, the combination of physical exercise with chitosan supplantation in the diet of treated animals was able to significantly reduce the levels of total cholesterol, triglycerides, LDL-c, VLDL-c, glucose, AST, and ALT to the established healthy thresholds ($p < 0.01$). The levels of lipid content both in the abdomen of animals and in faces were also influenced by the combined therapy attributed to improved nutrients' digestibility [54]. Although the precise mechanisms underlying the chitosan-decreased triglycerides, LDL-c, and VLDL-c are not fully clear, possible associations with the decrease of the ratios of surface lipids to core lipids of the VLDL particles [55], upregulation of hepatic LDL receptor mRNA expression [56], upregulation of lecithin cholesterol acyl transferase activity [57], and elevation of plasma angiopoietin-like 4 (ANGPTL4) protein and adiponectin expression [58] have been previously proposed. Such metabolic effects would lead not only to an increase in the hepatic metabolism of fatty acids, but also to elevated excretion of fecal bile acids. The regulation of the hepatic metabolism and excretion of lipids could also explain the improvement of the AST and ALT levels. In addition, the catecholamine response to exercise increases lipolysis of triacylglycerols in adipose tissue and increases the adipose tissue blood flow, decreasing fatty acid re-esterification in glycerol [59]. Therefore, the combination of treatments appears to act synergistically to reduce lipid constituents and improve the expression of liver enzymes in the blood.

4. Conclusions

In this study, we have demonstrated that oral administration of chitosan together with physical exercise had a hypolipidemic effect in a rodent model of dyslipidemia. Levels of total cholesterol, triglycerides, LDL-c, VLDL-c, glucose, and hepatic enzymes (AST and ALT) were significantly improved followed by improved histological features of hepatic parenchyma. A synergistic effect is therefore expected with the proposed therapy combining the effect of chitosan in reducing the risk of obesity and the reduction of oxidative stress promoted by physical exercise.

Author Contributions: J.P.G.P., C.R.M., F.M.A.C., P.S. and J.C.C. contributed to the conceptualization, methodology, validation, formal analysis, investigation, and writing—original draft preparation. J.L.S.C., A.C., E.B.S. and R.L.C.d.A.-J. contributed to the methodology, supervision, writing—review and editing, project administration, resources, and funding acquisition. All authors have made a substantial contribution to the work. All authors have read and agreed to the published version of the manuscript.

Funding: This research was funded by the National Council for Scientific and Technological Development (*Conselho Nacional de Desenvolvimento Científico e Tecnológico*—CNPq, Brazil), the Coordination for the Improvement of Higher Education Personnel (*Coordenação de Aperfeiçoamento de Pessoal de Nível Superior*—CAPES, Brazil), grant #2015/20630-4 São Paulo Research Foundation and grant #2021/05719-0 São Paulo Research Foundation, and by Fundação Carolina (*Movilidad de profesorado Brasil-España, Movilidad. Estancias de Investigación*, C.2020) granted to P.S.

Institutional Review Board Statement: The animal experiments were approved by the Research Ethics Committee of Universidade Tiradentes under the embodied opinion number 060209-1.

Informed Consent Statement: Not applicable.

Data Availability Statement: Not applicable.

Conflicts of Interest: The authors declare no conflict of interest.

References

1. Rychter, A.M.; Skrzypczak-Zielinska, M.; Zielinska, A.; Eder, P.; Souto, E.B.; Zawada, A.; Ratajczak, A.E.; Dobrowolska, A.; Krela-Kazmierczak, I. Is the Retinol-Binding Protein 4 a Possible Risk Factor for Cardiovascular Diseases in Obesity? *Int. J. Mol. Sci.* **2020**, *21*, 5229. [CrossRef] [PubMed]
2. Karczewski, J.; Zielińska, A.; Staszewski, R.; Eder, P.; Dobrowolska, A.; Souto, E.B. Obesity and the brain. *Int. J. Mol. Sci.* **2022**, submitted.
3. Kolb, H.; Martin, S. Environmental/lifestyle factors in the pathogenesis and prevention of type 2 diabetes. *BMC Med.* **2017**, *15*, 131. [CrossRef] [PubMed]
4. Galgani, J.E.; Fernández-Verdejo, R. Pathophysiological role of metabolic flexibility on metabolic health. *Obes. Rev.* **2021**, *22*, e13131. [CrossRef] [PubMed]
5. WHO (World Health Organization). Available online: https://www.who.int/ncds/prevention/physical-activity/inactivity-global-health-problem/en/ (accessed on 8 June 2021).
6. Stewart, J.; McCallin, T.; Martinez, J.; Chacko, S.; Yusuf, S. Hyperlipidemia. *Pediatr. Rev.* **2020**, *41*, 393–402. [CrossRef] [PubMed]
7. Chanoine, P.; Spector, N.D. Hyperlipidemia, eating disorders, and smoking cessation. *Curr. Opin. Pediatr.* **2008**, *20*, 734–739. [CrossRef] [PubMed]
8. Xi, Y.; Niu, L.; Cao, N.; Bao, H.; Xu, X.; Zhu, H.; Yan, T.; Zhang, N.; Qiao, L.; Han, K.; et al. Prevalence of dyslipidemia and associated risk factors among adults aged ≥35 years in northern China: A cross-sectional study. *BMC Public Health* **2020**, *20*, 1068. [CrossRef]
9. Dankner, R.; Ben Avraham, S.; Harats, D.; Chetrit, A. ApoE Genotype, Lipid Profile, Exercise, and the Associations With Cardiovascular Morbidity and 18-Year Mortality. *J. Gerontol. Ser. A Biol. Sci. Med. Sci.* **2020**, *75*, 1887–1893. [CrossRef]
10. Mendonça, M.A.A.; Ribeiro, A.R.S.; Lima, A.K.; Bezerra, G.B.; Pinheiro, M.S.; Albuquerque-Júnior, R.L.C.; Gomes, M.Z.; Padilha, F.F.; Thomazzi, S.M.; Novellino, E.; et al. Red Propolis and Its Dyslipidemic Regulator Formononetin: Evaluation of Antioxidant Activity and Gastroprotective Effects in Rat Model of Gastric Ulcer. *Nutrients* **2020**, *12*, 2951. [CrossRef]
11. Mendoza-Herrera, K.; Pedroza-Tobías, A.; Hernández-Alcaraz, C.; Ávila-Burgos, L.; Aguilar-Salinas, C.A.; Barquera, S. Attributable Burden and Expenditure of Cardiovascular Diseases and Associated Risk Factors in Mexico and other Selected Mega-Countries. *Int. J. Environ. Res. Public Health* **2019**, *16*, 4041. [CrossRef]
12. Gebreegziabiher, G.; Belachew, T.; Mehari, K.; Tamiru, D. Prevalence of dyslipidemia and associated risk factors among adult residents of Mekelle City, Northern Ethiopia. *PLoS ONE* **2021**, *16*, e0243510. [CrossRef]
13. Erem, C.; Hacihasanoglu, A.; Deger, O.; Kocak, M.; Topbas, M. Prevalence of dyslipidemia and associated risk factors among Turkish adults: Trabzon lipid study. *Endocrine* **2008**, *34*, 36–51. [CrossRef] [PubMed]
14. Opoku, S.; Gan, Y.; Fu, W.; Chen, D.; Addo-Yobo, E.; Trofimovitch, D.; Yue, W.; Yan, F.; Wang, Z.; Lu, Z. Prevalence and risk factors for dyslipidemia among adults in rural and urban China: Findings from the China National Stroke Screening and prevention project (CNSSPP). *BMC Public Health* **2019**, *19*, 1500. [CrossRef] [PubMed]
15. Gao, H.; Wang, H.; Shan, G.; Liu, R.; Chen, H.; Sun, S.; Liu, Y. Prevalence of dyslipidemia and associated risk factors among adult residents of Shenmu City, China. *PLoS ONE* **2021**, *16*, e0250573. [CrossRef] [PubMed]
16. Zhang, F.L.; Xing, Y.Q.; Wu, Y.H.; Liu, H.Y.; Luo, Y.; Sun, M.S.; Guo, Z.N.; Yang, Y. The prevalence, awareness, treatment, and control of dyslipidemia in northeast China: A population-based cross-sectional survey. *Lipids Health Dis.* **2017**, *16*, 61. [CrossRef] [PubMed]

17. Mosca, L. Management of Dyslipidemia in Women in the Post–hormone Therapy Era. *J. Gen. Intern. Med.* **2005**, *20*, 297–305. [CrossRef]
18. Yu, K.; Xue, Y.; He, T.; Guan, L.; Zhao, A.; Zhang, Y. Association of Spicy Food Consumption Frequency with Serum Lipid Profiles in Older People in China. *J. Nutr. Health Aging* **2018**, *22*, 311–320. [CrossRef]
19. Sobczak, A.I.S.; Blindauer, C.A.; Stewart, A.J. Changes in Plasma Free Fatty Acids Associated with Type-2 Diabetes. *Nutrients* **2019**, *11*, 2022. [CrossRef]
20. Guerra, R.L.F.; Prado, W.L.; Cheik, N.C.; Viana, F.P.; Botero, J.P.; Vendramini, R.C.; Carlos, I.Z.; Rossi, E.A.; Dâmaso, A.R. Effects of 2 or 5 consecutive exercise days on adipocyte area and lipid parameters in Wistar rats. *Lipids Health Dis.* **2007**, *6*, 16. [CrossRef]
21. Mann, S.; Beedie, C.; Jimenez, A. Differential effects of aerobic exercise, resistance training and combined exercise modalities on cholesterol and the lipid profile: Review, synthesis and recommendations. *Sports Med.* **2014**, *44*, 211–221. [CrossRef]
22. Bahijri, S.M.; Alsheikh, L.; Ajabnoor, G.; Borai, A. Effect of Supplementation With Chitosan on Weight, Cardiometabolic, and Other Risk Indices in Wistar Rats Fed Normal and High-Fat/High-Cholesterol Diets Ad Libitum. *Nutr. Metab. Insights* **2017**, *10*, 1178638817710666. [CrossRef]
23. Jemai, H.; Bouaziz, M.; Fki, I.; El Feki, A.; Sayadi, S. Hypolipidimic and antioxidant activities of oleuropein and its hydrolysis derivative-rich extracts from Chemlali olive leaves. *Chem.-Biol. Interact.* **2008**, *176*, 88–98. [CrossRef] [PubMed]
24. Silva, I.M.V.; Machado, F.; Moreno, M.J.; Nunes, C.; Coimbra, M.A.; Coreta-Gomes, F. Polysaccharide Structures and Their Hypocholesterolemic Potential. *Molecules* **2021**, *26*, 4559. [CrossRef] [PubMed]
25. Erickson, N.; Zafron, M.; Harding, S.V.; Marinangeli, C.P.F.; Rideout, T.C. Evaluating the Lipid-Lowering Effects of α-lipoic Acid Supplementation: A Systematic Review. *J. Diet. Suppl.* **2020**, *17*, 753–767. [CrossRef] [PubMed]
26. Poli, A.; Visioli, F. Pharmacology of Nutraceuticals with Lipid Lowering Properties. *High Blood Press. Cardiovasc. Prev.* **2019**, *26*, 113–118. [CrossRef]
27. Yang, M.; Hu, D.; Cui, Z.; Li, H.; Man, C.; Jiang, Y. Lipid-Lowering Effects of Inonotus obliquus Polysaccharide In Vivo and In Vitro. *Foods* **2021**, *10*, 3085. [CrossRef]
28. Derosa, G.; Colletti, A.; Maffioli, P.; D'Angelo, A.; Lupi, A.; Zito, G.B.; Mureddu, G.F.; Raddino, R.; Fedele, F.; Cicero, A.F.G. Lipid-lowering nutraceuticals update on scientific evidence. *J. Cardiovasc. Med.* **2020**, *21*, 845–859. [CrossRef]
29. Hadipour, E.; Taleghani, A.; Tayarani-Najaran, N.; Tayarani-Najaran, Z. Biological effects of red beetroot and betalains: A review. *Phytother. Res. PTR* **2020**, *34*, 1847–1867. [CrossRef]
30. Xiong, Z.; Cao, X.; Wen, Q.; Chen, Z.; Cheng, Z.; Huang, X.; Zhang, Y.; Long, C.; Zhang, Y.; Huang, Z. An overview of the bioactivity of monacolin K/lovastatin. *Food Chem. Toxicol.* **2019**, *131*, 110585. [CrossRef]
31. Gerards, M.C.; Terlou, R.J.; Yu, H.; Koks, C.H.; Gerdes, V.E. Traditional Chinese lipid-lowering agent red yeast rice results in significant LDL reduction but safety is uncertain—A systematic review and meta-analysis. *Atherosclerosis* **2015**, *240*, 415–423. [CrossRef]
32. Hosseini, Z.; Ghaedi, H.; Ahmadi, M.; Hosseini, S.A. Lipid-Lowering Effects of Concurrent Training and Green Tea Consumption in Overweight Women. *J. Obes. Metab. Syndr.* **2020**, *29*, 313–319. [CrossRef]
33. Conte, M.S.; Bradbury, A.W.; Kolh, P.; White, J.V.; Dick, F.; Fitridge, R.; Mills, J.L.; Ricco, J.B.; Suresh, K.R.; Murad, M.H. Global vascular guidelines on the management of chronic limb-threatening ischemia. *J. Vasc. Surg.* **2019**, *69*, 3S–125S.e140. [CrossRef] [PubMed]
34. Pearson, G.J.; Thanassoulis, G.; Anderson, T.J.; Barry, A.R.; Couture, P.; Dayan, N.; Francis, G.A.; Genest, J.; Grégoire, J.; Grover, S.A.; et al. 2021 Canadian Cardiovascular Society Guidelines for the Management of Dyslipidemia for the Prevention of Cardiovascular Disease in Adults. *Can. J. Cardiol.* **2021**, *37*, 1129–1150. [CrossRef] [PubMed]
35. Arocha Rodulfo, J.I. Sedentary lifestyle a disease from xxi century. *Clin. Investig. Arterioscler. Publ. Of. Soc. Esp. Arterioscler.* **2019**, *31*, 233–240. [CrossRef]
36. Naumann, S.; Schweiggert-Weisz, U.; Eglmeier, J.; Haller, D.; Eisner, P. In Vitro Interactions of Dietary Fibre Enriched Food Ingredients with Primary and Secondary Bile Acids. *Nutrients* **2019**, *11*, 1424. [CrossRef] [PubMed]
37. Maezaki, Y.; Tsuji, K.; Nakagawa, Y.; Kawai, Y.; Akimoto, M.; Tsugita, T.; Takekawa, W.; Terada, A.; Hara, H.; Mitsuoka, T. Hypocholesterolemic Effect of Chitosan in Adult Males. *Biosci. Biotechnol. Biochem.* **1993**, *57*, 1439–1444. [CrossRef]
38. Pan, H.; Yang, Q.; Huang, G.; Ding, C.; Cao, P.; Huang, L.; Xiao, T.; Guo, J.; Su, Z. Hypolipidemic effects of chitosan and its derivatives in hyperlipidemic rats induced by a high-fat diet. *Food Nutr. Res.* **2016**, *60*, 31137. [CrossRef]
39. Choi, C.R.; Kim, E.K.; Kim, Y.S.; Je, J.Y.; An, S.H.; Lee, J.D.; Wang, J.H.; Ki, S.S.; Jeon, B.T.; Moon, S.H.; et al. Chitooligosaccharides decreases plasma lipid levels in healthy men. *Int. J. Food Sci. Nutr.* **2012**, *63*, 103–106. [CrossRef]
40. Caffall, K.H.; Mohnen, D. The structure, function, and biosynthesis of plant cell wall pectic polysaccharides. *Carbohydr. Res.* **2009**, *344*, 1879–1900. [CrossRef]
41. Naveed, M.; Phil, L.; Sohail, M.; Hasnat, M.; Baig, M.; Ihsan, A.U.; Shumzaid, M.; Kakar, M.U.; Mehmood Khan, T.; Akabar, M.D.; et al. Chitosan oligosaccharide (COS): An overview. *Int. J. Biol. Macromol.* **2019**, *129*, 827–843. [CrossRef]
42. Swiatkiewicz, S.; Swiatkiewicz, M.; Arczewska-Wlosek, A.; Jozefiak, D. Chitosan and its oligosaccharide derivatives (chito-oligosaccharides) as feed supplements in poultry and swine nutrition. *J. Anim. Physiol. Anim. Nutr.* **2015**, *99*, 1–12. [CrossRef]
43. Zhang, J.; Xia, W.; Liu, P.; Cheng, Q.; Tahirou, T.; Gu, W.; Li, B. Chitosan modification and pharmaceutical/biomedical applications. *Mar. Drugs* **2010**, *8*, 1962–1987. [CrossRef] [PubMed]

44. Ngo, D.H.; Kim, S.K. Antioxidant effects of chitin, chitosan, and their derivatives. *Adv. Food Nutr. Res.* **2014**, *73*, 15–31. [CrossRef] [PubMed]
45. Riaz Rajoka, M.S.; Zhao, L.; Mehwish, H.M.; Wu, Y.; Mahmood, S. Chitosan and its derivatives: Synthesis, biotechnological applications, and future challenges. *Appl. Microbiol. Biotechnol.* **2019**, *103*, 1557–1571. [CrossRef] [PubMed]
46. Chiu, C.Y.; Yen, T.E.; Liu, S.H.; Chiang, M.T. Comparative Effects and Mechanisms of Chitosan and Its Derivatives on Hypercholesterolemia in High-Fat Diet-Fed Rats. *Int. J. Mol. Sci.* **2019**, *21*, 92. [CrossRef]
47. Tong, A.J.; Hu, R.K.; Wu, L.X.; Lv, X.C.; Li, X.; Zhao, L.N.; Liu, B. Ganoderma polysaccharide and chitosan synergistically ameliorate lipid metabolic disorders and modulate gut microbiota composition in high fat diet-fed golden hamsters. *J. Food Biochem.* **2020**, *44*, e13109. [CrossRef]
48. Dos Reis, I.G.M.; Martins, L.E.B.; de Araujo, G.G.; Gobatto, C.A. Forced Swim Reliability for Exercise Testing in Rats by a Tethered Swimming Apparatus. *Front. Physiol.* **2018**, *9*, 1839. [CrossRef]
49. Gonçalves, R.P.; Ferreira, W.H.; Gouvêa, R.F.; Andrade, C.T. Effect of Chitosan on the Properties of Electrospun Fibers From Mixed Poly(Vinyl Alcohol)/ Chitosan Solutions. *Mater. Res.* **2017**, *20*, 984–993. [CrossRef]
50. Shi, P.; Chen, J.; Lin, J.; Zhang, L. High-throughput fat quantifications of hematoxylin-eosin stained liver histopathological images based on pixel-wise clustering. *Sci. China Inf. Sci.* **2017**, *60*, 092108. [CrossRef]
51. Jull, A.B.; Ni Mhurchu, C.; Bennett, D.A.; Dunshea-Mooij, C.A.; Rodgers, A. Chitosan for overweight or obesity. *Cochrane Database Syst. Rev.* **2008**, *16*, CD003892. [CrossRef]
52. Trivedi, V.R.; Satia, M.C.; Deschamps, A.; Maquet, V.; Shah, R.B.; Zinzuwadia, P.H.; Trivedi, J.V. Single-blind, placebo controlled randomised clinical study of chitosan for body weight reduction. *Nutr. J.* **2016**, *15*, 3. [CrossRef]
53. Tungland, B.C.; Meyer, D. Nondigestible Oligo- and Polysaccharides (Dietary Fiber): Their Physiology and Role in Human Health and Food. *Compr. Rev. Food Sci. Food Saf.* **2002**, *1*, 90–109. [CrossRef] [PubMed]
54. Razdan, A.; Pettersson, D. Effect of chitin and chitosan on nutrient digestibility and plasma lipid concentrations in broiler chickens. *Br. J. Nutr.* **1994**, *72*, 277–288. [CrossRef] [PubMed]
55. Yao, H.T.; Chiang, M.T. Plasma lipoprotein cholesterol in rats fed a diet enriched in chitosan and cholesterol. *J. Nutr. Sci. Vitaminol.* **2002**, *48*, 379–383. [CrossRef] [PubMed]
56. Xu, G.; Huang, X.; Qiu, L.; Wu, J.; Hu, Y. Mechanism study of chitosan on lipid metabolism in hyperlipidemic rats. *Asia Pac. J. Clin. Nutr.* **2007**, *16* (Suppl. 1), 313–317.
57. Wang, D.; Han, J.; Yu, Y.; Li, X.; Wang, Y.; Tian, H.; Guo, S.; Jin, S.; Luo, T.; Qin, S. Chitosan oligosaccharide decreases very-low-density lipoprotein triglyceride and increases high-density lipoprotein cholesterol in high-fat-diet-fed rats. *Exp. Biol. Med.* **2011**, *236*, 1064–1069. [CrossRef]
58. Liu, S.-H.; Cai, F.-Y.; Chiang, M.-T. Long-Term Feeding of Chitosan Ameliorates Glucose and Lipid Metabolism in a High-Fructose-Diet-Impaired Rat Model of Glucose Tolerance. *Mar. Drugs* **2015**, *13*, 7302–7313. [CrossRef]
59. Muscella, A.; Stefàno, E.; Lunetti, P.; Capobianco, L.; Marsigliante, S. The Regulation of Fat Metabolism During Aerobic Exercise. *Biomolecules* **2020**, *10*, 1699. [CrossRef]

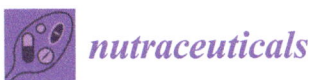

Article

Anti-Allergic Effect of Aqueous Extract of Coriander (*Coriandrum sativum* L.) Leaf in RBL-2H3 Cells and Cedar Pollinosis Model Mice

Yurika Kitamura [1], Kosuke Nishi [1,2], Momoko Ishida [1], Sogo Nishimoto [3] and Takuya Sugahara [1,2,*]

[1] Department of Bioscience, Graduate School of Agriculture, Ehime University, Matsuyama 790-8566, Japan; e652005y@mails.cc.ehime-u.ac.jp (Y.K.); nishi.kosuke.mx@ehime-u.ac.jp (K.N.); ishida.momoko.vb@ehime-u.ac.jp (M.I.)
[2] Food and Health Sciences Research Center, Ehime University, Matsuyama 790-8566, Japan
[3] Department of Food Science, Faculty of Bioresources and Environmental Sciences, Ishikawa Prefectural University, Nonoichi 921-8836, Japan; niss@ishikawa-pu.ac.jp
* Correspondence: mars95@agr.ehime-u.ac.jp; Tel.: +81-89-946-9863

Abstract: Coriander (*Coriandrum sativum* L.) is classified in the Apiaceae family and used as an herb. Coriander leaf has been reported to possess various health functions. Here, we report the anti-allergic effect of aqueous coriander leaf extract (ACLE). ACLE with 1.0 mg/mL or higher concentration significantly inhibited degranulation of RBL-2H3 cells in a concentration-dependent manner with no cytotoxicity. ACLE suppressed the increase in the intracellular Ca^{2+} concentration in response to antigen-specific stimulation. Immunoblot analysis demonstrated that ACLE significantly downregulates phosphorylation of phosphatidylinositol 3-kinase and tends to downregulate phosphorylation of Syk kinase in the signaling pathways activated by antigen-mediated stimulation. Oral administration of ACLE did not alter the sneezing frequency of pollinosis model mice stimulated with cedar pollen, but significantly reduced the serum IgE level. Our data show anti-allergic effects of coriander leaf in both cultured cells and pollinosis mice. These results suggest that coriander leaf has the potential to be a functional foodstuff with anti-allergy effects.

Keywords: anti-allergy; *Coriandrum sativum* L.; cedar pollen; degranulation; RBL-2H3 cell; coriander leaf

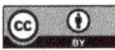

1. Introduction

An allergy means to immunize excessively against antigens invading from the outside of the body. Allergy falls into four types, among which type I allergy, including allergic rhinitis, asthma, atopic dermatitis, and hay fever, is increasing in the number of patients in recent years worldwide. The number of patients with pollinosis is approximately 30% of the population and is still increasing in Japan [1,2]. Type I allergy, also called immediate hypersensitivity or anaphylactoid type, is attributed to immunoglobulin E (IgE) [3]. Antigen-specific IgE antibodies are secreted by plasma cells and bind to FcεRI receptor on mast cells. Upon crosslinking of antigens to IgE antibody bound on FcεRI, various chemical mediators contained in granules are released from the cells. This phenomenon is called degranulation, and the secreted chemical mediators cause smooth muscle contraction, hypervascular permeability, hyperactivity, etc. Suppressing degranulation can therefore be an effective strategy for relieving allergy symptoms, and the research on the substance that alleviates allergic symptoms is considered crucially important.

Coriander (*Coriandrum sativum* L.), an aromatic herb commonly used for cooking in southeast Asia thanks to its unique aroma and flavor, belongs to the Apiaceae family. Coriander is well known to possess several biological activities [4–8]. For example, antimicrobial activities of *C. sativum* essential oil have been well reported [9–11]. *C. sativum* seeds exhibit antidiabetic effects in streptozotocin-induced diabetic mice [12,13], in rats fed a high-fat diet [14], and in obese–hyperglycemic–hyperlipidemic *Meriones shawi* rats [15]. *C. sativum* seeds also show anxiolytic [16] and sedative [17] activities. We then tried to find a novel biological activity of *C. sativum*. After screening using various cell-based assays, we found an anti-allergic effect of a water-soluble extract from leaves of *C. sativum* in a mast cell degranulation assay using RBL-2H3 cells, although an allergen is present in coriander [18,19]. Herein, we report a suppressive activity of an aqueous extract of coriander leaf on degranulation of RBL-2H3 cells. We also aimed to elucidate the mechanism of action of the extract. We further hypothesized that the extract is effective in a mouse model of type I allergy.

2. Materials and Methods

2.1. Reagents

Triton X-100, anti-dinitrophenyl (DNP) IgE, DNP-human serum albumin (HSA), bovine serum albumin (BSA), Trizma base, and *p*-coumaric acid were obtained from Sigma-Aldrich (St. Louis, MO, USA). Cedar pollen allergen (purified Cry j1 and Cry j2) was obtained from Hayashibara (Okayama, Japan). Horseradish peroxidase (HRP)-labeled anti-goat IgG antibody and goat anti-actin antibody were obtained from Santa Cruz Biotechnology (Santa Cruz, CA, USA). Anti-Syk antibody, anti-phosphorylated Syk (Tyr525/526) antibody, anti-phosphoinositide 3-kinase (PI3K) p55 antibody, anti-phosphorylated PI3K p85 (Tyr458)/p55 (Tyr199) antibody, and anti-rabbit IgG antibody labeled with HRP were purchased from Cell Signaling Technology (Danvers, MA, USA).

2.2. Sample Preparation

C. sativum L. leaf was obtained from S&B Foods Inc. (Tokyo, Japan). First, raw leaves of *C. sativum* L. were lyophilized and pulverized into powders. The powder was suspended in 10 mM Na phosphate buffer (pH 7.4) for 24 h and was centrifuged at $15,000 \times g$ for 20 min at 4 °C. After adjusting the pH to 7.4 and filtrating through a 0.45 μm membrane, the supernatant was used as aqueous coriander leaf extract (ACLE).

2.3. Cells and Cell Culture

Rat basophilic leukemia RBL-2H3 cells were obtained from American Type Culture Collection (Rockville, MD, USA). Dulbecco's modified Eagle's medium (DMEM, Sigma-Aldrich) supplemented with 100 U/mL of penicillin (Sigma-Aldrich), 100 μg/mL of streptomycin (Sigma-Aldrich), and 5% fetal bovine serum (FBS, Sigma-Aldrich) was used for propagation of RBL-2H3 cells in a monolayer culture at 37 °C under humidified 5% CO_2 [20]. RBL-2H3 cells were detached using a trypsin/EDTA solution at approximately 80% confluence. RBL-2H3 cells with a viability of >90% before 15 passages were used for the experiments described below.

2.4. Mice

Female BALB/c mice were acquired from Japan SLC (Hamamatsu, Japan) and were kept at 24 ± 1 °C under a 12 h light/dark cycle. Animals freely received water and standard laboratory chow. Animal experiments were approved by the Animal Experiment Committee of Ehime University and were performed in accordance with the Guidelines of Animal Experiments of Ehime University (approval number: 08U13-1).

2.5. β-Hexosaminidase Release Assay

The assay was conducted as previously described [21] with some modifications. RBL-2H3 cells (4.0×10^4 cells/well) seeded in each well of a 96-well culture plate (Corning, Corning, NY, USA) were precultured for 18 h. The cells were next sensitized with 50 ng/mL of anti-DNP IgE for 2 h and were subsequently treated with the indicated concentration of ACLE for 10 min. Degranulation was then induced with 50 ng/mL of DNP-HSA for 30 min. Following the collection of the medium from each well, the cells were sonicated on ice. After preincubating the collected medium and cell lysate for 5 min at 37 °C, the β-hexosaminidase substrate (*p*-nitrophenyl 2-acetamido-2-deoxy-β-D-glucopyranoside) was added and incubated at 37 °C for 25 min. After terminating the enzymatic reaction, the absorbance (405 nm) was measured using an SH-8000Lab microplate reader (Corona Electric, Hitachinaka, Japan). β-Hexosaminidase release rate (%) was calculated as follows:

$$100 \times [(A_{supernatant} - A_{blank\ of\ supernatant}) / \{(A_{supernatant} - A_{blank\ of\ supernatant}) + (A_{cell\ lysate} - A_{blank\ of\ cell\ lysate})\}]$$

where "A" is the absorbance of each well.

2.6. Cell Viability

Cytotoxicity of ACLE to RBL-2H3 cells was assessed by WST-8 assay described previously [22]. RBL-2H3 cells were seeded at 4.0×10^4 cells/well into each well of a 96-well culture plate (Corning). After treatment with 0, 1.0, 2.0, and 4.0 mg/mL of ACLE for 10 min, the cells were incubated with a WST-8 reagent for 15 min at 37 °C, and the absorbance (450 nm) was measured using a Model 550 microplate reader (Bio-Rad Laboratories, Hercules, CA, USA). The absorbance of wells with the cells treated with ACLE was compared to the absorbance of wells with the cells untreated. The assay was conducted in triplicate.

2.7. Monitoring of Intracellular Ca^{2+} Concentration ($[Ca^{2+}]_i$)

$[Ca^{2+}]_i$ was monitored using a fluorescent calcium indicator Fluo 3-AM (Dojindo Laboratories, Mashiki, Japan) as described previously [23]. RBL-2H3 cells were seeded and sensitized as described in Section 2.5. The cells were next incubated in the loading buffer containing Fluo 3-AM for 1 h. After washing with phosphate-buffered saline (PBS, pH 7.4), the cells were incubated in the recording buffer containing ACLE (4.0 mg/mL) for 10 min at 37 °C. The cells were subsequently stimulated with DNP-HSA at a final concentration of 2.5 µg/mL, and the fluorescence intensity was immediately monitored using the SH-8000Lab microplate reader (excitation wavelength: 480 nm; emission wavelength: 530 nm).

2.8. Immunoblot Analysis

Immunoblot analysis was conducted as described previously [24]. RBL-2H3 cells seeded at 5.0×10^5 cells/dish in 3.5 cm culture dishes (Corning) were precultured for 18 h. After sensitizing with 50 ng/mL of anti-DNP IgE for 2 h, the cells were subsequently treated with 980 µL of modified Tyrode's buffer containing 4.0 mg/mL of ACLE for 10 min. The cells were next stimulated with DNP-HSA at a final concentration of 50 ng/mL for 5 min. After the added reagents were removed, the cells were lysed and centrifuged at $12,000 \times g$ for 15 min at 4 °C. Proteins were then separated by sodium dodecyl sulfate-polyacrylamide gel electrophoresis and were transferred onto a polyvinylidene fluoride membrane (GE Healthcare, Buckinghamshire, UK). After blocking with 20 mM Tris-buffered saline (TBS, pH 7.6) containing 5% skim milk for 1 h at room temperature, the membrane was reacted with anti-actin antibody (1:200 dilution), anti-Syk antibody (1:1000 dilution), anti-phosphorylated Syk antibody (1:1000 dilution), anti-PI3K p55 antibody (1:1000 dilution), or anti-phosphorylated PI3K p85/p55 antibody (1:1000 dilution) as a primary antibody at 4 °C overnight. After washing with TBS containing 0.1% Tween 20 thrice, the membrane was reacted with HRP-labeled anti-rabbit IgG antibody (1:2000 dilution) or HRP-labeled anti-goat IgG antibody (1:2000 dilution) as a secondary antibody for 1 h at room temperature. After washing the membrane with TBS containing 0.05% Tween 20 thrice, the blot was developed with ImmunoStar LD chemiluminescence detection reagent (Fujifilm Wako Pure Chemical, Osaka, Japan), and bands were visualized using a ChemiDoc XRS system (Bio-Rad Laboratories).

2.9. A Mouse Model of Japanese Cedar Pollinosis

Japanese cedar pollinosis model mice were developed as described previously [25,26]. Following an adaptation period for 1 week, 6-week-old female BALB/c mice were randomly assigned to two groups as follows: the control group (9 mice) and the ACLE group (8 mice). The mice were intranasally sensitized with 10 µL of PBS containing 2.0 µg of purified cedar pollen allergen on days 0, 7, 14, and 21, as shown in Figure 1. The mice were next intranasally challenged with 10 µL of PBS containing 0.4 µg of cedar pollen allergen for seven consecutive days from day 28 to 34. The mice in the ACLE group were orally administered 20 µL of ACLE at 50 mg/kg/day for six consecutive days from day 28 to 33, while the mice in the control group were with 20 µL of the vehicle alone. On day 34, all the mice were intranasally challenged with 0.4 µg of cedar pollen allergen. Sneezing frequency was counted for 15 min immediately after the final nasal treatment. On day 35, serum was obtained to determine their serum IgE levels.

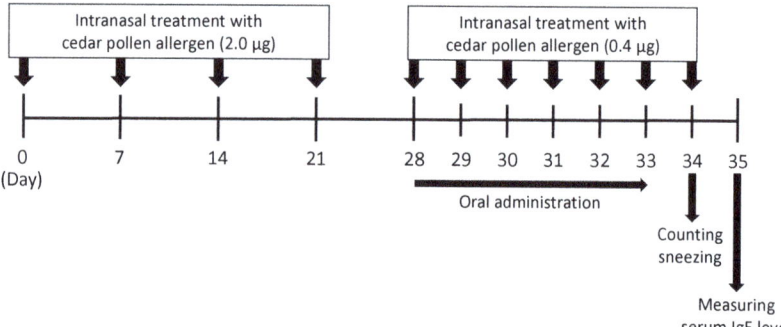

Figure 1. Schedule of the in vivo experiment using Japanese cedar pollinosis mice.

2.10. Enzyme-Linked Immunosorbent Assay (ELISA)

Serum IgE levels were measured by in-house-developed ELISA as previously described [27]. The absorbance (415 nm) was measured using the SH-8000Lab microplate reader after adding 1.5% oxalic acid (100 µL/well) to terminate the enzymatic reaction.

2.11. High-Performance Liquid Chromatography (HPLC) Analysis

Reversed-phase HPLC analysis of ACLE was performed on a LaChrom Elite HPLC system (Hitachi, Tokyo, Japan) with an XBridge C18 column (100 × 4.6 mm, 3.5 µm, Waters, Milford, MA, USA). A linear gradient elution program was applied as follows: 0–6 min (20% acetonitrile + 0.1% formic acid); 6–9 min (20–95% acetonitrile + 0.1% formic acid); 9–12 min (95% acetonitrile + 0.1% formic acid). The flow rate was maintained at 1.0 mL/min, and the temperature of the column was set at 35 °C. The chromatogram was monitored at a wavelength of 220 nm.

2.12. Statistical Analysis

Data obtained are shown as mean ± SEM. Statistical analysis was conducted using GraphPad Prism version 7.02 (GraphPad Software, La Jolla, CA, USA). Mann-Whitney U test or Dunnett's test was used to assess the statistical significance of the treatments against control. Values of * $p < 0.05$, ** $p < 0.01$ and *** $p < 0.001$ were considered statistically significant.

3. Results and Discussion

3.1. Effect of ACLE on Degranulation of RBL-2H3 Cells

We first investigated whether ACLE possesses a suppressive effect on degranulation. RBL-2H3 cells sensitized with anti-DNP IgE were treated with the indicated concentration of ACLE, and degranulation was induced with the antigen. Secreted β-hexosaminidase was utilized as a degranulation marker. ACLE with 1.0 mg/mL or higher concentration significantly inhibited the degranulation in a concentration-dependent manner, as shown in Figure 2A. This result indicates that water-soluble, bioactive substance exist in coriander leaf, which exhibits anti-allergic activity by suppressing degranulation. We next examined by the WST-8 assay whether ACLE affects the viability of RBL-2H3 cells. As shown in

Figure 2B, the viability of RBL-2H3 cells was unaffected by ACLE with the concentration tested. These data indicated that ACLE suppresses the degranulation of RBL-2H3 cells with no cytotoxicity.

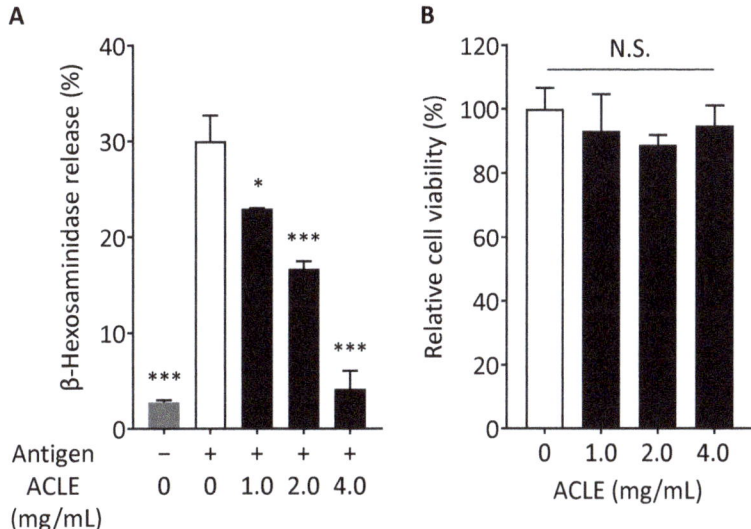

Figure 2. Effects of aqueous coriander leaf extract (ACLE) on degranulation and viability of RBL-2H3 cells. (**A**) Effect of ACLE on the degranulation. (**B**) Effect of ACLE on the cell viability. Data are represented as mean ± SEM (n = 3). * p < 0.05, *** p < 0.001 against control (an open bar) by Dunnett's test. N.S. indicates not significant.

3.2. Effect of ACLE on the Elevation of $[Ca^{2+}]_i$ Induced by Antigen

Degranulation occurs upon the antigen binding to IgE on mast cells, thereby initiating intracellular signal transduction and increasing Ca^{2+} concentration in the cell. The elevation of intracellular concentration of Ca^{2+}, the major second messenger in intracellular signaling, is the critical process in mast cell degranulation. The effect of ACLE on the elevation of intracellular calcium concentration was hence evaluated using Fluo 3-AM. Relative fluorescence intensity of Fluo 3 reflects the intracellular Ca^{2+} concentration. RBL-2H3 cells sensitized with anti-DNP IgE antibody were treated with ACLE (4.0 mg/mL), and $[Ca^{2+}]_i$ was monitored for 6 min. $[Ca^{2+}]_i$ rapidly rose upon stimulation with antigen, as shown in Figure 3. However, the increase in intracellular calcium ion concentration was significantly suppressed in the presence of 4.0 mg/mL of ACLE. It was supposed from this result that ACLE inhibits degranulation by downregulating the intracellular signaling pathway leading to the elevation of $[Ca^{2+}]_i$.

3.3. Effect of ACLE on Intracellular Signaling Pathways Leading to Degranulation

The onset of the signaling pathways resulting in degranulation is regulated by phosphorylation of Syk kinase located close to FcεRI, accompanied by phosphorylation of downstream signaling factors, leading to the increase in intracellular calcium ion concentration. We examined by immunoblot analysis how ACLE affects the signaling pathways related to degranulation (Figure 4A). As shown in Figure 4B, treating cells with ACLE tended to decrease the phosphorylation of Syk kinase (p = 0.0795 vs. control), and phosphorylation of PI3K was significantly inhibited by ACLE treatment (Figure 4C).

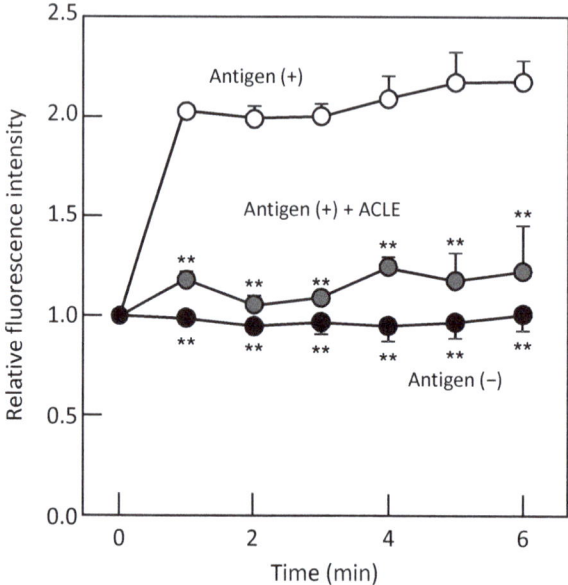

Figure 3. Effect of aqueous coriander leaf extract (ACLE) on the elevation in intracellular Ca^{2+} concentration in RBL-2H3 cells. Relative fluorescence intensity of Fluo 3 reflects intracellular Ca^{2+} concentration. RBL-2H3 cells were treated with ACLE (4.0 mg/mL). Open circle, the cells not treated with ACLE but stimulated with antigen (control); gray circle, the cells treated with ACLE and stimulated with antigen; closed circle, the cells not treated with ACLE nor stimulated with antigen. Data are shown as mean ± SEM (n = 3). ** $p < 0.01$ against control by Dunnett's test.

There are two pathways for mast cell degranulation: calcium-dependent and calci-um-independent pathways [28,29]. The calcium-dependent pathway is activated by the tyrosine kinase Lyn located proximal to FcεRI, thereby activating another tyrosine kinase Syk [30]. Phosphorylated Syk activates a signaling cascade including phospholipase Cγ. As a result, Ca^{2+} inflow into the interior of cells through the Ca^{2+} channel is induced, which causes degranulation by increased $[Ca^{2+}]_i$. On the other hand, tyrosine kinase Fyn is activated by cross-linking of antigen to IgE on FcεRI, which results in the activation of the calcium-independent pathway [31]. Phosphorylation of PI3K leads to microtubule reorganization that causes degranulation by migrating granules [32]. In the degranulation process, the calcium-dependent pathway plays a crucial role, while the calcium-independent pathway has been reported to be given priority under weak stimulation when cells were stimulated with a low concentration of antigen [33]. Our results indicated that downregulated phosphorylation of Syk kinase and PI3K is a key process for the suppressive activity of ACLE on degranulation. As PI3K is located downstream of Syk kinase, downregulated phosphorylation of PI3K, as shown in Figure 4C, might be attributed to reduced phosphorylation of Syk. Our data suggested that an inhibitory effect of ACLE on the calcium-dependent pathway causes the reduced elevation of $[Ca^{2+}]_i$ induced with antigen (Figure 3), resulting in suppressed degranulation.

PI3K plays a crucial role in certain tumor progression [34,35]. Because ACLE inhibits phosphorylation of PI3K, it might exhibit antitumor activity. Indeed, the *C. sativum* leaf has been reported to possess antitumor effect [36,37]. Syk is expressed in various cells and is a potential target for treating several diseases, such as liver fibrosis [38], acute myeloid leukemia [39], and autoimmune diseases [40]; ACLE might therefore be effective in attenuating the symptoms of these diseases by inhibiting phosphorylation of Syk. In addition, because a Syk inhibitor can attenuate allergen-induced symptoms in patients with allergic rhinitis exposed to pollens [41], we further investigated whether ACLE is capable of reducing allergic symptoms in pollinosis mice.

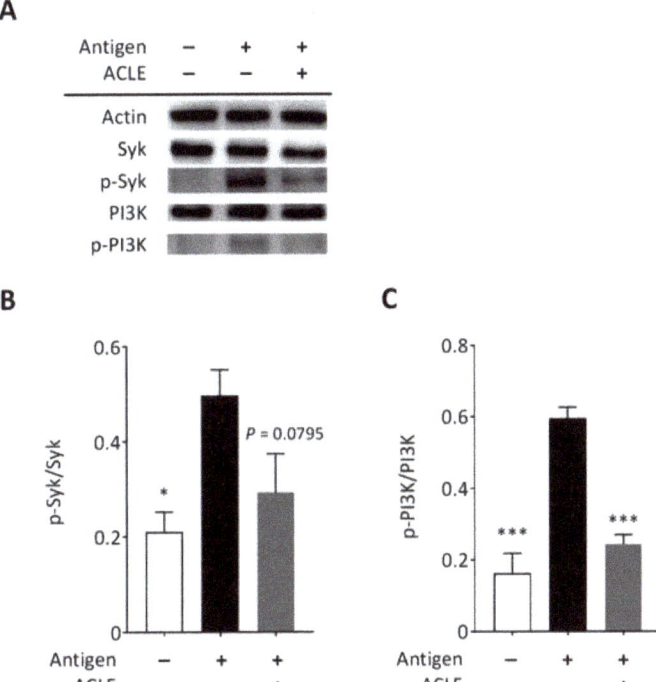

Figure 4. Effect of aqueous coriander leaf extract (ACLE) on the intracellular signaling molecules participating in the degranulation of RBL-2H3 cells. p-Syk and p-PI3K represent phosphorylated Syk and phosphorylated phosphoinositide 3-kinase (PI3K), respectively. (**A**) A representative blot from four independent experiments. (**B**) The ratio of phosphorylated protein to the whole protein of Syk. (**C**) The ratio of phosphorylated protein to the whole protein of PI3K. Data are shown as mean ± SEM ($n = 4$). * $p < 0.05$, *** $p < 0.001$ against control (a closed bar) by Dunnett's test.

3.4. Effect of ACLE on a Mouse Model of Japanese Cedar Pollinosis

Cedar pollinosis mice were used to investigate the in vivo effect of ACLE. Mice were sensitized with Cry j1 and Cry j2, the main allergens of Japanese cedar pollen. Cedar pollinosis was induced by intranasal treatment of cedar pollen allergen 11 times for 5 weeks. The ACLE group was orally administered ACLE for the last six days. Oral administration of ACLE unaffected the body weight of mice (data not shown), indicating that ACLE is not toxic to mice. The sneezing frequency was counted for 15 min on day 34. As a result, ACLE administration did not alter sneezing frequency (Figure 5A). This result indicated that the water-soluble, bioactive ingredient in ACLE seems to be inefficiently absorbed into the mouse body or to be readily metabolized after the absorption into the body. ACLE thus did not alleviate the allergic symptom.

On day 35, sera were collected to measure the serum IgE level by ELISA. Unexpectedly, the serum IgE level of the ACLE group was significantly reduced compared with that of the control group (Figure 5B). This result suggested that ACLE could suppress the IgE production as well as mast cell degranulation. This result also implied that ACLE might possess the potential to prevent sensitization with an allergen by inhibiting IgE production. The bioavailability of ACLE in mice is now under investigation to elucidate why ACLE did not mitigate the allergic symptom but decreased IgE levels in pollinosis mice. In addition, the mechanism of ACLE underlying the decrease in IgE production is also under exploration. It might be possible that ACLE affects lymphocytes, such as T lymphocytes and B lymphocytes, to inhibit the class switching to IgE antibody.

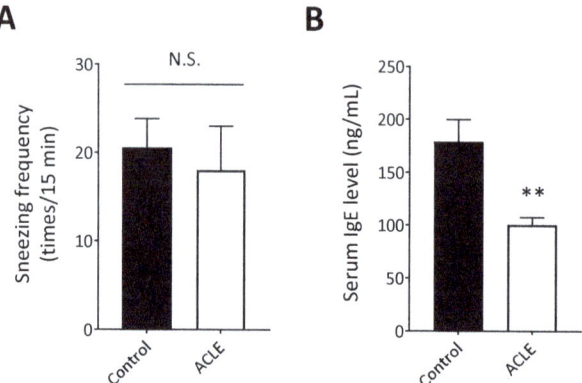

Figure 5. Effect of aqueous coriander leaf extract (ACLE) on pollinosis model mice. BALB/c mice were assigned randomly to two groups: the control group (9 mice) and the ACLE group (8 mice). (**A**) Sneezing frequency was counted for 15 min following the final challenge with pollen allergen. (**B**) Serum IgE level in each group. Data are shown as mean ± SEM. ** $p < 0.01$ against control by Mann-Whitney U test. N.S. indicates not significant.

3.5. HPLC Analysis of ACLE

Finally, a reversed-phase HPLC analysis of ACLE was conducted. The chemical composition of essential oils of *C. sativum* has been well reported, and various secondary metabolites in aerial part of *C. sativum*, such as flavonoids and coumarins, have been also identified [42,43]; however, papers reporting the chemical composition of water-soluble molecules in *C. sativum* is limited [44], although several papers have reported estimated total phenolic contents.

ACLE (20 µL) was subjected to an XBridge C18 column. Figure 6 shows an HPLC chromatogram of ACLE. The result showed that coumaric acid was present at 6.8 µg/mL in ACLE. Other peaks have not been identified yet. Zeković et al. [45] identified ferulic acid and sinapic acid, in addition to coumaric acid, in an aqueous coriander seeds extract; however, ferulic acid and sinapic acid were not found in ACLE in this study. This seems to result from the differences in the part of the plant used for extraction (seeds vs. leaves) and in the extraction solvent (water vs. sodium phosphate buffer.) Chen et al. [46] have reported that coumaric acid exhibits a suppressive effect on the degranulation of RBL-2H3 cells. Coumaric acid, a secondary metabolite of this plant, thus might be partially attributed to the suppressive effect of ACLE on degranulation of RBL-2H3 cells; however, the coumaric acid concentration (6.8 µg/mL) found in ACLE seems too low to exhibit the suppressive effect of ACLE by itself, as shown in Figure 2A. We thus assume that there is another bioactive ingredient in ACLE in addition to coumaric acid. Identification of the peaks shown in Figure 6 is now under investigation to explore the water-soluble bioactives contained in coriander leaf.

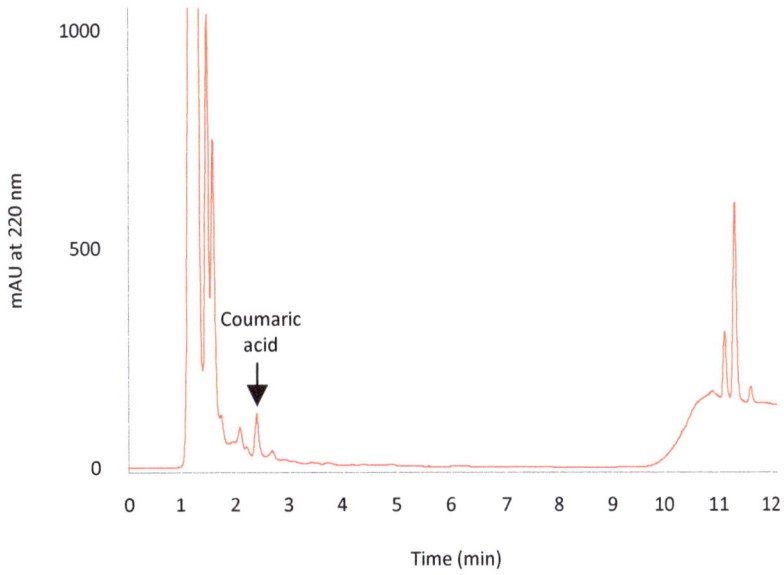

Figure 6. Reversed-phase high-performance liquid chromatography fingerprint of aqueous coriander leaf extract. A linear gradient elution program was as follows: 0–6 min (20% CH$_3$CN + 0.1% formic acid); 6–9 min (20–95% CH$_3$CN + 0.1% formic acid); 9–12 min (95% CH$_3$CN + 0.1% formic acid). The chromatogram was monitored at 220 nm. The retention time of coumaric acid was 2.4 min.

4. Conclusions

ACLE inhibited degranulation of RBL-2H3 cells with no cytotoxicity by suppressing the elevation of intracellular Ca^{2+} concentration resulting from downregulated phosphorylation of the intracellular signal transduction pathways. In addition, oral administration of ACLE significantly decreased the serum IgE level in pollinosis model mice. These findings suggest that coriander leaf possesses the potential to be a functional foodstuff with anti-allergic effects.

Author Contributions: Conceptualization, T.S.; data curation, Y.K., K.N., M.I., S.N. and T.S.; investigation, Y.K. and K.N.; supervision, K.N. and T.S.; writing—original draft, Y.K. and K.N.; writing—review and editing, K.N. and T.S. All authors have read and agreed to the published version of the manuscript.

Funding: This research received no external funding.

Institutional Review Board Statement: The animal study protocol was conducted in accordance with the Guidelines of Animal Experiments of Ehime University and approved by the Animal Experiment Committee of Ehime University (approval number: 08U13-1).

Informed Consent Statement: Not applicable.

Data Availability Statement: The data that support the findings in this study are available from the corresponding author upon reasonable request.

Acknowledgments: Animal experiments were conducted at the Division of Genetic Research of the Advanced Research Support Center (ADRES), Ehime University.

Conflicts of Interest: Ehime University has filed a patent application related to a new anti-allergic agent, and T.S. is an inventor of the patent application. The remaining authors declare no conflict of interest.

References

1. Yamada, T.; Saito, H.; Fujieda, S. Present state of Japanese cedar pollinosis: The national affliction. *J. Allergy Clin. Immunol.* **2014**, *133*, 632–639. [CrossRef] [PubMed]
2. Nishihata, S.; Murata, T.; Inoue, S.; Okubo, K.; Sahashi, N.; Takahashi, H.; Hirooka, J.; Hoshiyama, Y.; Murayama, K.; Mezawa, A.; et al. Prevalence of Japanese cedar pollinosis in Tokyo: A survey conducted by the Tokyo Metropolitan Government. *Clin. Exp. Allergy Rev.* **2010**, *10*, 8–11. [CrossRef]
3. Galli, S.J.; Tsai, M.; Piliponsky, A.M. The development of allergic inflammation. *Nature* **2008**, *454*, 445–454. [CrossRef] [PubMed]
4. Laribi, B.; Kouki, K.; M'Hamdi, M.; Bettaieb, T. Coriander (*Coriandrum sativum* L.) and its bioactive constituents. *Fitoterapia* **2015**, *103*, 9–26. [CrossRef] [PubMed]
5. Sahib, N.G.; Anwar, F.; Gilani, A.H.; Hamid, A.A.; Saari, N.; Alkharfy, K.M. Coriander (*Coriandrum sativum* L.): A potential source of high-value components for functional foods and nutraceuticals—A review. *Phytother. Res.* **2013**, *27*, 1439–1456. [CrossRef] [PubMed]
6. Wei, J.N.; Liu, Z.H.; Zhao, Y.P.; Zhao, L.L.; Xue, T.K.; Lan, Q.K. Phytochemical and bioactive profile of *Coriandrum sativum* L. *Food Chem.* **2019**, *286*, 260–267. [CrossRef]
7. Prachayasittikul, V.; Prachayasittikul, S.; Ruchirawat, S.; Prachayasittikul, V. Coriander (*Coriandrum sativum*): A promising functional food toward the well-being. *Food Res. Int.* **2018**, *105*, 305–323. [CrossRef]
8. Sobhani, Z.; Mohtashami, L.; Amiri, M.S.; Ramezani, M.; Emami, S.A.; Simal-Gandara, J. Ethnobotanical and phytochemical aspects of the edible herb *Coriandrum sativum* L. *J. Food Sci.* **2022**, *87*, 1386–1422. [CrossRef]
9. Matasyoh, J.C.; Maiyo, Z.C.; Ngure, R.M.; Chepkorir, R. Chemical composition and antimicrobial activity of the essential oil of *Coriandrum sativum*. *Food Chem.* **2009**, *113*, 526–529. [CrossRef]
10. Begnami, A.F.; Duarte, M.C.T.; Furletti, V.; Rehder, V.L.G. Antimicrobial potential of *Coriandrum sativum* L. against different *Candida* species in vitro. *Food Chem.* **2010**, *118*, 74–77. [CrossRef]
11. Silva, F.; Domingues, F.C. Antimicrobial activity of coriander oil and its effectiveness as food preservative. *Crit. Rev. Food Sci. Nutr.* **2017**, *57*, 35–47. [CrossRef] [PubMed]
12. Gray, A.M.; Flatt, P.R. Insulin-releasing and insulin-like activity of the traditional anti-diabetic plant *Coriandrum sativum* (coriander). *Br. J. Nutr.* **1999**, *81*, 203–209. [CrossRef] [PubMed]
13. Eidi, M.; Eidi, A.; Saeidi, A.; Molanaei, S.; Sadeghipour, A.; Bahar, M.; Bahar, K. Effect of coriander seed (*Coriandrum sativum* L.) ethanol extract on insulin release from pancreatic beta cells in streptozotocin-induced diabetic rats. *Phytother. Res.* **2009**, *23*, 404–406. [CrossRef] [PubMed]
14. Chithra, V.; Leelamma, S. *Coriandrum sativum*—Mechanism of hypoglycemic action. *Food Chem.* **1999**, *67*, 229–231. [CrossRef]
15. Aissaoui, A.; Zizi, S.; Israili, Z.H.; Lyoussi, B. Hypoglycemic and hypolipidemic effects of *Coriandrum sativum* L. in *Meriones shawi* rats. *J. Ethnopharmacol.* **2011**, *137*, 652–661. [CrossRef]
16. Emamghoreishi, M.; Khasaki, M.; Aazam, M.F. *Coriandrum sativum*: Evaluation of its anxiolytic effect in the elevated plus-maze. *J. Ethnopharmacol.* **2005**, *96*, 365–370. [CrossRef]
17. Gastón, M.S.; Cid, M.P.; Vázquez, A.M.; Decarlini, M.F.; Demmel, G.I.; Rossi, L.I.; Aimar, M.L.; Salvatierra, N.A. Sedative effect of central administration of *Coriandrum sativum* essential oil and its major component linalool in neonatal chicks. *Pharm. Biol.* **2016**, *54*, 1954–1961. [CrossRef]
18. Suhonen, R.; Keskinen, H.; Björkstén, F.; Vaheri, E.; Zitting, A. Allergy to coriander a case report. *Allergy* **1979**, *34*, 327–330. [CrossRef]
19. Jensen-Jarolim, E.; Leitner, A.; Hirschwehr, R.; Kraet, D.; Wüthrich, B.; Scheiner, O.; Graf, J.; Ebner, C. Characterization of allergens in *Apiaceae* spices: Anise, fennel, coriander and cumin. *Clin. Exp. Allergy* **1997**, *27*, 1299–1306. [CrossRef]
20. Morita, Y.; Siraganian, R.P. Inhibition of IgE-mediated histamine release from rat basophilic leukemia cells and rat mast cells by inhibitors of transmethylation. *J. Immunol.* **1981**, *127*, 1339–1344.
21. Kim, I.H.; Kanayama, Y.; Nishiwaki, H.; Sugahara, T.; Nishi, K. Structure-activity relationships of fish oil derivatives with antiallergic activity in vitro and in vivo. *J. Med. Chem.* **2019**, *62*, 9576–9592. [CrossRef]
22. Nugrahini, A.D.; Ishida, M.; Nakagawa, T.; Nishi, K.; Sugahara, T. Anti-degranulation activity of caffeine: In vitro and in vivo study. *J. Funct. Foods* **2019**, *60*, 103422. [CrossRef]
23. Nugrahini, A.D.; Ishida, M.; Nakagawa, T.; Nishi, K.; Sugahara, T. Trigonelline: An alkaloid with anti-degranulation properties. *Mol. Immunol.* **2020**, *118*, 201–209. [CrossRef]
24. Hada, M.; Nishi, K.; Ishida, M.; Onda, H.; Nishimoto, S.; Sugahara, T. Inhibitory effect of aqueous extract of *Cuminum cyminum* L. seed on degranulation of RBL-2H3 cells and passive cutaneous anaphylaxis reaction in mice. *Cytotechnology* **2019**, *71*, 599–609. [CrossRef]
25. Nomiya, R.; Okano, M.; Fujiwara, T.; Maeda, M.; Kimura, Y.; Kino, K.; Yokoyama, M.; Hirai, H.; Nagata, K.; Hara, T.; et al. CRTH2 plays an essential role in the pathophysiology of Cry j 1-induced pollinosis in mice. *J. Immunol.* **2008**, *180*, 5680–5688. [CrossRef]
26. Nishi, K.; Kanayama, Y.; Kim, I.H.; Nakata, A.; Nishiwaki, H.; Sugahara, T. Docosahexaenoyl ethanolamide mitigates IgE-mediated allergic reactions by inhibiting mast cell degranulation and regulating allergy-related immune cells. *Sci. Rep.* **2019**, *9*, 16213. [CrossRef]
27. Kondo, M.; Nishi, K.; Sugahara, T. Ishizuchi dark tea suppresses IgE-mediated degranulation of RBL-2H3 cells and nasal rubbing behavior of pollinosis in mice. *J. Funct. Foods* **2015**, *14*, 659–669. [CrossRef]

28. Nishida, K.; Yamasaki, S.; Ito, Y.; Kabu, K.; Hattori, K.; Tezuka, T.; Nishizumi, H.; Kitamura, D.; Goitsuka, R.; Geha, R.S.; et al. FcεRI-mediated mast cell degranulation requires calcium-independent microtubule-dependent translocation of granules to the plasma membrane. *J. Cell Biol.* **2005**, *170*, 115–126. [CrossRef]
29. Kopeć, A.; Panaszek, B.; Fal, A.M. Intracellular signaling pathways in IgE-dependent mast cell activation. *Arch. Immunol. Ther. Exp.* **2006**, *54*, 393–401. [CrossRef]
30. Siraganian, R.P.; Zhang, J.; Suzuki, K.; Sada, K. Protein tyrosine kinase Syk in mast cell signaling. *Mol. Immunol.* **2002**, *38*, 1229–1233. [CrossRef]
31. Parravicini, V.; Gadina, M.; Kovarova, M.; Odom, S.; Gonzalez-Espinosa, C.; Furumoto, Y.; Saitoh, S.; Samelson, L.E.; O'Shea, J.J.; Rivera, J. Fyn kinase initiates complementary signals required for IgE-dependent mast cell degranulation. *Nat. Immunol.* **2002**, *3*, 741–748. [CrossRef]
32. Ménasché, G.; Longé, C.; Bratti, M.; Blank, U. Cytoskeletal transport, reorganization, and fusion regulation in mast cell-stimulus secretion coupling. *Front. Cell Dev. Biol.* **2021**, *9*, 652077. [CrossRef]
33. Furumoto, Y.; Gonzalez-Espinosa, C.; Gomez, G.; Kovarova, M.; Odom, S.; Parravicini, V.; Ryan, J.J.; Rivera, J. Rethinking the role of Src family protein tyrosine kinases in the allergic response. *Immunol. Res.* **2004**, *30*, 241–253. [CrossRef]
34. Goncalves, M.D.; Hopkins, B.D.; Cantley, L.C. Phosphatidylinositol 3-kinase, growth disorders, and Cancer. *N. Engl. J. Med.* **2018**, *379*, 2052–2062. [CrossRef]
35. Alzahrani, A.S. PI3K/Akt/mTOR inhibitors in cancer: At the bench and bedside. *Semin. Cancer Biol.* **2019**, *59*, 125–132. [CrossRef]
36. Cortés-Eslava, J.; Gómez-Arroyo, S.; Villalobos-Pietrini, R.; Espinosa-Aguirre, J.J. Antimutagenicity of coriander (*Coriandrum sativum*) juice on the mutagenesis produced by plant metabolites of aromatic amines. *Toxicol. Lett.* **2004**, *153*, 283–292. [CrossRef]
37. Huang, H.; Nakamura, T.; Yasuzawa, T.; Ueshima, S. Effects of *Coriandrum sativum* on migration and invasion abilities of cancer cells. *J. Nutr. Sci. Vitaminol.* **2020**, *66*, 468–477. [CrossRef]
38. Qu, C.; Zheng, D.; Li, S.; Liu, Y.; Lidofsky, A.; Holmes, J.A.; Chen, J.; He, L.; Wei, L.; Liao, Y.; et al. Tyrosine kinase SYK is a potential therapeutic target for liver fibrosis. *Hepatology* **2018**, *68*, 1125–1139. [CrossRef]
39. Bartaula-Brevik, S.; Lindstad Brattås, M.K.; Tvedt, T.H.A.; Reikvam, H.; Bruserud, Ø. Splenic tyrosine kinase (SYK) inhibitors and their possible use in acute myeloid leukemia. *Expert Opin. Investig. Drugs* **2018**, *27*, 377–387. [CrossRef] [PubMed]
40. Tang, S.; Yu, Q.; Ding, C. Investigational spleen tyrosine kinase (SYK) inhibitors for the treatment of autoimmune diseases. *Expert Opin. Investig. Drugs* **2022**, *31*, 291–303. [CrossRef]
41. Denyer, J.; Patel, V. Syk kinase inhibitors in allergic diseases. *Drug News Perspect.* **2009**, *22*, 146–150. [CrossRef]
42. Burdock, G.A.; Carabin, I.G. Safety assessment of coriander (*Coriandrum sativum* L.) essential oil as a food ingredient. *Food Chem. Toxicol.* **2009**, *47*, 22–34. [CrossRef]
43. Shoko, T.; Manhivi, V.E.; Mtlhako, M.; Sivakumar, D. Changes in functional compounds, volatiles, and antioxidant properties of culinary herb coriander leaves (*Coriandrum sativum*) stored under red and blue LED light for different storage times. *Front. Nutr.* **2022**, *9*, 856484. [CrossRef]
44. Ishikawa, T.; Kondo, K.; Kitajima, J. Water-soluble constituents of coriander. *Chem. Pharm. Bull.* **2003**, *51*, 32–39. [CrossRef]
45. Zeković, Z.; Kaplan, M.; Pavlić, B.; Olgun, E.O.; Vladić, J.; Canlı, O.; Vidović, S. Chemical characterization of polyphenols and volatile fraction of coriander (*Coriandrum sativum* L.) extracts obtained by subcritical water extraction. *Ind. Crops Prod.* **2016**, *87*, 54–63. [CrossRef]
46. Chen, H.J.; Shih, C.K.; Hsu, H.Y.; Chiang, W. Mast cell-dependent allergic responses are inhibited by ethanolic extract of adlay (*Coix lachryma-jobi* L. var. *ma-yuen* Stapf) testa. *J. Agric. Food Chem.* **2010**, *58*, 2596–2601. [CrossRef]

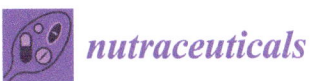 *nutraceuticals*

Article

European Black Elderberry Fruit Extract Inhibits Replication of SARS-CoV-2 In Vitro

Christian Setz [1], Maria Fröba [1], Maximilian Große [1], Pia Rauch [1], Janina Auth [1], Alexander Steinkasserer [2], Stephan Plattner [3,*] and Ulrich Schubert [1,*]

[1] Institute of Virology, Friedrich-Alexander University Erlangen-Nürnberg (FAU), 91054 Erlangen, Germany
[2] Department of Immune Modulation, Universitätsklinikum Erlangen, 91054 Erlangen, Germany
[3] IPRONA AG/SPA, Industriestraße 1/6, 39011 Lana, Italy
* Correspondence: stephan.plattner@iprona.com (S.P.); ulrich.schubert@fau.de (U.S.); Tel.: +39-0473-552900 (S.P.); +49-9131-85-26478 (U.S.)

Abstract: Coronavirus disease-19 (COVID-19) is still affecting the lives of people round the globe and remains a major public health threat. The emergence of new variants more efficiently transmitted, more virulent and more capable of escaping naturally acquired and vaccine-induced immunity creates a long-term negative outlook for the management of the pandemic. The development of effective and viable prevention and treatment options to reduce viral transmission is of the utmost importance. The fruits of the European black elderberry and extracts thereof have been traditionally used to treat viral infections such as coughs, cold and flu. Specifically, its efficacy against the Influenza A virus has been shown in vitro as well as in human clinical trials. In the current project, we investigated the antiviral activity of a black elderberry extract, mainly containing anthocyanins and phenolic compounds, against SARS-CoV-2 and its variants of concern and explored the possible mode of action by performing time of addition experiments. The results revealed that the extract displayed a strong anti-SARS-CoV-2 activity against the Wuhan type as well as the variants of concern Alpha, Beta, Gamma, Delta and Omicron with a comparable antiviral activity. Based on cytotoxicity data, a 2-log theoretical therapeutic window was established. The data accumulated so far suggest that the viral replication cycle is inhibited at later stages, inasmuch as the replication process was affected after virus entry. Therefore, it would be legitimate to assume that black elderberry extract might have the potential to be an effective treatment option for SARS-CoV-2 infections.

Keywords: European black elderberry extract; natural substance; anthocyanins; phenolic compounds; SARS-CoV-2; antiviral; COVID-19; coronavirus; SARS-CoV-2 variants of concern

Citation: Setz, C.; Fröba, M.; Große, M.; Rauch, P.; Auth, J.; Steinkasserer, A.; Plattner, S.; Schubert, U. European Black Elderberry Fruit Extract Inhibits Replication of SARS-CoV-2 In Vitro. *Nutraceuticals* **2023**, *3*, 91–106. https://doi.org/10.3390/nutraceuticals3010007

Academic Editors: Ivan Cruz-Chamorro and Luisa Tesoriere

Received: 9 December 2022
Revised: 3 January 2023
Accepted: 6 January 2023
Published: 13 January 2023

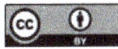

Copyright: © 2023 by the authors. Licensee MDPI, Basel, Switzerland. This article is an open access article distributed under the terms and conditions of the Creative Commons Attribution (CC BY) license (https:// creativecommons.org/licenses/by/ 4.0/).

1. Introduction

The Coronavirus disease 2019 (COVID-19), caused by the Severe Acute Respiratory Syndrome Coronavirus 2 (SARS-CoV-2), is responsible for short- and long-term complications, e.g., the need for respiratory support or persistent cardiovascular complications. To date, the pandemic has resulted in around 647 million global cases and over 6.6 million deaths [1]. An ongoing major problem is the continuous emergence and spread of SARS-CoV-2 variants determined as "Variants of Concern" (VoCs) by the WHO. These variants are able to evade vaccine- or infection-induced antiviral immune response [2,3].

Mutations in SARS-CoV-2 VoCs are mainly located within the spike glycoprotein and generally change the interaction with host receptors and thus affect the infectivity, transmissibility or pathogenicity of the virus [4–7]. The VoCs described to date include SARS-CoV-2 Alpha [8], SARS-CoV-2 Beta [9], SARS-CoV-2 Gamma [10], SARS-CoV-2 Delta [11] as well as SARS-CoV-2 Omicron [12]. The latter is subdivided in the sub-lineages BA.1, BA.2, BA.3, BA.4 and BA.5 [13], with BA.5 being predominant worldwide at the moment. With BQ.1.1 a new sub-lineage increases, especially in Europe and USA. This Omicron variant is resistant against all clinically available monoclonal antibodies [14]. In comparison to the other VoCs,

Omicron variants contain a high number of deletions, insertions and mutations, especially in the spike protein [13,15]. Generally, VoCs were reported to show higher transmissibility and infectivity [4,16–20]. In light of the continuing COVID-19 pandemic and the ongoing occurrence of new SARS-CoV-2 variants, the development of broadly effective prophylactic and therapeutic countermeasures remains of the utmost importance.

At the beginning of 2022, the first antiviral small molecule drugs were approved for high risk patients and only for use at early stages following infection with SARS-CoV-2 [21]. Nirmatrelvir, an inhibitor of the 3-Chymotrypsin-like protease of SARS-CoV-2 combined with Ritonavir, an HIV-1-protease inhibitor, were distributed under the label Paxlovid® [22,23]. However, a recent study revealed that the use of Paxlovid® exhibits only beneficiary effects for patients >65 years following infection with the VoC Omicron [24]. In addition, Molnupiravir targeting the RNA-dependent RNA-Polymerase of SARS-CoV-2 received approval for high-risk COVID-19 patients [25]. Despite some severe side effects of these drugs, they also target mutation-prone viral components leading to a high risk of the development of drug-resistance.

Although several vaccines have been authorized to this point [26,27], herd-immunity might be difficult to achieve, as the vaccines do not confer complete immunity [28]. All these points underline that there is still an unmet need to develop prophylactically active as well as safe therapeutic agents, which should ideally be rapidly available and broadly acting against different viral strains of SARS-CoV-2. Regarding the time- and cost-consuming path for the development of new therapeutics, the investigation of natural substances for their antiviral activity against various SARS-CoV-2 VoCs represent a fast and promising alternative. Natural products have been shown repeatedly to have antiviral effects against a variety of viruses. Since the beginning of the SARS-CoV-2 pandemic, several natural substances have been tested for their potential effects against SARS-CoV-2 with promising results [29–32].

European black elderberries and extracts thereof have been used for centuries in traditional medicine to treat upper respiratory infections [33]. The antiviral effects of black elderberries have been evaluated in several in vivo and in vitro studies. Thereby, it was shown that liquid black elderberry extract has an inhibitory effect on the propagation of the human pathogenic Influenza A virus (IAV) lines KAN-1 and H5N1 [34]. In addition, elderberry extracts exhibit strong antiviral activity against Feline Immunodeficiency Virus (FIV) [35] as well as IAV by inhibiting hemagglutinin [36]. An ethanolic *Sambucus Formosana Nakai* (also known as *Sambucus javanica*) extract, a species of elderberry rich in phenolic acid components, exhibited antiviral activity against human coronavirus HCoV-NL63 in vitro [37]. Moreover, human clinical trials have shown that black elderberry extracts reduce symptom severity as well as the duration of viral infections, especially IAV and the Influenza B virus (IBV) [36,38–40]. A juice concentrate of black elderberry suppressed viral replication in the bronchoalveolar lavage fluids of mice infected with human IAV [41].

Although black elderberry has been tested against a variety of different viruses, there are no data available regarding an inhibitory activity on the replication of SARS-CoV-2 and its VoCs. Here, it is described for the first time that black elderberry fruit extracts exhibit antiviral activity not only against the SARS-CoV-2 Wuhan type but also the VoCs Alpha, Beta, Gamma, Delta and Omicron with comparable IC_{50} values in different human cell lines. Moreover, time of addition experiments revealed that the viral replication cycle is inhibited at later stages, as virus entry was not affected by the addition of the extracts. To characterize the main compounds present in the elderberry extracts, HPLC analysis was performed identifying the anthocyanins cyanidin-3-glucoside, cyanidin-3-sambubioside, cyanidin-3-sambubioside-5-glucoside as well as the phenolic compounds chlorogenic acid, rutin and isoquercitrin as the main components of the extract.

2. Materials and Methods

2.1. Inhibitors

Liquid and dry European black elderberry (*Sambucus nigra* L.) extract (brand name ElderCraft®) was provided by IPRONA AG/SPA, Italy, and was designated as EC 3.2 and EC 14, respectively. EC 3.2 is a water extract in liquid format, standardized to a minimum of 3.2% anthocyanin while EC 14 is a spray-dried water extract standardized to minimum of 14% anthocyanin. To compare the activity of the EC 3.2 and EC 14, the EC 14 powder was diluted in water and set to the same anthocyanin content as EC 3.2.

2.2. Viruses

The "Wuhan type" virus SARS-CoV-2$_{PR-1}$, isolated from a 61-year-old patient, was amplified in Vero B4 cells as described in [29]. The virus strains SARS-CoV-2 Alpha, Beta, Gamma and Delta were obtained from Michael Schindler (University Hospital, Tübingen, Germany). The SARS-CoV-2 Alpha variant (210416_UKv) was generated as described in [31]. SARS-CoV-2 Beta was generated as described in [42]. The Gamma variant (210504_BRv) and the Delta variant (210601_INv) were isolated from throat swabs collected in May 2021 at the Institute for Medical Virology and Epidemiology of Viral Diseases, University Hospital, Tübingen, from PCR-positive patients and generated as described in [32]. The clinical SARS-CoV-2 Omicron variant was generated as described in [43]. SARS-CoV-2 Viral titers of each variant were determined by an endpoint titration assay. For the generation of new virus stock, virus-containing cell culture supernatant was harvested 72 h post-infection (hpi) and passed through a 0.45 μm pore-size filter. All virus stocks were stored at −80 °C until further usage.

2.3. Infection Experiments

For infection experiments, cells were inoculated with SARS-CoV-2$_{PR-1}$ (Wuhan type) or the VoCs Alpha, Beta, Gamma, Delta and SARS-CoV-2 Omicron (multiplicity of infection (MOI): 2×10^{-2}) for 1 h, washed and further treated with interventions. At 72 hpi, virus-containing cell culture supernatants were incubated for 10 min at 95 °C and finally used for qRT-PCR analysis. For titer determination of SARS-CoV-2 virus stocks, A549-ACE2/TMPRSS2 and Calu-3 cells were infected with serial dilutions of the virus stock over 72 h. Afterwards, cells were fixed (4% PFA), permeabilized (0.5% Triton/PBS), blocked (1% BSA/PBS-T) and finally stained with a SARS-CoV-2 NP antibody (Biozol, Eching, Germany). Endpoint of virus infection was analyzed via fluorescence microscopy and viral titer was calculated by the method of Reed and Muench [44].

For preincubation experiments, cells were preincubated either with or without inhibitors for 2 h at 37 °C. After 1 h of infection, the inoculum was removed and cells were incubated without treatment for another 3 days. At 72 hpi, supernatants were harvested and analyzed as described above. For the co-treatment experiments, inhibitors were present during the 1 h of infection, following removement of the inoculum and incubation of the cells for another 3 days without treatment. At 72 hpi, supernatants were harvested and analyzed as described above.

2.4. Cell Culture

Calu-3 cells were maintained in Minimal Essential Medium (MEM) containing 20% (v/v) inactivated fetal calf serum (FCS), 1 mM l-glutamine, 100 U/mL penicillin and 100 μg/mL streptomycin and 1 mM sodium pyruvate. Caco-2 (human colorectal adenocarcinoma) cells were cultured at 37 °C with 5% CO_2 in DMEM containing 10% FCS, with 2 mM l-glutamine, 100 μg/mL penicillin-streptomycin and 1% non-essential amino acids. A549-cells expressing ACE2 and TMPRSS2 were generated by retroviral transduction as described in [29] and cultivated in RPMI 1640 medium containing 10% (v/v) inactivated FCS, 2 mM l-glutamine, 100 U/mL penicillin, 100 μg/mL streptomycin and 100 μg/mL blastomycin.

2.5. Assessment of Cell Viability

Viability of infected and treated cells was assessed by the water-soluble tetrazolium salt (WST)-1 assay (Cat.: 5015944001, Roche, Penzberg, Germany) according to the manufacturer's instructions.

2.6. Determination of the Amount of Viral RNA Copies from Released Viruses by qRT-PCR

The amount of viral RNA copies in the virus–containing samples was quantified by real-time PCR Luna Universal Probe One-Step RT-PCR Kit from New England Biolabs (Cat: E3006L, Ipswich, MA, USA). This kit allows reverse transcription, cDNA synthesis and PCR amplification in a single step. Samples were analyzed by 7500 software v2.3 (Applied Biosystems, Waltham, MA, USA). As described previously in [45], PCR primers were designed and used. Thereby, the polynucleotide sequence contains parts of the SARS-CoV-2 Envelope (E) and RNA-dependent RNA-polymerase (RdRp) genes and was used as standard for the determination of viral RNA copies in the experiments. The sequences of the used primers were: RdRp_forward (fwd): 5′-GTG-ARA-TGG-TCA-TGT-GTG-GCG-G-3′ and RdRp_reverse (rev) 5′-CAR-ATG-TTA-AAS-ACA-CTA-TTA-GCA-TA-C-3′. Probe was 5′-CAG-GTG-GAA-/ZEN/CCT-CAT-CAG-GAG-ATG-C-3′ (Label: FAM/IBFQ Iowa Black FQ). A dsDNA-polynucleotide sequence (Integrated DNA Technologies, Coralville, IA, USA) was used as a positive control: 5′-TAA-TAC-GAC-TCA-CTA-TAG-GGT-ATT-GAG-TGA-AAT-GGT-CAT-GTG-TGG-CGG-TTC-ACT-ATA-TGT-TAA-ACC-AGG-TGG-AAC-CTC-ATC-AGG-AGA-TGC-CAC-AAC-TGC-TTA-TGC-TAA-TAG-TGT-TTT-TAA-CAT-TTG-GAA-GAG-ACA-GGT-ACG-TTA-ATA-GTT-AAT-AGC-GTA-CTT-CTT-TTT-CTT-GCT-TTC-GTG-GTA-TTC-TTG-CTA-GTT-ACA-CTA-GCC-ATC-CTT-ACT-GCG-CTT-CGA-TTG-TGT-GCG-TAC-TGC-TGC-AAT-ATT-GTT-3′. Generating a series of dilutions (10^4, 10^5, 10^6 and 10^7 copies/mL) of this standard, the experiments were quantified using a standard curve to obtain absolute values of RNA copies in the sample.

2.7. Software and Statistics

Microsoft Word and Excel were used. GraphPad Prism 9.0 was used for statistical analyses and to generate graphs. Figures were generated with CorelDrawX7. The 7500 software v2.3 was used to evaluate the results obtained by qRT-PCR. The HPLC analysis data were captured and evaluated using Chromeleon 7 (Thermo Fisher Scientific Inc., Waltham, MA, USA).

2.8. High Performance Liquid Chromatography (HPLC) Analysis of Elderberry Extracts

The HPLC analysis was performed as published by IFU No. 71 as established by International Fruit and Vegetable Juice Association with modifications [46]. The analysis was performed on an UltiMate 3000 HPLC device coupled with a diode array detector DAD-3000 (Thermo Fisher Scientific Inc., Waltham, MA, USA). For phenolic compounds, a wavelength of 350 nm and for anthocyanins a wavelength of 520 nm was used. Total anthocyanin content was calculated using cyanidin-chloride as standard with conversion factor of 1.393 to convert the result from cyanidin-chloride into cyanidin-3-glucoside.

3. Results

3.1. European Black Elderberry Extract Compositional Analysis

Initially, the main components of European black elderberry extract (EC 3.2) and European black elderberry extract dried power (EC 14; resolved in water), both used in this study, were determined. Therefore, the anthocyanin and polyphenol content of the extracts were analyzed using High Performance Liquid Chromatography (HPLC). The main anthocyanins were identified in both extracts as cyanidin-3-sambubioside-5-glucoside, cyanidin-3-sambubioside and cyanidin-3-glucoside (chromatogram of liquid extract EC 3.2 shown in Figure 1).

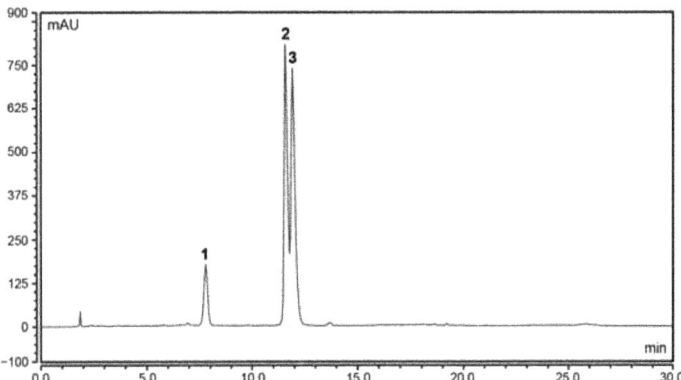

Figure 1. The HPLC chromatogram of anthocyanins in EC 3.2. Peak 1: cyanidin-3-sambubioside-5-glucoside; peak 2: cyanidin-3-sambubioside; peak 3: cyanidin-3-glucoside. Absorbance (mAU) measured at 520 nm.

The analysis of the content of phenolic compounds revealed that, among others, mainly rutin, chlorogenic acid and isoquercitirin were present in both black elderberry extracts (chromatogram of liquid extract EC 3.2 shown in Figure 2).

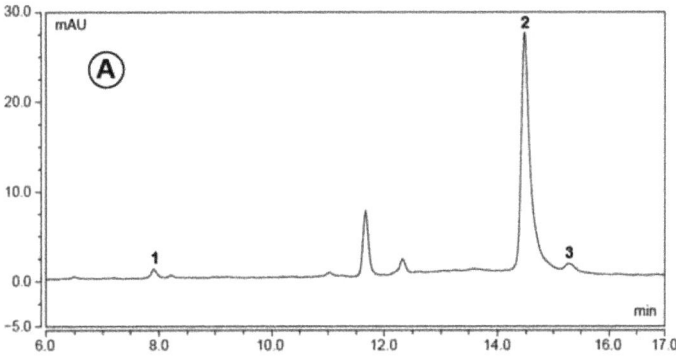

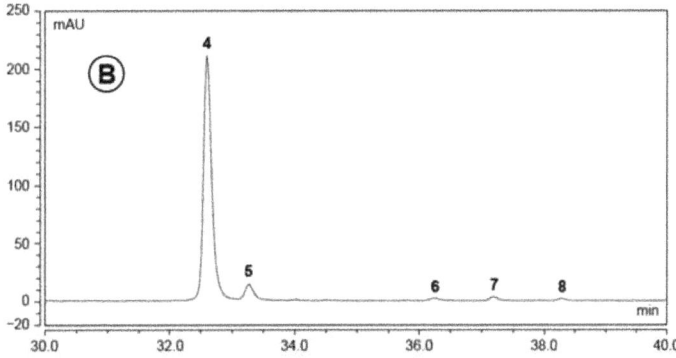

Figure 2. The HPLC chromatogram of phenolic compounds in EC 3.2. (**A**): peak 1: neochlorogenic acid; peak 2: chlorogenic acid; peak 3: cryptochlorogenic acid. (**B**): peak 4: rutin; peak 5: isoquercitrin; peak 6: kaempferol-3-rutinoside; peak 7: isorhamnetin-3-rutinoside; peak 8: isorhamnetin-3-glucoside.

Table 1 summarizes the total amounts of the identified compounds of EC 3.2 and EC 14.

Table 1. Quantitative analysis of compounds in black elderberry extracts EC 3.2 and EC 14.

Compound	EC 3.2 (mg/kg)	EC 14 (mg/kg)
Cyanidin-3-glucoside	14,889	58,336
Cyanidin-3-sambubioside	16,584	77,507
Cyanidin-3-sambubioside-5-glucoside	3558	13,682
Neochlorogenic acid	42	151
Chlorogenic acid	1890	5953
Cryptochlorogenic acid	72	359
Rutin	8419	31,999
Isoquercitrin	507	1784
Kaempferol-3-rutinoside	69	195
Isorhamnetin-3-rutinoside	67	221
Isorhamnetin-3-glucoside	48	215

3.2. European Black Elderberry Extract Exhibits Efficient Antiviral Activity against SARS-CoV-2 in Different Cell Lines

In order to determine whether liquid European black elderberry extract (EC 3.2) exhibits antiviral activity against SARS-CoV-2, human Caco-2 colon carcinoma-derived epithelial cells [47] and Calu-3 human lung cells, the most extensively studied surrogate lung cell infection model that expresses ACE2 and TMPRSS2 endogenously [48], were infected with SARS-CoV-2 Wuhan type (Figure 3).

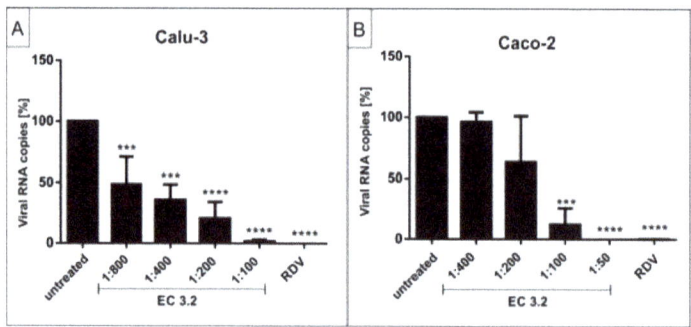

Figure 3. Liquid European black elderberry (EC 3.2) extract inhibits replication of SARS-CoV-2 Wuhan type in Calu-3 and Caco-2 cells. Calu-3 (**A**) and Caco-2 cells (**B**) were infected with the clinical isolate SARS-CoV-2$_{PR-1}$ at a MOI of 2×10^{-2}. One hour after infection and removal of input virus, cells were treated with indicated dilution steps of EC 3.2. A total of 1 µM Remdesivir (RDV) was included as a positive control. Cell culture supernatants were harvested at 3 dpi. The virions were purified and analyzed by qRT-PCR. Bars show mean values of three independent experiments ± standard deviation. Statistical analysis was performed using a multiple comparison Kruskal–Wallis test (Anova) followed by Dunn's post hoc test (*** $p < 0.001$; **** $p < 0.0001$ versus the untreated control).

One hour post-infection, different dilutions of EC 3.2 were added to the cell cultures. Three days post-infection (dpi), cell culture supernatants were harvested and virus production was analyzed by quantitative RT-PCR (qRT-PCR) (Figure 3).

Treatment with EC 3.2 led to a dose dependent reduction of virus replication in all infected cell lines. At a dilution of 1:100, EC 3.2 almost completely blocked the production of progeny virions, which was comparable to 1 µM Remdesivir. Thereby, the IC_{50} values varied between ~1:800 in Calu-3 cells and ~1:200 in Caco-2 cells (Figure 3).

To control for the potential unspecific effects of EC 3.2 treatment on cell viability, water-soluble tetrazolium salt (WST)-1 assays were performed in uninfected Caco-2 or Calu-3 cells under otherwise identical conditions as for the virus infection experiments. The results, summarized in Figure 4, demonstrate that treatment with EC 3.2 at dilutions up to 1:100, and thus in a concentration range where the replication of SARS-CoV-2 was completely blocked, had no impact on cell viability in both investigated cell types (Figure 4). The TD_{50} values for EC 3.2 were ~1:25 in Caco-2 and 1:50 in Calu-3 cells. Staurosporine (StS) was used as a positive control at a concentration of 1 µM.

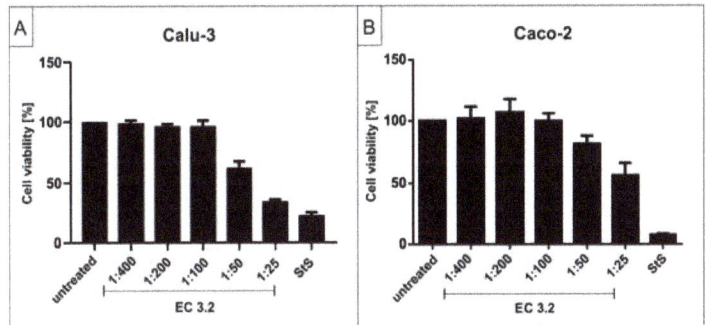

Figure 4. Influence of EC 3.2 on the cell viability of Calu-3 (**A**) and Caco-2 cells (**B**). Following treatment with different dilutions of EC 3.2 (indicated at the x-axis) for three days, the influence on cell viability was measured by water-soluble tetrazolium salt (WST)-1 assay. Bars represent means of 3 independent experiments ± SD. Staurosprine (StS, 1 µM) was used as a positive control.

Next, it was determined if European black elderberry dried power (EC 14) resolved in water also showed a similar antiviral activity to EC 3.2. As this dried powder is commonly used in food supplements, it is of interest whether the drying process has any negative influence on its antiviral activity.

Therefore, Calu-3 cells were infected with the SARS-CoV-2 Wuhan type as described before and qRT-PCR analysis was performed (Figure 5). Similarly to EC 3.2, EC 14 also inhibits the replication of SARS-CoV-2 in a dose-dependent manner with a comparable IC_{50} value of ~1:800 (Figure 5).

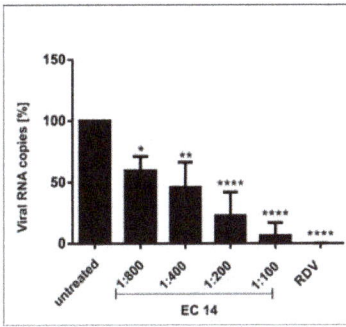

Figure 5. European black elderberry dried powder (EC 14) resolved in water inhibits replication of SARS-CoV-2 Wuhan type. Calu-3 cells were infected with the clinical isolate SARS-CoV-2$_{PR-1}$ at a MOI of 2×10^{-2}. One hour after infection and removal of input virus, cells were treated with indicated dilution steps of EC 14. A total of 1 µM RDV was included as a positive control. Cell culture

supernatants were harvested at 3 dpi. The virions were purified and analyzed by qRT-PCR. Bars show mean values of three independent experiments ± standard deviation. Statistical analysis was performed using a multiple comparison Kruskal–Wallis test (Anova) followed by Dunn's post hoc test (* $p < 0.05$; ** $p < 0.01$; **** $p < 0.0001$ versus the untreated control).

3.3. EC 3.2 Exhibits Comparable Antiviral Activity against All SARS-CoV-2 Variants of Concern

In order to determine if EC 3.2 exhibits a comparable, broad antiviral activity against all described VoCs of SARS-CoV-2, Calu-3 human lung cells were infected with the VoCs Alpha, Beta, Gamma, Delta and Omicron (Figure 6).

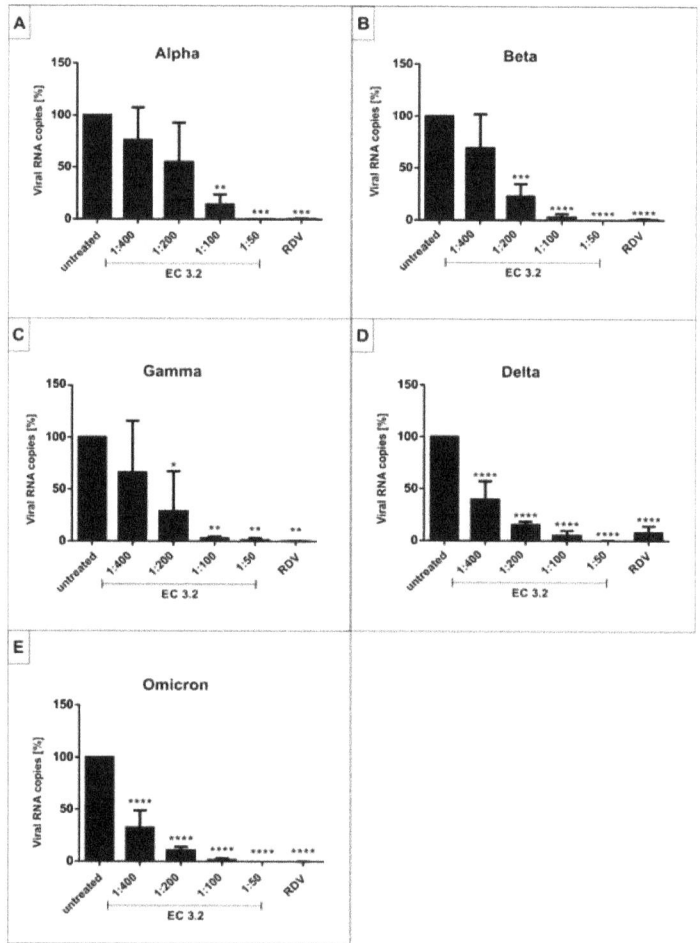

Figure 6. EC 3.2 inhibits replication of the SARS-CoV-2 Variants of Concern (VoCs) Alpha, Beta, Gamma, Delta and Omicron with comparable antiviral efficacy. Calu-3 cells were infected with clinical isolates of the SARS-CoV-2 VoCs Alpha (**A**), Beta (**B**), Gamma (**C**), Delta (**D**) or Omicron (**E**) at a MOI of 2×10^{-2}. One hour after infection and removal of input virus, cells were treated with the indicated dilutions of EC 3.2. A total of 1 µM RDV was included as a positive control. Cell culture supernatants were harvested at 3 dpi. The virions were purified and analyzed by qRT-PCR. Bars show mean values of three independent experiments ± standard deviation. Statistical analysis was performed using a multiple comparison Kruskal–Wallis test (Anova) followed by Dunn's post hoc test (* $p < 0.05$; ** $p < 0.01$; *** $p < 0.001$; **** $p < 0.0001$ versus the untreated control).

One hour post-infection, different dilutions of EC 3.2 were added to the cells. Three dpi cell culture supernatants were harvested and virus production was analyzed by qRT-PCR (Figure 6).

Treatment with EC 3.2 led to a dose-dependent reduction of virus replication that occurred with comparable efficacy for all VoCs (Figure 6). The IC_{50} values varied between ~1:800 for the Wuhan type (Figure 3) and ~1:200 for Alpha (Figure 6). However, the IC_{90} was ~1:100 for all VoCs and thus in a similar range (Figure 6).

The IC_{50} and IC_{90} values for EC 3.2 following infection with the Wuhan type and respective VoCs are summarized in Table 2.

Table 2. IC_{50} and IC_{90} values of EC 3.2 against SARS-CoV-2 Wuhan type and VoCs in Calu-3 cells.

	EC 3.2	
	IC_{50}	IC_{90}
Wuhan Type	~1:800	~1:100
Alpha	~1:200	~1:100
Beta	~1:300	~1:100
Gamma	~1:300	~1:100
Delta	~1:400	~1:100
Omicron	~1:400	~1:100

Next, we calculated the IC_{50} values for the main compounds of EC 3.2, based on the results of the HPLC analysis (Figures 1 and 2 and Table 1). The results are summarized in Table 3.

Table 3. The IC_{50} values [µM] of the main compounds of EC 3.2 following infection of Calu-3 cells with SARS-CoV-2 Wuhan Type and VoCs.

	IC_{50} [µM]					
	Wuhan Type	Alpha	Beta	Gamma	Delta	Omicron
Cyanidin-3-sambubioside-5-glucoside	6	24	18	18	12	12
Cyanidin-3-sambubioside	35	142	107	107	71	71
Cyanidin-3-glucoside	41	165	123	123	82	82
Chlorogenic acid	6.6	27	20	20	13	13
Rutin	17	68	51	51	34	34
Isoquercitrin	1.3	5.4	4	4	2.7	2.7

3.4. Treatment with EC 3.2 Does Not Affect Early Steps of the Replication of SARS-CoV-2

Next, it was analyzed if EC 3.2 blocks the replication of SARS-CoV-2 by interfering with the early steps of the viral replication cycle. Therefore, time of addition (TOA) experiments were performed. First, Calu-3 cells were preincubated with different concentrations of EC 3.2 for 2 h at 37 °C (see treatment scheme Figure 7A). Following two washing steps with PBS to remove EC 3.2, cells were infected with SARS-CoV-2 Wuhan type and cell culture supernatants were harvested after 3 days and analyzed by qRT-PCR.

The data revealed that the preincubation of the cells without further treatment during the infection and post-infection period does not interfere with SARS-CoV-2 replication (Figure 7A). Remdesivir, an inhibitor of RNA metabolism [49], was used as a control and also exhibit no antiviral activity in this experimental setup (Figure 7A).

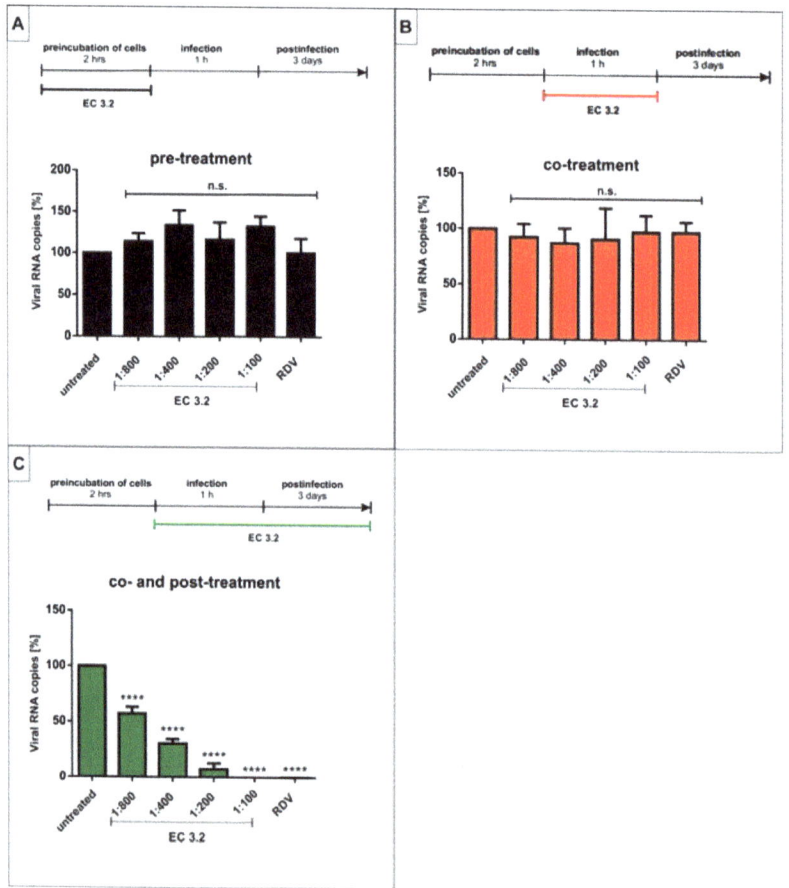

Figure 7. Treatment with EC 3.2 before or during the infection with SARS-CoV-2 has no influence on viral replication. (**A**) Time of addition (TOA) of EC 3.2 with the indicated dilutions. Calu-3 cells were preincubated with EC 3.2 for 2 h following two washing steps with PBS. (**B**) The TOA of EC 3.2 was only during infection of Calu-3 cells for 1 h. (**C**) The TOA of EC 3.2 was during infection of cells for 1 h and following removal of input virus, for 3 days post-infection. (**A–C**) Cells were infected with the clinical isolate SARS-CoV-2$_{PR-1}$ at a MOI of 2×10^{-2} for 1 h. A total of 1 µM RDV was included as a positive control. Cell culture supernatants were harvested at 3 dpi. The virions were purified and analyzed by qRT-PCR. Bars show mean values of three independent experiments ± standard deviation. Statistical analysis was performed using a multiple comparison Kruskal–Wallis test (Anova) followed by Dunn's post hoc test (n.s. = not significant; **** $p < 0.0001$ versus the untreated control).

Next, EC 3.2 was added to Calu-3 cells only during the time of infection with SARS-CoV-2 Wuhan type for 1 h and without applying further treatment to the cells afterwards (treatment scheme Figure 7B). After 1 h, the infectious supernatants were removed and the cells were incubated without further treatment for three days, followed by q RT-PCR analysis of the supernatants. As described for the pre-treatment, the co-treatment with EC 3.2 also has no influence on the replication capacity of SARS-CoV-2 (Figure 7B).

Within a final setup, Calu-3 cells were treated during the 1 h infection period with SARS-CoV-2 Wuhan type and, additionally, during three days post-infection with EC 3.2 (treatment scheme Figure 7C). Thereby, a similar dose-dependent reduction of viral replication (Figure 7C) was detected as with the post-treatment alone (Figure 3A). The IC_{50} was ~1:800; thus, the additional co-treatment with EC 3.2 has no further influence on the replication capacity of SARS-CoV-2 (Figure 7C). In summary, the TOA experiments revealed that EC 3.2 does not influence early steps in the replication cycle of SARS-CoV-2 but rather exerts its antiviral activity effect during the later steps of viral replication.

4. Discussion

COVID-19, caused by SARS-CoV-2, is still responsible for the ongoing worldwide pandemic that led to a global health and socioeconomic crisis. Similar to the occurrence of SARS-CoV, Middle East respiratory syndrome-related coronavirus (MERS-CoV) and SARS-CoV-2, it can be expected that in the future new coronaviruses will emerge by zoonotic transmission from animals to humans potentially leading to new threats. This demonstrates the need for pandemic preparedness.

Regarding viral infections, vaccines are valuable but have limitations due to the high mutation rate of viruses, especially for RNA viruses such as SARS-CoV-2. This causes the continuous appearance of escape mutants, which are able to evade vaccine-induced immunity. Thus, there is an urgent need for new therapeutics that are available within a short period of time, broadly active, safe, cost-effective and easily distributable for patients all over the world when compared to standard antivirals.

In this study, an antiviral effect of European black elderberry fruit extract against SARS-CoV-2 and its VoCs was shown for the first time. In order to analyze whether black elderberry extract exhibits antiviral activity against various VoCs, Calu-3 cells were infected with SARS-CoV-2 Alpha, Beta, Gamma, Delta and Omicron. The results showed that the replication of these variants could be blocked in a comparable concentration range (Figure 6). This suggests an effective inhibition of viral replication independent of the current and possibly future variants of SARS-CoV-2.

Fruit extracts and juices have previously been shown to be a potential source of antiviral agents (for review, see [50]). Thereby, fruit extracts from, e.g., blackberry, blackcurrant, mulberry and pomegranate exhibit antiviral properties against various viruses such as the Dengue virus, IAV, Zika, Hepatitis C virus (HCV), Human immunodeficiency virus 1 (HIV-1) and the polio virus [50]. For black elderberry extracts, several in vitro studies show an antiviral activity against IAV and IBV, as well as FIV [34–36,51,52]. Moreover, an ethanolic *Sambucus Formosana Nakai* extract exhibits antiviral activity against the endemic human coronavirus HCoV-NL63 [37]. Most importantly, human clinical trials have shown that a *Sambucus nigra* extract significantly reduces the total duration and severity of upper respiratory symptoms following common cold or IAV infections [38]. In addition, black elderberry extracts exhibit an immunomodulatory effect, which seems to be attributed to the polysaccharide fraction. In this context, it was shown that *Sambucus nigra* fruits contain peptic polysaccharides influencing the immune system via the activation of macrophages and dendritic cells [53–55], which might also contribute to the therapeutic effects seen in human clinical trials.

The black elderberry extract used in this study is a standardized European black elderberry fruit extract (*Sambucus nigra*, variety 'Haschberg') with a total polyphenol content of 4.6% and a total anthocyanin content of 3.5%. The used extract in this study consists of a mixture of organic compounds including but not limited to polyphenols, anthocyanin, mono- and disaccharides, proteins, lipids and carbohydrates. Therefore, the observed antiviral effect of the whole elderberry extract cannot be attributed to single compounds. Further studies including the identified main compounds of the used black elderberry fruit extract are necessary to designate the anti-SARS-CoV-2 effect to specific compounds of the whole extract.

The antiviral activities of polyphenols as well as anthocyanins against various viruses were extensively described previously (for review, see [56,57]). The phenolic compounds of various plants are discussed to be effective against SARS-CoV-2 [58]. For the extracts of some plants, not including black elderberry, an antiviral activity of phenolic compounds against SARS-CoV-2 was shown in vitro [58]. In this study, we identified as the main anthocyanins cyanidin-3-sambubioside-5-glucoside, cyanidin-3-sambubioside and cyanidin-3-glucoside (Figure 1). The main polyphenols were identified as chlorogenic acid, rutin and isoquercetin (Figure 2). This is consistent with previous reports on the phenolic content of elderberry fruits [59–61]. For some of these identified compounds, an antiviral activity was reported previously. For instance, isoquercitrin displayed potent antiviral activity against the Varicella Zoster virus (VZV) and human Cytomegalovirus (hCMV) [62]. In addition, a very recent study shows that isoquercitrin inhibits the replication of IAV [63]. Moreover, it was proposed that the combinational treatment of quercetin and vitamin C might be an effective therapy for the prevention and treatment of COVID-19 [64]. For chlorogenic acid, an antiviral activity was described against different viral strains of IAV as well as for Enterovirus 71 [65,66]. However, to our knowledge, the specific anti-SARS-CoV-2 activities of these compounds have not been reported yet.

Analyzing the potential antiviral mode of action of phenolic compounds, it was shown that the flavonoids present in elderberry fruits can directly bind to H1N1 Influenza virus particles, thereby inhibiting the entry of the virus into the host cells [52]. Another study indicates that an ethanolic extract of *Sambucus nigra* fruits can inhibit the infectious bronchitis virus (IBV), a pathogenic chicken coronavirus, at early points during replication [67]. By performing time of addition experiments, Cho et al. showed that isoquercetin inhibits viral attachment and the entry of IAV [63]. Such a mechanism inhibiting the early stages of the replication of SARS-CoV-2 is unlikely to be the case for European black elderberry extract inasmuch as the time of addition experiments performed in this study displayed antiviral activity only for the later stages of virus replication. Treatment before or during the infection with SARS-CoV-2 had no influence on the replication capacity (Figure 7), strongly indicating an inhibitory effect after virus entry.

However, there are also several reports showing an antiviral effect of anthocyanins or phenolic compounds at later stages in the viral replication cycle. For instance, the main anthocyanin present in European black elderberry fruits, i.e., cyanidin-3-sambubiocide, can bind and inhibit the active pocket of the IAV neuraminidase [51]. In another study, it was demonstrated that natural phenolic compounds are able to inhibit the papain-like protease (PLpro) of SARS-CoV-2 with an IC_{50} of 4–10 µM [68]. The papain-like protease is a viral protease with multiple functions and is crucial for the virus replication of SARS-CoV-2. Such a mechanism might also be responsible for the observed antiviral effect of black elderberry fruit extract (Figures 3, 5 and 6 and Tables 1 and 2) and will be the subject of further investigations. For rutin, which is also a main phenolic compound in the black elderberry extract used in this study (Figure 2 and Table 1), an inhibition of the second SARS-CoV-2 protease 3CLpro was shown in a low micromolar range [69–71], which might also, at least partially, be responsible for the antiviral effect of European black elderberry fruit extract.

Due to the history of using European black elderberry, it can be considered as safe for ingestion. The unripe berries of black elderberry can contain cyanogenic compounds such as sambunigrin, which is readily degraded during a short heat treatment. Thus, both extracts used in this study, EC 3.2 and EC 14, undergo a short heat treatment during production. This is in concert with the data in this study, which showed no toxic effect on Caco-2 and Calu-3 cells when treated with different concentrations of black elderberry extract up to a dilution of 1:50, which points towards a broad therapeutic window (Figure 4).

The results of this study suggest that European black elderberry fruit extracts could provide beneficial effects in therapeutic settings following a SARS-CoV-2 infection. Their low cytotoxicity and wide availability in nature would make them a readily distributable treatment option for current and future pandemics.

5. Patents

IPRONA AG/SPA has filed a PCT and EP patent entitled "Elderberry extract for use in a method of preventing or treating a SARS-CoV-2 infection" claiming the priority date of 06.12.2021.

Author Contributions: Conceptualization, C.S., U.S., A.S. and S.P.; methodology, C.S., M.F., P.R., M.G. and J.A.; validation, C.S., M.F., S.P. and U.S.; investigation, C.S., M.F., M.G., J.A. and P.R.; data curation, U.S.; writing—original draft preparation, C.S., S.P., A.S. and U.S.; writing—review and editing, C.S., S.P., A.S. and U.S.; visualization, C.S., M.F. and J.A.; supervision, U.S. and S.P.; project administration, C.S., S.P. and U.S.; funding acquisition, S.P. and U.S. All authors have read and agreed to the published version of the manuscript.

Funding: This research was funded by the Deutsche Forschungsgemeinschaft (DFG, German Research Foundation)—401821119/GRK2504 to U.S and supported by the Interdisciplinary Center for Clinical Research (IZKF) at the University Hospital of the University of Erlangen-Nuremberg to J.A. and M.F. (MD-Thesis Scholarship Programme). Additional funding was received by the Autonomous Province of Bozen/Bolzano (Italy)—File 106/2021, decree 14449.

Institutional Review Board Statement: Not applicable.

Informed Consent Statement: Not applicable.

Data Availability Statement: Data are included in the article.

Acknowledgments: The present work was performed in partial fulfillment of the requirements for obtaining Dr. med. degree at the Friedrich-Alexander University Erlangen-Nuremberg for M.F. and J.A.

Conflicts of Interest: The authors have read the journal's policy and declare that the author Stephan Plattner is employed by IPRONA AG/SPA. Stephan Plattner, Ulrich Schubert, Christian Setz and Alexander Steinkasserer are inventors of a patent submission related to the content of the manuscript; the number of this patent application is EP21212602. The funders had no role in the design of the study; in the collection, analyses, or interpretation of data; in the writing of the manuscript, or in the decision to publish the results. All other authors declare no conflict of interest.

References

1. Medicine, J.H.U. COVID-19 Dashboard by the Center for Systems Science and Engineering (CSSE) at Johns Hopkins University. Available online: https://coronavirus.jhu.edu/map.html (accessed on 8 December 2022).
2. Collier, D.A.; De Marco, A.; Ferreira, I.; Meng, B.; Datir, R.P.; Walls, A.C.; Kemp, S.A.; Bassi, J.; Pinto, D.; Silacci-Fregni, C.; et al. Sensitivity of SARS-CoV-2 B.1.1.7 to mRNA vaccine-elicited antibodies. *Nature* **2021**, *593*, 136–141. [CrossRef] [PubMed]
3. Wibmer, C.K.; Ayres, F.; Hermanus, T.; Madzivhandila, M.; Kgagudi, P.; Oosthuysen, B.; Lambson, B.E.; de Oliveira, T.; Vermeulen, M.; van der Berg, K.; et al. SARS-CoV-2 501Y.V2 escapes neutralization by South African COVID-19 donor plasma. *Nat. Med.* **2021**, *27*, 622–625. [CrossRef] [PubMed]
4. Korber, B.; Fischer, W.M.; Gnanakaran, S.; Yoon, H.; Theiler, J.; Abfalterer, W.; Hengartner, N.; Giorgi, E.E.; Bhattacharya, T.; Foley, B.; et al. Tracking Changes in SARS-CoV-2 Spike: Evidence that D614G Increases Infectivity of the COVID-19 Virus. *Cell* **2020**, *182*, 812–827.e19. [CrossRef] [PubMed]
5. Galloway, S.E.; Paul, P.; MacCannell, D.R.; Johansson, M.A.; Brooks, J.T.; MacNeil, A.; Slayton, R.B.; Tong, S.; Silk, B.J.; Armstrong, G.L.; et al. Emergence of SARS-CoV-2 B.1.1.7 Lineage—United States, December 29, 2020–January 12, 2021. *MMWR Morb. Mortal. Wkly. Rep.* **2021**, *70*, 95–99. [CrossRef] [PubMed]
6. Meng, B.; Kemp, S.A.; Papa, G.; Datir, R.; Ferreira, I.; Marelli, S.; Harvey, W.T.; Lytras, S.; Mohamed, A.; Gallo, G.; et al. Recurrent emergence of SARS-CoV-2 spike deletion H69/V70 and its role in the Alpha variant B.1.1.7. *Cell Rep.* **2021**, *35*, 109292. [CrossRef]
7. Tegally, H.; Wilkinson, E.; Giovanetti, M.; Iranzadeh, A.; Fonseca, V.; Giandhari, J.; Doolabh, D.; Pillay, S.; San, E.J.; Msomi, N.; et al. Detection of a SARS-CoV-2 variant of concern in South Africa. *Nature* **2021**, *592*, 438–443. [CrossRef]
8. Public Health England Investigation of SARS-CoV-2 Variants of Concern: Technical Briefings. Available online: https://www.gov.uk/government/publications/investigation-of-novel-sars-cov-2-variant-variant-of-concern-20201201 (accessed on 13 April 2022).
9. Mwenda, M.; Saasa, N.; Sinyange, N.; Busby, G.; Chipimo, P.J.; Hendry, J.; Kapona, O.; Yingst, S.; Hines, J.Z.; Minchella, P.; et al. Detection of B.1.351 SARS-CoV-2 Variant Strain—Zambia, December 2020. *MMWR Morb. Mortal. Wkly. Rep.* **2021**, *70*, 280–282. [CrossRef]

10. National Institute of Infectious Diseases (NIID) of Japan Brief Report: New Variant Strain of SARS-CoV-2 Identified in Travelers from Brazil. Available online: https://www.niid.go.jp/niid/en/2019-ncov-e/10108-covid19-33-en.html (accessed on 29 July 2022).
11. Cherian, S.; Potdar, V.; Jadhav, S.; Yadav, P.; Gupta, N.; Das, M.; Rakshit, P.; Singh, S.; Abraham, P.; Panda, S.; et al. SARS-CoV-2 Spike Mutations, L452R, T478K, E484Q and P681R, in the Second Wave of COVID-19 in Maharashtra, India. *Microorganisms* **2021**, *9*, 1542. [CrossRef]
12. WHO. *Classification of Omicron (B. 1.1. 529): SARS-CoV-2 Variant of Concern*; World Health Organization: Geneva, Switzerland, 2021; Available online: https://www.who.int/news/item/26-11-2021-classification-of-omicron-(b.1.1.529)-sars-cov-2-variant-of-concern (accessed on 28 November 2021).
13. Ke, H.; Chang, M.R.; Marasco, W.A. Immune Evasion of SARS-CoV-2 Omicron Subvariants. *Vaccines* **2022**, *10*, 1545. [CrossRef]
14. Arora, P.; Kempf, A.; Nehlmeier, I.; Schulz, S.R.; Jäck, H.M.; Pöhlmann, S.; Hoffmann, M. Omicron sublineage BQ.1.1 resistance to monoclonal antibodies. *Lancet Infect. Dis.* **2022**, *23*, 22–23. [CrossRef]
15. Karim, S.S.A.; Karim, Q.A. Omicron SARS-CoV-2 variant: A new chapter in the COVID-19 pandemic. *Lancet* **2021**, *398*, 2126–2128. [CrossRef] [PubMed]
16. Volz, E.; Mishra, S.; Chand, M.; Barrett, J.C.; Johnson, R.; Geidelberg, L.; Hinsley, W.R.; Laydon, D.J.; Dabrera, G.; O'Toole, Á.; et al. Assessing transmissibility of SARS-CoV-2 lineage B.1.1.7 in England. *Nature* **2021**, *593*, 266–269. [CrossRef] [PubMed]
17. Davies, N.G.; Abbott, S.; Barnard, R.C.; Jarvis, C.I.; Kucharski, A.J.; Munday, J.D.; Pearson, C.A.B.; Russell, T.W.; Tully, D.C.; Washburne, A.D.; et al. Estimated transmissibility and impact of SARS-CoV-2 lineage B.1.1.7 in England. *Science* **2021**, *372*, eabg3055. [CrossRef]
18. Kim, Y.J.; Jang, U.S.; Soh, S.M.; Lee, J.Y.; Lee, H.R. The Impact on Infectivity and Neutralization Efficiency of SARS-CoV-2 Lineage B.1.351 Pseudovirus. *Viruses* **2021**, *13*, 633. [CrossRef] [PubMed]
19. Planas, D.; Veyer, D.; Baidaliuk, A.; Staropoli, I.; Guivel-Benhassine, F.; Rajah, M.M.; Planchais, C.; Porrot, F.; Robillard, N.; Puech, J.; et al. Reduced sensitivity of SARS-CoV-2 variant Delta to antibody neutralization. *Nature* **2021**, *596*, 276–280. [CrossRef] [PubMed]
20. Wang, P.; Casner, R.G.; Nair, M.S.; Wang, M.; Yu, J.; Cerutti, G.; Liu, L.; Kwong, P.D.; Huang, Y.; Shapiro, L.; et al. Increased Resistance of SARS-CoV-2 Variant P.1 to Antibody Neutralization. *bioRxiv* **2021**. [CrossRef] [PubMed]
21. WHO Therapeutics and COVID-19: Living Guideline. Available online: https://www.who.int/publications/i/item/WHO-2019-nCoV-therapeutics-2022.1 (accessed on 8 February 2022).
22. EMA EMA Issues Advice on Use of Paxlovid (PF-07321332 and Ritonavir) for the Treatment of COVID-19: Rolling Review Starts in Parallel. Available online: https://www.ema.europa.eu/en/news/ema-issues-advice-use-paxlovid-pf-07321332-ritonavir-treatment-covid-19-rolling-review-starts (accessed on 8 February 2022).
23. National Insitutes of Health COVID-19 Treatment Guidelines—Therapeutic Management of Nonhospitalized Adults with COVID-19. Available online: https://www.covid19treatmentguidelines.nih.gov/management/clinical-management/nonhospitalized-adults--therapeutic-management/ (accessed on 28 July 2022).
24. Arbel, R.; Wolff Sagy, Y.; Hoshen, M.; Battat, E.; Lavie, G.; Sergienko, R.; Friger, M.; Waxman, J.G.; Dagan, N.; Balicer, R.; et al. Nirmatrelvir Use and Severe COVID-19 Outcomes during the Omicron Surge. *N. Engl. J. Med.* **2022**, *387*, 790–798. [CrossRef]
25. Singh, A.K.; Singh, A.; Singh, R.; Misra, A. Molnupiravir in COVID-19: A systematic review of literature. *Diabetes Metab. Syndr.* **2021**, *15*, 102329. [CrossRef]
26. Creech, C.B.; Walker, S.C.; Samuels, R.J. SARS-CoV-2 Vaccines. *JAMA* **2021**, *325*, 1318–1320. [CrossRef]
27. European Medicines Agency. COVID-19 Vaccines: Authorised. Available online: https://www.ema.europa.eu/en/human-regulatory/overview/public-health-threats/coronavirus-disease-covid-19/treatments-vaccines/vaccines-covid-19/covid-19-vaccines-authorised#authorised-covid-19-vaccines-section (accessed on 22 March 2022).
28. European Centre for Disease Prevention and Control Risk of SARS-CoV-2 Transmission from Newly-Infected Individuals with Documented Previous Infection or Vaccination. Available online: https://www.ecdc.europa.eu/en/publications-data/sars-cov-2-transmission-newly-infected-individuals-previous-infection#copy-to-clipboard (accessed on 18 August 2022).
29. Große, M.; Ruetalo, N.; Layer, M.; Hu, D.; Businger, R.; Rheber, S.; Setz, C.; Rauch, P.; Auth, J.; Fröba, M.; et al. Quinine Inhibits Infection of Human Cell Lines with SARS-CoV-2. *Viruses* **2021**, *13*, 647. [CrossRef]
30. Mani, J.S.; Johnson, J.B.; Steel, J.C.; Broszczak, D.A.; Neilsen, P.M.; Walsh, K.B.; Naiker, M. Natural product-derived phytochemicals as potential agents against coronaviruses: A review. *Virus Res.* **2020**, *284*, 197989. [CrossRef] [PubMed]
31. Auth, J.; Fröba, M.; Große, M.; Rauch, P.; Ruetalo, N.; Schindler, M.; Morokutti-Kurz, M.; Graf, P.; Dolischka, A.; Prieschl-Grassauer, E.; et al. Lectin from Triticum vulgaris (WGA) Inhibits Infection with SARS-CoV-2 and Its Variants of Concern Alpha and Beta. *Int. J. Mol. Sci.* **2021**, *22*, 10355. [CrossRef] [PubMed]
32. Fröba, M.; Große, M.; Setz, C.; Rauch, P.; Auth, J.; Spanaus, L.; Münch, J.; Ruetalo, N.; Schindler, M.; Morokutti-Kurz, M.; et al. Iota-Carrageenan Inhibits Replication of SARS-CoV-2 and the Respective Variants of Concern Alpha, Beta, Gamma and Delta. *Int. J. Mol. Sci.* **2021**, *22*, 13202. [CrossRef]
33. Roxas, M.; Jurenka, J. Colds and influenza: A review of diagnosis and conventional, botanical, and nutritional considerations. *Altern. Med. Rev. J. Clin. Ther.* **2007**, *12*, 25–48.

34. Krawitz, C.; Mraheil, M.A.; Stein, M.; Imirzalioglu, C.; Domann, E.; Pleschka, S.; Hain, T. Inhibitory activity of a standardized elderberry liquid extract against clinically-relevant human respiratory bacterial pathogens and influenza A and B viruses. *BMC Complement. Altern. Med.* **2011**, *11*, 16. [CrossRef] [PubMed]
35. Uncini Manganelli, R.E.; Zaccaro, L.; Tomei, P.E. Antiviral activity in vitro of *Urtica dioica* L. *Parietaria diffusa* M. et K. and *Sambucus nigra* L. *J. Ethnopharmacol.* **2005**, *98*, 323–327. [CrossRef] [PubMed]
36. Zakay-Rones, Z.; Varsano, N.; Zlotnik, M.; Manor, O.; Regev, L.; Schlesinger, M.; Mumcuoglu, M. Inhibition of several strains of influenza virus in vitro and reduction of symptoms by an elderberry extract (*Sambucus nigra* L.) during an outbreak of influenza B Panama. *J. Altern. Complement. Med.* **1995**, *1*, 361–369. [CrossRef]
37. Weng, J.R.; Lin, C.S.; Lai, H.C.; Lin, Y.P.; Wang, C.Y.; Tsai, Y.C.; Wu, K.C.; Huang, S.H.; Lin, C.W. Antiviral activity of Sambucus FormosanaNakai ethanol extract and related phenolic acid constituents against human coronavirus NL63. *Virus Res.* **2019**, *273*, 197767. [CrossRef]
38. Hawkins, J.; Baker, C.; Cherry, L.; Dunne, E. Black elderberry (*Sambucus nigra*) supplementation effectively treats upper respiratory symptoms: A meta-analysis of randomized, controlled clinical trials. *Complement. Ther. Med.* **2019**, *42*, 361–365. [CrossRef]
39. Tiralongo, E.; Wee, S.S.; Lea, R.A. Elderberry Supplementation Reduces Cold Duration and Symptoms in Air-Travellers: A Randomized, Double-Blind Placebo-Controlled Clinical Trial. *Nutrients* **2016**, *8*, 182. [CrossRef]
40. Zakay-Rones, Z.; Thom, E.; Wollan, T.; Wadstein, J. Randomized study of the efficacy and safety of oral elderberry extract in the treatment of influenza A and B virus infections. *J. Int. Med. Res.* **2004**, *32*, 132–140. [CrossRef] [PubMed]
41. Kinoshita, E.; Hayashi, K.; Katayama, H.; Hayashi, T.; Obata, A. Anti-influenza virus effects of elderberry juice and its fractions. *Biosci. Biotechnol. Biochem.* **2012**, *76*, 1633–1638. [CrossRef] [PubMed]
42. Becker, M.; Dulovic, A.; Junker, D.; Ruetalo, N.; Kaiser, P.D.; Pinilla, Y.T.; Heinzel, C.; Haering, J.; Traenkle, B.; Wagner, T.R.; et al. Immune response to SARS-CoV-2 variants of concern in vaccinated individuals. *Nat. Commun.* **2021**, *12*, 3109. [CrossRef] [PubMed]
43. Setz, C.; Große, M.; Auth, J.; Fröba, M.; Rauch, P.; Bausch, A.; Wright, M.; Schubert, U. Synergistic Antiviral Activity of Pamapimod and Pioglitazone against SARS-CoV-2 and Its Variants of Concern. *Int. J. Mol. Sci.* **2022**, *23*, 6830. [CrossRef]
44. Reed, L.J.M. A Simple Method of Estimating Fifty Per Cent Endpoints. *Am. J. Epidemiol.* **1936**, *27*, 493–497. [CrossRef]
45. Corman, V.M.; Landt, O.; Kaiser, M.; Molenkamp, R.; Meijer, A.; Chu, D.K.; Bleicker, T.; Brünink, S.; Schneider, J.; Schmidt, M.L.; et al. Detection of 2019 novel coronavirus (2019-nCoV) by real-time RT-PCR. *Euro Surveill.* **2020**, *25*, 2000045. [CrossRef]
46. Anon, M. Determination of Anthocyanins by HPLC No. 71. In *Handbook of Analytical Methods*; The international Fruit Juice Union: Paris, France, 1999.
47. Bertram, S.; Glowacka, I.; Blazejewska, P.; Soilleux, E.; Allen, P.; Danisch, S.; Steffen, I.; Choi, S.Y.; Park, Y.; Schneider, H.; et al. TMPRSS2 and TMPRSS4 facilitate trypsin-independent spread of influenza virus in Caco-2 cells. *J. Virol.* **2010**, *84*, 10016–10025. [CrossRef]
48. Aguiar, J.A.; Tremblay, B.J.; Mansfield, M.J.; Woody, O.; Lobb, B.; Banerjee, A.; Chandiramohan, A.; Tiessen, N.; Cao, Q.; Dvorkin-Gheva, A.; et al. Gene expression and in situ protein profiling of candidate SARS-CoV-2 receptors in human airway epithelial cells and lung tissue. *Eur. Respir. J.* **2020**, *56*, 2001123. [CrossRef]
49. Kokic, G.; Hillen, H.S.; Tegunov, D.; Dienemann, C.; Seitz, F.; Schmitzova, J.; Farnung, L.; Siewert, A.; Höbartner, C.; Cramer, P. Mechanism of SARS-CoV-2 polymerase stalling by remdesivir. *Nat. Commun.* **2021**, *12*, 279. [CrossRef]
50. Santhi, V.P.; Sriramavaratharajan, V.; Murugan, R.; Masilamani, P.; Gurav, S.S.; Sarasu, V.P.; Parthiban, S.; Ayyanar, M. Edible fruit extracts and fruit juices as potential source of antiviral agents: A review. *J. Food Meas. Charact.* **2021**, *15*, 5181–5190. [CrossRef]
51. Swaminathan, K.; Dyason, J.C.; Maggioni, A.; von Itzstein, M.; Downard, K.M. Binding of a natural anthocyanin inhibitor to influenza neuraminidase by mass spectrometry. *Anal. Bioanal. Chem.* **2013**, *405*, 6563–6572. [CrossRef] [PubMed]
52. Roschek, B., Jr.; Fink, R.C.; McMichael, M.D.; Li, D.; Alberte, R.S. Elderberry flavonoids bind to and prevent H1N1 infection in vitro. *Phytochemistry* **2009**, *70*, 1255–1261. [CrossRef] [PubMed]
53. Ho, G.T.; Ahmed, A.; Zou, Y.F.; Aslaksen, T.; Wangensteen, H.; Barsett, H. Structure-activity relationship of immunomodulating pectins from elderberries. *Carbohydr. Polym.* **2015**, *125*, 314–322. [CrossRef] [PubMed]
54. Ho, G.T.; Wangensteen, H.; Barsett, H. Elderberry and Elderflower Extracts, Phenolic Compounds, and Metabolites and Their Effect on Complement, RAW 264.7 Macrophages and Dendritic Cells. *Int. J. Mol. Sci.* **2017**, *18*, 584. [CrossRef]
55. Stich, L.; Plattner, S.; McDougall, G.; Austin, C.; Steinkasserer, A. Polysaccharides from European Black Elderberry Extract Enhance Dendritic Cell Mediated T Cell Immune Responses. *Int. J. Mol. Sci.* **2022**, *23*, 3949. [CrossRef]
56. Badshah, S.L.; Faisal, S.; Muhammad, A.; Poulson, B.G.; Emwas, A.H.; Jaremko, M. Antiviral activities of flavonoids. *Biomed. Pharmacother.* **2021**, *140*, 111596. [CrossRef]
57. Mohammadi Pour, P.; Fakhri, S.; Asgary, S.; Farzaei, M.H.; Echeverría, J. The Signaling Pathways, and Therapeutic Targets of Antiviral Agents: Focusing on the Antiviral Approaches and Clinical Perspectives of Anthocyanins in the Management of Viral Diseases. *Front. Pharmacol.* **2019**, *10*, 1207. [CrossRef]
58. Tirado-Kulieva, V.A.; Hernández-Martínez, E.; Choque-Rivera, T.J. Phenolic compounds versus SARS-CoV-2: An update on the main findings against COVID-19. *Heliyon* **2022**, *8*, e10702. [CrossRef]
59. Młynarczyk, K.; Walkowiak-Tomczak, D.; Łysiak, G.P. Bioactive properties of *Sambucus nigra* L. as a functional ingredient for food and pharmaceutical industry. *J. Funct. Foods* **2018**, *40*, 377–390. [CrossRef]
60. Mocanu, M.L.; Amariei, S. Elderberries-A Source of Bioactive Compounds with Antiviral Action. *Plants* **2022**, *11*, 740. [CrossRef]

61. Lee, J.; Finn, C.E. Anthocyanins and other polyphenolics in American elderberry (*Sambucus canadensis*) and European elderberry (*S. nigra*) cultivars. *J. Sci. Food Agric.* **2007**, *87*, 2665–2675. [CrossRef] [PubMed]
62. Kim, C.H.; Kim, J.E.; Song, Y.J. Antiviral Activities of Quercetin and Isoquercitrin against Human Herpesviruses. *Molecules* **2020**, *25*, 2379. [CrossRef] [PubMed]
63. Cho, W.K.; Lee, M.M.; Ma, J.Y. Antiviral Effect of Isoquercitrin against Influenza a Viral Infection via Modulating Hemagglutinin and Neuraminidase. *Int. J. Mol. Sci.* **2022**, *23*, 13112. [CrossRef] [PubMed]
64. Colunga Biancatelli, R.M.L.; Berrill, M.; Catravas, J.D.; Marik, P.E. Quercetin and Vitamin C: An Experimental, Synergistic Therapy for the Prevention and Treatment of SARS-CoV-2 Related Disease (COVID-19). *Front. Immunol.* **2020**, *11*, 1451. [CrossRef] [PubMed]
65. Li, X.; Liu, Y.; Hou, X.; Peng, H.; Zhang, L.; Jiang, Q.; Shi, M.; Ji, Y.; Wang, Y.; Shi, W. Chlorogenic acid inhibits the replication and viability of enterovirus 71 in vitro. *PLoS ONE* **2013**, *8*, e76007. [CrossRef]
66. Ding, Y.; Cao, Z.; Cao, L.; Ding, G.; Wang, Z.; Xiao, W. Antiviral activity of chlorogenic acid against influenza A (H1N1/H3N2) virus and its inhibition of neuraminidase. *Sci. Rep.* **2017**, *7*, 45723. [CrossRef]
67. Chen, C.; Zuckerman, D.M.; Brantley, S.; Sharpe, M.; Childress, K.; Hoiczyk, E.; Pendleton, A.R. Sambucus nigra extracts inhibit infectious bronchitis virus at an early point during replication. *BMC Vet. Res.* **2014**, *10*, 24. [CrossRef]
68. Srinivasan, V.; Brognaro, H.; Prabhu, P.R.; de Souza, E.E.; Günther, S.; Reinke, P.Y.A.; Lane, T.J.; Ginn, H.; Han, H.; Ewert, W.; et al. Antiviral activity of natural phenolic compounds in complex at an allosteric site of SARS-CoV-2 papain-like protease. *Commun. Biol.* **2022**, *5*, 805. [CrossRef]
69. Agrawal, P.K.; Agrawal, C.; Blunden, G. Rutin: A Potential Antiviral for Repurposing as a SARS-CoV-2 Main Protease (Mpro) Inhibitor. *Nat. Prod. Commun.* **2021**, *16*, 1934578X21991723. [CrossRef]
70. Rahman, F.; Tabrez, S.; Ali, R.; Alqahtani, A.S.; Ahmed, M.Z.; Rub, A. Molecular docking analysis of rutin reveals possible inhibition of SARS-CoV-2 vital proteins. *J. Tradit. Complement. Med.* **2021**, *11*, 173–179. [CrossRef]
71. Rizzuti, B.; Grande, F.; Conforti, F.; Jimenez-Alesanco, A.; Ceballos-Laita, L.; Ortega-Alarcon, D.; Vega, S.; Reyburn, H.T.; Abian, O.; Velazquez-Campoy, A. Rutin Is a Low Micromolar Inhibitor of SARS-CoV-2 Main Protease 3CLpro: Implications for Drug Design of Quercetin Analogs. *Biomedicines* **2021**, *9*, 375. [CrossRef] [PubMed]

Disclaimer/Publisher's Note: The statements, opinions and data contained in all publications are solely those of the individual author(s) and contributor(s) and not of MDPI and/or the editor(s). MDPI and/or the editor(s) disclaim responsibility for any injury to people or property resulting from any ideas, methods, instructions or products referred to in the content.

nutraceuticals

Review

Almond, Hazelnut, and Pistachio Skin: An Opportunity for Nutraceuticals

Tariq A. Alalwan [1,*,†], Duha Mohammed [1,†], Mariam Hasan [1], Domenico Sergi [2], Cinzia Ferraris [3], Clara Gasparri [4], Mariangela Rondanelli [5,6] and Simone Perna [1,*]

1. Department of Biology, College of Science, University of Bahrain, Sakhir Campus, Zallaq P.O. Box 32038, Bahrain
2. Department of Translational Medicine, University of Ferrara, 44121 Ferrara, Italy
3. Laboratory of Food Education and Sport Nutrition, Department of Public Health, Experimental and Forensic Medicine, University of Pavia, 27100 Pavia, Italy
4. Endocrinology and Nutrition Unit, Azienda di Servizi alla Persona "Istituto Santa Margherita", University of Pavia, 27100 Pavia, Italy
5. IRCCS Mondino Foundation, 27100 Pavia, Italy
6. Unit of Human and Clinical Nutrition, Department of Public Health, Experimental and Forensic Medicine, University of Pavia, 27100 Pavia, Italy
* Correspondence: talalwan@uob.edu.bh (T.A.A.); simoneperna@hotmail.it (S.P.)
† These authors contributed equally to this work.

Abstract: Nuts are dry, single-seeded fruits, with a combination of beneficial compounds that aid in disease prevention and treatment. This review aims to summarize the antioxidant components and the nutraceutical properties and applications of hazelnut, almond, and pistachio skins, as well as discuss their ability to prevent and treat specific diseases based on in vitro and in vivo studies. The search strategy included searching PubMed database and Google Scholar for relevant articles published in English. Research articles focusing on hazelnut, pistachio, and almond were included. The nut skin extracts were considered and other by-products were excluded from this search. Pistachio and almond skin hydroalcoholic extracts have antibacterial effects and decrease the risk of liver cancer by eliminating reactive oxygen species. Moreover, hazelnut skin can lower plasma against low-density lipoprotein-cholesterol, thus reducing the risk of colon cancer, and its polyphenolic extract can also decrease the formation of advanced glycation end products in vitro with multidimensional effects. Overall, hazelnut, pistachio, and almond skins are a great source of antioxidants, making them suitable for nutraceuticals' development.

Keywords: anti-inflammation; antioxidant activity; chronic disease; diabetes; fruit; oxidative stress; phenols; testa

1. Introduction

Nuts are used to describe dry, single-seeded fruits growing on trees. They are generally composed of leaf, green leafy cover, hull, hard shell, and skin. They are nutrient-dense foods, widely consumed as components of healthy diets worldwide and in both raw and processed forms [1].

There are many types of edible tree nuts such as almonds (*Prunus amigdalis*), hazelnuts (*Corylus avellana*), walnuts (*Juglans regia*), pistachios (*Pistachia vera*), pine nuts (*Pinus pinea*), cashews (*Anacardium occidentale*), pecans (*Carya illinoiensis*), macadamias (*Macadamia integrifolia*), and Brazil nuts (*Bertholletia excelsa*). Peanuts (*Arachis hypogea*) are botanically groundnuts or legumes, but are identified as part of the nut food group from a consumer's perspective. Moreover, chestnuts (*Castanea sativa*) are considered nuts, although they differ from common nuts in terms of nutrient profile, having a higher starch content than others [2].

Tree nuts' production worldwide varies according to a recent statistic from the International Nut and Dried Fruits Council (INC) showing the evolution of the world's production of different nuts. For instance, the United States (US) is the leading country for almond production (79%), followed by both Australia and Spain (7%). Moreover, China is the world's biggest walnut producer (47%) followed by the United States and Chile, at 31% and 7%, respectively. Australia and Western Africa are considered the leading countries for producing macadamias (25%), followed by China (14%) [3].

In Western countries, individuals consume whole nuts (fresh or roasted) as a snack, in desserts, or as part of a meal. Additionally, nuts oils are added as a versatile food ingredient to commercial products including sauces, pastries, ice creams, and baked goods. The consumption of nuts has increased in recent years because they are considered as a good energy source and beneficial to include in the daily diet. Nuts have an optimal nutritional density regarding healthy minerals and contain high amounts of vegetable protein and fat, especially unsaturated fatty acids (UFAs) [4]. Nuts also contain various nutrients and provide dietary fibers, vitamins, minerals, and other bioactive compounds [5].

Nuts' skins are a good source of antioxidants thanks to the presence of polyphenolic compounds and other phytochemicals that can delay or inhibit lipid oxidation and neutralization of free radicals, contributing to disease prevention and treatments [1]. Antioxidant activity (AO) can be detected by several chemical or biological methods such as ferric reducing antioxidant power (FRAP) assay, 2,2-diphenyl-1-picrylhydrazyl (DPPH) radical scavenging activity, and 2,2'-azino-bis 3-ethylbenzothiazoline-6-sulphonic acid (ABTS) [1]. Naturally, antioxidants are nutrient and non-nutrient (phytochemicals) compounds with various types and properties. Nutrient antioxidants possess a weak AO (e.g., vitamin A, vitamin C, and selenium). Regarding non-nutrient antioxidants, they are considered much stronger in their activity, especially phenolic compounds [5].

1.1. Characteristics and Compositions of Pistachio Nut and Skin

Pistachio nut (*Pistacia vera*) is one of the world's most popular tree nuts, belonging to the *Anacardiaceae* family, which comprises about 70 genera and over 600 species. *P. vera* is considered the only species of the genus commercially cultivated, while the other species are mostly used as rootstocks [6]. The pistachio fruits are drupe and grape-like clusters, containing a single seed covered with a soft and thin seed coat (skin/testa), the edible part (Figure 1a). The seed is covered with an inedible, smooth, hard, and cream-colored shell, which is alternatively covered by a thin and pale green colored hull, forming a blush of red color during maturity (Figure 1b) [7]. Production of pistachios is highly concentrated in the United States, with a percentage of 47% in comparison with other countries such as Turkey (30%) and Iran (19%) according to the INC 2021 statistics [3].

Pistachio skin (testa) is the soft, thin, and edible seed coat that appears in red-purple. It is the main by-product, reaching more than 60%, with Iran producing around 400,000 tons of pistachio skin annually. Furthermore, various processing methods such as roasting and bleaching can cause destruction of bioactive compounds in pistachio skins [8].

Pistachio skin has value; although limited, it can be used in appropriate methods by different industries and fields. Testa is a rich source of phenolic or antioxidant compounds such as flavonoids (e.g., myricetin), gallotannins, and other phenolic compounds. In addition, the skin is used to prepare natural polymers thanks to its cellulose content [8]. Furthermore, it can be used in food and food processing, cosmetics, and pharmaceutical industries [7,8]. Moreover, the presence of various beneficial bioactive compounds in pistachio skin makes them valuable to add to an individual's daily diet, which can contribute to disease prevention, as many studies have reported [5,7].

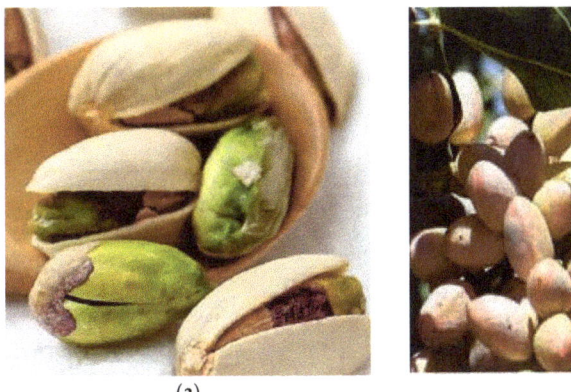

Figure 1. *Pistacia vera* L. open hard shell showing the red-purple skin (**a**); pistachio ripe fruit (hull) (**b**) [7].

1.2. Characteristics and Compositions of Almond Nut and Skin

Prunus dulcis or almonds are a stone fruit under the *Rosaceae* family, and their trees require sustainable irrigation practices for cultivation and development, specifically in arid and dry regions [9]. As previously stated, the United States is the world's largest producer of almonds, surpassing 1.3 million metric tons (MT) according to the INC statistical yearbook 2020/21 [3]. Almond nut consists of five main parts including the outer cover or hull with a greenish appearance, the intermediate shell, the edible brown skin coating, and the seed or kernel produced after the full ripening cycle of the fruit (Figure 2) [9]. The almond's hull is the heaviest part of the kernel with a total fresh weight of around 52%, affected by the variable ripening cycle that changes according to cultivation conditions [10].

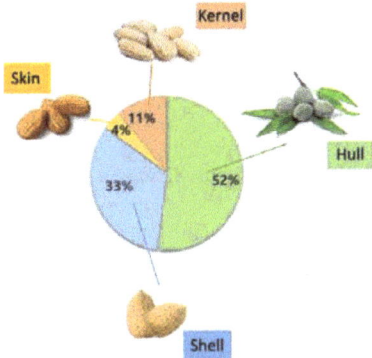

Figure 2. Weight proportion of the main structural parts of almond fruit [9].

Almond skin serves as a protective layer for the kernel against microbial contamination and oxidation. It appears as a brown leathery coating and represents 4% of the total weight (Figure 2). It contains many beneficial phytochemicals properties, comprising between 70% and 100% of the total phenols in the whole almond fruit [9].

Moreover, compounds have synergistic effects when linked with vitamins C and E, protecting against low-density lipoprotein-cholesterol (LDL-C) oxidation and improving the AO. Furthermore, the skin contains different quantities of triterpenoids, especially betulinic acid, oleanoic acid, and ursolic acid, which have anti-inflammatory, anticancer, and antiviral activities against human immunodeficiency virus (HIV) [9].

Almond skins are used in various products, including as a base component in wheat flour and as coloring for altering biscuits color [11]. A recent study proposed using almond skin extract for patients with intestinal inflammatory diseases [12]. In addition, the skin is a great source of fiber that serves as a prebiotic, affecting the gut microbiome [13].

1.3. Characteristics and Compositions of Hazelnut and Its Skin

Hazelnuts (*Corylus avellana* L.) belong to the Betulaceae family and are one of the most famous types of nuts worldwide. They are ranked third in the global nut market, as its production reaches over 863,000 MT per year. The largest producer of hazelnuts is Turkey (60%), estimated at 320,000 MT in 2020/21 statistics (Figure 3) [3]. The hazelnut consists of the green shell, the hard shell, leaves, skin, and the edible kernel [14].

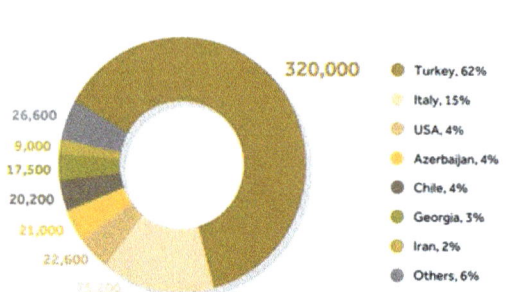

Figure 3. INC 2020/21 statistics for hazelnut production in kernel bases (metric tons) [3].

Hazelnuts are used in a wide range of applications with increased demands for them in the global markets. They are used mainly as a feedstock in the food industry, especially in the sweet sector such as chocolate bars, ice creams, dairy products, and coffee. Furthermore, it can be added to many other products, from cereals and bread to yogurts and salads [14]. Moreover, hazelnut oil is used in cosmetic, medicinal, massaging, and cooking products. Hazelnut also contains filbert, which is a flavoring compound added in per-fumes [15]. Recently, the use of hazelnuts in other fields has increased, where hazelnut oil is considered a source of biodiesel fuel, as its chemical content is approximately similar to natural oil [16].

Hazelnut skin is a by-product of the roasting process and contains 7.5% moisture, 8% protein, 14.5% fat, and 1.7% ash. Dietary fiber represents the most abundant constituent of hazelnut skin (67.7%), of which 57.7% is insoluble fiber [17]. Moreover, the skin has a good AO compared with other food items [18]. According to Özdemir et al., the total phenolic content expressed as mg gallic acid equivalents per gram (mg GAE/g) is 233 mg GAE/g in skin. The skin of hazelnuts is used as a coloring agent in foods because of its natural brown color [17]. Similarly, it is an ingredient in different processed foods, especially bakery and confectionery products [18]. Skins can be used as an enrichment ingredient to produce functional yogurt [19] and can be added in freshly made pasta, increasing the total fiber content and AO [20]. The current review aims to explore the benefits of hazelnut, almond, and pistachio skins and their ability to prevent and treat diseases.

2. Materials and Methods

2.1. Search Strategy

Studies published from 1 January 2010 through 31 March 2022 were involved in the research based on the most related papers and subjects published within this period. Articles published in English were used by searching the PubMed database and manual search using Google Scholar. The search strategy was based on the following items: "hazelnut", "almond" AND "pistachio" OR "skin" OR "disease prevention" OR "antioxidant activity".

2.2. Inclusion and Exclusion Criteria

For all of the relevant abstracts, full publications were retrieved for evaluation based on criteria established a priori. In vitro and in vivo studies were included, while in-silico-based research articles were excluded. Research articles focusing on hazelnut, pistachio, and almond were included; however, the whole nuts and their skin extract were considered and other by-products were excluded.

3. Results and Discussion

Owing to all of the beneficial compounds found in the skins of pistachios, almonds, and hazelnuts, they are proved to have potential roles in the prevention and treatment of diseases by various studies shown in Table 1.

Table 1. Studies on the effect of pistachio, almond, and hazelnut skin in health treatment.

Type of Nuts Skin	Type of Study	Sample	Dosage of Treatment	Main Results	Paper
Pistachio skin	Laboratory study	Gram-positive bacteria (*Staphylococcus aureus*, *Streptococcus pyogenes*, and *Bacillus cereus*)	15 µL of methanolic extracted fresh pistachio skin.	Strong antibacterial effect of fresh pistachio skin extract against (*S.aureus, S. pyogenes,* and *B. cereus*)	Sadeghpour and Noorbakhsh [21]
	Laboratory study	Liver cancer cells (HepG2 cell line)	Hydroalcoholic extract of pistachio skin (0 to 4 mg/mL in 24 h and 48 h)	Decrease variability of cancer cells since ROS are eliminated by phenolic compounds	Harandi et al. [22]
Almond skin	Laboratory study	*S. aureus* ATCC 6538P, *S. aureus* ATCC 43300 (MRSA), four clinical strains of *S. aureus* obtained from pharynges, two clinical strains of *S. aureus* from duodenal ulcers, three clinical strains *of S. aureus* from hip prostheses (strains 6, 32, 84), and HSV-1 prototype	HSV-1 infected cells treated with 0.4 mg/mL of NS MIX for 1 h. Cells infected with *S. aureus* strains treated with 0.6–1.6 mg/mL of NS MIX of 72 h	Antimicrobial and antiviral activity against *S.aureus* and HSV-1, respectively	Musarra-Pizzo et al. [23]
	Randomized, parallel, double-blind, placebo-controlled pilot study of 8 weeks	Adults with moderate hypercholesterolemia, aged from 18 to 65 years old	7.5 mg hydroxytyrosol from olives and 210 mg and polyphenols from almond skin per day for 8 weeks	Protect LDL-C from oxidation and prevent inflammatory status in subjects with moderate hypercholesterolemia	Fonollá et al. [24]
Hazelnut skin	*In vivo* (animal study)	10-week-old male hamsters	123 g of hazelnut skin extract Fiberox™ (FBX) was added to the high-fat diet	Lower plasma LDL-C, triglycerides, and non-esterified free fatty acids reduced the risk factor of colon cancer	Caimari et al. [25]
	Laboratory study	Bovine serum albumin (BSA) and methylglyoxal (MGO)	0.5 g of hazelnut skins	Polyphenolic extract of hazelnut skins can reduce formation of AGEs in vitro	Spagnuolo et al. [26]

3.1. Antioxidant Effects of Pistachio and Its Skin

Pistachios contain many phenolic compounds such as flavonoids and its subclasses (flavan-3-ols, flavanones, isoflavones, and flavones), which can reach up to 16–70 mg/100 g depending on the type [7,27]. A study performed by Moreno-Rojas et al. analyzed the antioxidant potential of 11 pistachio cultivars by different methods with significant differences ($p < 0.01$) in the AO values measured by ABTS (2.51 mmol/100 g) and DPPH (1.97 mmol/100 g) on average in 2020 [28]. Variations seen in AO between cultivars are due to different climatic conditions between years [28].

A study by performed by Nuzzo et al. shows the importance of AO in pistachio, indicating that the regular intake of pistachio can decrease the deleterious effects of a high-fat diet in the brain of obese mice [29]. Phenolic compounds in pistachios can attenuate the reactive oxygen species (ROS) generated in the mitochondria and induced by redox stress in the mouse brain, leading to neuroprotective effects (e.g., decreased brain apoptosis, decreased brain lipid, and improvement in mitochondrial function) (Figure 4) [29].

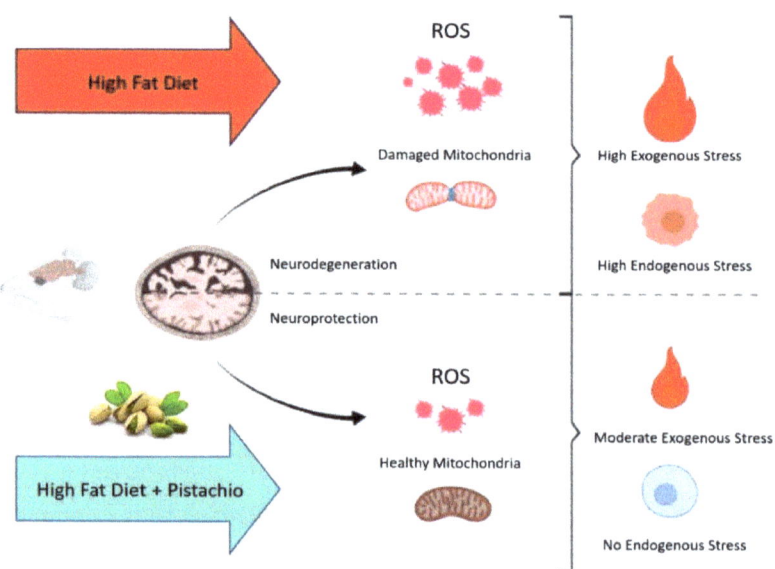

Figure 4. The neurodegenerated effects of a high-fat diet in comparison with the neuroprotective effects of regular consumption of pistachio [29].

Pistachios can contribute to disease prevention, as many studies have reported. For instance, it has been found in a randomized trial that adults with type 2 diabetes on a pistachio diet had a significant reduction in systolic ambulatory blood pressure by 3.5 ± 2.2 mmHg. These effects may be mediated by their high concentrations of magnesium and low concentrations of sodium [30]. Additionally, pistachios are a rich source of dietary fiber, which promotes satiety and likely favors adherence in weight reduction programs. This is supported by clinical data by Fantino et al., who demonstrated that daily intake of 44 g of pistachios during a 12-week period did not adversely affect body weight control in healthy French women [31]. Furthermore, Sari et al. demonstrated that consuming (30–80 g/day) pistachios can lower the total cholesterol to 10.1% and LDL-C to 8.6% [32]. London et al. also reported improvements in blood glucose levels, in endothelial function, and in some indices of inflammation and oxidative status among healthy young men following increased intake of pistachios [33].

Meanwhile, another study indicated that the consumption of high-carbohydrate foods in addition to pistachios reduces the absorption of carbohydrate as well as postprandial glucose levels [34]. On the other hand, there is epidemiological evidence showing pistachios' biological mechanisms and potential in reducing the risk of cancer and the effects of anticancer drugs, including that pistachios incorporated into the diet with anticancer drugs will lessen the disruptions in motor and cognitive functions [27]. Moreover, the study of Sadeghpour and Noorbakhsh reported the therapeutic potential of pistachio skin extract and its antibacterial effect on gram-positive bacteria [21].

In particular, positive effects were observed by Harandi et al. using the skin of pistachios' hydroalcoholic extract and its liposomal form on human liver cancer cells

(HepG2) cell line, as their viability decreased [22]. This reduction occurred as phenolic compounds found in pistachio and their high AO can eliminate ROS, which promote cancer cell proliferation. Nonetheless further research and clinical applications need to be conducted to examine the role of pistachio skin in the treatment and prevention of cancer.

3.2. Antioxidant, Antiviral, and Antibacterial Effects of Almond and Its Skin

Almonds contain high amounts of phenolic compounds, but the total content detected by studies varies owing to the cultivars selected, protocol of extraction, and detection method used for analyzing these compounds [9]. For example, Čolić et al. confirmed the presence of 28 polyphenols in almonds grown in Serbia, with catechin predominating up to 46.3% of total phenols in addition to chlorogenic acid, naringenin, rutin, apigenin, and astragalin [35]. Another study identified several other polyphenolic compounds including stilbenes (the least polyphenol found), polydatin in kernels (0.7 ng/g), skins (1.8 ng/g), blanch water (72 ng/g), and oxyresveratrol with piceatannol in blanch water (17 ng/g) [36]. AO was detected by several methods in almonds and their by-products. Various almond cultivars displayed high radical scavenging activity (SA) rates with high DPPH-SA reaching up to 90%. Similarly, the skin showed variations regarding DPPH-SA due to processing, as dehydration has the ability to promote higher activities in dried almond skins (40.4 μmol of Trolox equivalents). Similarly, the skin showed variations regarding DPPH-SA due to processing, as dehydration has the ability to promote higher activities in dried almond skins (40.4 μmol of Trolox equivalents (TE)/g almond skin) in comparison with non-dried skins [11].

Almond nuts and their skins have been used for disease treatment since ancient times, and studies have reported their beneficial effects [9]. A study has recently proposed using almond skin extract for patients with intestinal inflammatory diseases [12]. In addition, the skin is a great source of fiber that serves as a prebiotic, affecting the gut microbiome [13]. Regular consumption of almonds can reduce cardiovascular disease (CVD) risk factors. A randomized controlled trial carried out by Jamshed et al. concluded that eating 10 g/day of almonds before breakfast can reduce serum uric acid in coronary artery disease (CAD) patients, thus protecting against vascular and kidney damage [37]. Concerning the anti-inflammation feature of almonds, a crossover study reported that high monounsaturated fatty acids (MUFAs) and other components present in almonds were responsible for reducing E-selectin and C-reactive protein levels, which mediate inflammation [38]. Almond-derived compounds are also reported to possess other activities including anticancer (e.g., preventing the development of breast cancer), antimicrobial, and antiviral activities with polyphenolic compounds tested in vitro [23,39]. A study tested the antibacterial and antiviral effect of a mix of polyphenols present in natural almond skin (NS MIX) on different clinical strains of *Staphylococcus aureus* and Herpes simplex virus type I (HSV-1). Upon evaluation, almond skin polyphenolic extracts exhibited antimicrobial activity against *S. aureus* and antiviral activity observed by a decrease in the viral titer and viral DNA accumulation in the cells of HSV-1. However, further studies are required to establish possible synergistic effects with antibiotics or antivirals [23].

A randomized, double-blind, placebo-controlled study by Fonollá et al. on adults with moderate hypercholesterolemia, aged from 18 to 65 years old, was carried out to evaluate the effect of supplementation with a combination of almond and olive extracts [24]. It concluded that daily consumption of both extracts has a protective ability against LDL-C oxidation and prevents inflammatory status in subjects with moderate hypercholesterolemia [24].

3.3. Antioxidant Effects of Hazelnut and Its Skin

Like all nuts, hazelnuts have high AO, containing 291–875 mg/100 g of polyphenols. The main phenolic compounds present in hazelnut skin are phenolic acids (e.g., hydroxybenzoic acids, gallic acid, protocatechuic acid, salicylic acid, vanillic acid, and many others), flavonoids (e.g., quercetin, quercetin glucuronide, quercetin hexoside isomer, quercetin-3-O-glucoside, and others), hydrolysable tannins (e.g., ellagic acid hexoside isomer, ellagic acid pentoside isomer, flavogallonic acid dilactone isomer, bis (hexahydroxydiphenoyl)-glucose (HHDP-glucose) isomer, and valoneic acid dilactone/sanguisorbic acid dilactone), and other phenolics (e.g., dihydroxycoumarin and procyanidin dimer) [40].

A study performed by Pycia et al. analyzed the antioxidant potential of hazelnut fruit with various cultivars during its progress through maturation [41]. They reported that, as maturation progresses, the antioxidant potential of nuts harvested was lower than the previously harvested batch, reaching an average of 95% for ABTS, 86% for DPPH, and 89% for FRAP [41]. In another study, a total of 31 polyphenolic subclass flavan-3-ols were identified and quantified with an average content of total polyphenols of about 675 mg/100 g. Additionally, 3.5% of flavonols and dihydrochalcones were represented in the different hazelnut samples, with phenolic acids being the least amount of total polyphenolics found in the skin (<1%) [18].

In a randomized controlled trial by Guaraldi et al. that evaluated the effects of short-term consumption of hazelnuts on oxidative stress and DNA damage in children and adolescents with primary hyperlipidemia, an improvement was detected in cell DNA protection and resistance against oxidative stress [42]. The authors concluded that the consumption of hazelnut is associated with reduced levels of DNA strand breaks, formamidopyrimidine DNA glycosylase sensitive site, and hydrogen peroxide-induced DNA strand breaks [42].

Hazelnuts can prevent many chronic diseases such as CAD, strokes, Alzheimer's (reducing its symptoms), cancer, and atherosclerosis [43]. Generally, a diet containing a high dose of nuts lowers cholesterol. For example, a previous study showed that ingesting three various forms of hazelnuts leads to an equally enhanced lipoprotein profile and α-tocopherol concentrations in mildly hypercholesterolemic individuals, reducing the risk for CVDs [44]. Moreover, as hazelnuts are high in polyphenols, they contribute to high antioxidant potential, antimicrobial activities, and decrease the risk of inflammatory diseases when they act synergistically with phytochemicals present in nuts [41].

A systematic review by Perna et al. showed an analysis of nine studies about hazelnut addition in diets and evaluated its effect on blood lipids and body weight [45]. Subsequently, the analysis indicated that hazelnut intake reduced LDL-C, while the high-density lipoprotein-cholesterol, triglycerides, and body mass index remained unchanged. These findings support the fact that hazelnut consumption may prevent the risk of suffering from a CVD [45].

The important action of hazelnut skin is demonstrated in an in vivo animal study in improving the plasma profile of the lithocholic/deoxycholic bile acid fecal ratio in hamsters fed a high-fat diet, which included hazelnut skin. The results found that hazelnut skin has lipid-lowering blood effects, specifically LDL-C, triglycerides, and non-esterified free fatty acids (FAs), thus reducing the risk factor of colon cancer [25].

Non-enzymatic reactions of sugar with protein side chains in cells can produce advanced glycation end-products (AGEs), some of which are oxidoreductive in nature. AGEs at higher amounts can cause diabetic complications such as renal failure, oxidative stress, and chronic inflammation. Thus, a study was performed to evaluate the antiglycation effects of polyphenol compounds extracted from hazelnut skin, resulting in reduced AGEs' formation [26].

4. Future Directions

As shown in Table 1 and Figure 5, pistachio skin properties are based on a strong antibacterial effect and decreased variability of cancer cells, as ROS are eliminated by phenolic compounds [38,39]. This is a very interesting study because, in 2018, Seffadinipour et al. demonstrated the potential effects of pistachios on the inhibition of angiogenesis [46]. Although the almond skin did not show high AO, clear effects on antimicrobial and antiviral activity against *S. aureus* and HSV-1, respectively, have been demonstrated [23]. Hazelnuts provide potential protective effects against LDL oxidation and prevent inflammatory status in subjects with moderate hypercholesterolemia, as concluded by a recent meta-analysis [45].

Moreover, hazelnuts showed an effect on triglycerides and non-esterified free FAs, thus reducing the risk factor of colon cancer [25]. The potential effects of the polyphenolic extract of hazelnut skins can reduce the formation of AGEs in vitro [26]. It is worth mentioning that AGEs contribute to the pathogenesis of several chronic diseases, like cancer and diabetes. For this reason, natural bioactive molecules present in hazelnut skin that are able to inhibit their production could be an interesting new strategy for supporting therapeutic approaches with a positive effect on human health.

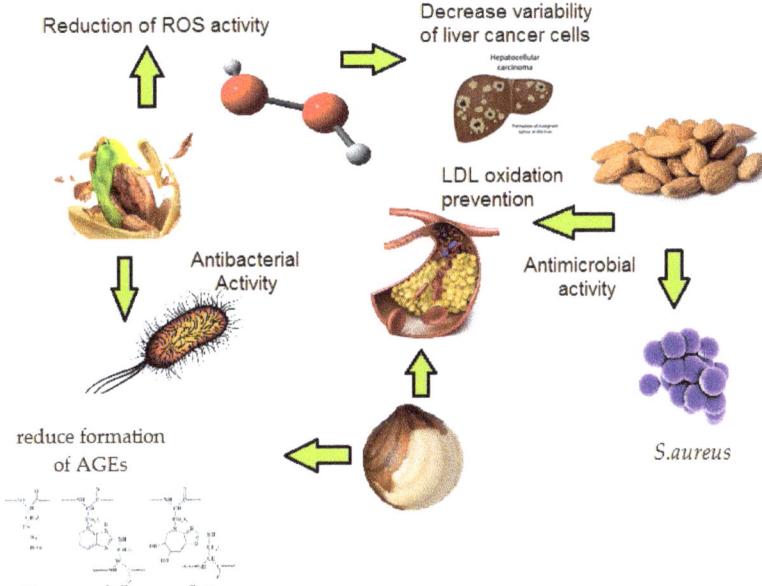

Figure 5. Mechanisms of action of almond, hazelnut, and pistachio skin on cancer cells, LDL oxidation, and antimicrobial activity.

5. Conclusions

To conclude, nuts are nutrient-dense foods that are widely consumed as components of healthy diets globally, in both raw and roasted forms. These nuts may have the potential to be developed as nutraceuticals or dietary supplements in the foreseeable future, as research has shown nut skins to possess high AOs owing to the high amounts of phenolic compounds present in them. Ultimately, the bioactive compounds in nut skins could be optimized and validated for the prevention and treatment of many pathological conditions, including mental disorders, CVDs, cancer, and diabetes.

Author Contributions: Conceptualization, S.P., C.F. and T.A.A.; methodology, D.M., M.R. and M.H.; validation, S.P., D.M. and C.G.; data curation, M.H., D.M. and M.R.; writing—original draft preparation, S.P., D.M., T.A.A. and M.H.; writing—review and editing, D.M. and T.A.A.; visualization, S.P. and M.H.; supervision, S.P. and D.S.; project administration, S.P. All authors have read and agreed to the published version of the manuscript.

Funding: This research received no external funding.

Conflicts of Interest: The authors declare no conflict of interest.

References

1. Chang, S.K.; Alasalvar, C.; Bolling, B.W.; Shahidi, F. Nuts and their co-products: The impact of processing (roasting) on phenolics, bioavailability, and health benefits—A comprehensive review. *J. Funct. Foods* **2016**, *26*, 88–122. [CrossRef]
2. Ros, E. Health Benefits of Nut Consumption. *Nutrients* **2010**, *2*, 652–682. [CrossRef] [PubMed]

3. The International Nut and Dried Fruits Council (INC). Available online: https://www.nutfruit.org/files/tech/1621253983_INC_Statistical_Yearbook_2020-_2021.pdf (accessed on 12 March 2022).
4. Martínez-González, M.Á.; Hershey, M.S.; Zazpe, I.; Trichopoulou, A. Transferability of the Mediterranean diet to non-Mediterranean countries. What is and what is not the Mediterranean diet. *Nutrients* **2017**, *9*, 1226. [CrossRef]
5. Alasalvar, C.; Bolling, B.W. Review of nut phytochemicals, fat-soluble bioactives, antioxidant components and health effects. *Br. J. Nutr.* **2015**, *113*, S68–S78. [CrossRef] [PubMed]
6. Noguera-Artiaga, L.; García-Romo, S.J.; Rosas-Burgos, C.E.; Cinco-Moroyoqui, J.F.; Vidal-Quintanar, L.R.; Carbonell-Barrachina, A.A.; Burgos-Hernández, A. Antioxidant, Antimutagenic and Cytoprotective Properties of Hydrosos Pistachio Nuts. *Molecules* **2019**, *24*, 4362. [CrossRef] [PubMed]
7. Mandalari, G.; Barreca, D.; Gervasi, T.; Roussell, M.A.; Klein, B.; Feeney, M.J.; Carughi, A. Pistachio Nuts (*Pistacia vera* L.): Production, Nutrients, Bioactives and Novel Health Effects. *Plant* **2021**, *11*, 18. [CrossRef]
8. Tomaino, A.; Martorana, M.; Arcoraci, T.; Monteleone, D.; Giovinazzo, C.; Saija, A. Antioxidant activity and phenolic profile of pistachio (*Pistacia vera* L., variety Bronte) seeds and skins. *Biochimie* **2010**, *92*, 1115–1122. [CrossRef]
9. Ros, E.; Singh, A.; O'Keefe, J.H. Nuts: Natural Pleiotropic Nutraceuticals. *Nutrients* **2021**, *13*, 3269. [CrossRef]
10. Prgomet, I.; Gonçalves, B.; Domínguez-Perles, R.; Santos, R.; Saavedra, M.J.; Aires, A.; Pascual-Seva, N.; Barros, A. Irrigation deficit turns almond by-products into a valuable source of antimicrobial (poly)phenols. *Ind. Crops Prod.* **2019**, *132*, 186–196. [CrossRef]
11. Pasqualone, A.; Laddomada, B.; Spina, A.; Todaro, A.; Guzmàn, C.; Summo, C.; Mita, G.; Giannone, V. Almond by-products: Extraction and characterization of phenolic compounds and evaluation of their potential use in composite dough with wheat flour. *LWT- Food Sci. Technol.* **2018**, *89*, 299–306. [CrossRef]
12. Lauro, M.R.; Marzocco, S.; Rapa, S.F.; Musumeci, T.; Giannone, V.; Picerno, P.; Aquino, R.P.; Puglisi, G. Recycling of Almond By-Products for Intestinal Inflammation: Improvement of Physical-Chemical, Technological and Biological Characteristics of a Dried Almond Skins Extract. *Pharmaceutics* **2020**, *12*, 884. [CrossRef] [PubMed]
13. Liu, Z.; Lin, X.; Huang, G.; Zhang, W.; Ra, P.; Ni, L. Prebiotic effects of almonds and almond skins on intestinal microbiota in healthy adult humans. *Anaerobe* **2014**, *26*, 1–6. [CrossRef] [PubMed]
14. Król, K.; Gantner, M. Morphological Traits and Chemical Composition of Hazelnut from Different Geographical Origins: A Review. *Agriculture* **2020**, *10*, 375. [CrossRef]
15. Kornsteiner, K.M.; Wagner, K.H.; Elmadfa, I. Phytosterol content and fatty acid pattern of ten different nut types. *Int. J. Vitam. Nutr. Res.* **2013**, *83*, 263–270. [CrossRef] [PubMed]
16. Saydut, A.; Erdogan, S.; Kafadar, A.B.; Kaya, C.; Aydin, F.; Hamamci, C. Process optimization for production of biodiesel from hazelnut oil, sunflower oil, and their hybrid feedstock. *Fuel* **2016**, *183*, 512–517. [CrossRef]
17. Özdemir, K.S.; Yılmaz, C.; Durmaz, G.; Gökmen, V. Hazelnut skin powder: A new brown colored functional ingredient. *Food Res. Int.* **2014**, *65*, 291–297. [CrossRef]
18. Del Rio, D.; Calani, L.; Dall'Asta, M.; Brighenti, F. Polyphenolic Composition of Hazelnut Skin. *J. Agric. Food Chem.* **2011**, *59*, 9935–9941. [CrossRef]
19. Dinkçi, N.; Aktaş, M.; Akdeniz, V.; Sirbu, A. The Influence of Hazelnut Skin Addition on Quality Properties and Antioxidant Activity of Functional Yogurt. *Foods* **2021**, *10*, 2855. [CrossRef]
20. Zeppa, G.; Belviso, S.; Bertolino, M.; Cavallero, M.C.; Dal Bello, B.; Ghirardello, D.; Giordano, M.; Giorgis, M.; Grosso, A.; Rolle, L.; et al. The effect of hazelnut roasted skin from different cultivars on the quality attributes, polyphenol content and texture of fresh egg pasta. *J. Sci. Food Agric.* **2014**, *95*, 1678–1688. [CrossRef]
21. Sadeghpour, M.; Noorbakhsh, F. The effect of the fresh peel extract pistachio (*Pistacia Atlantica*) on the growth of staphylococcus aureus, streptococcus pyogenes and bacillus cereus isolated from clinical specimens in vitro. *Stud. Med. Sci.* **2015**, *26*, 813–823.
22. Harandi, H.; Majd, A.; Khanamani Falahati-Pour, S.; Mahmoodi, M. Toxicity Effect of Hydro-Alcoholic Extract of Pistachio Hull and Its Liposomal Form on Liver Cancer Cells (HepG2). *J. Rafsanjan UMS* **2020**, *18*, 1035–1048.
23. Musarra-Pizzo, M.; Ginestra, G.; Smeriglio, A.; Pennisi, R.; Sciortino, T.M.; Mandalari, G. The Antimicrobial and Antiviral Activity of Polyphenols from Almond (*Prunus dulcis* L.) skin. *Nutrients* **2019**, *11*, 2355. [CrossRef] [PubMed]
24. Fonollá, J.; Maldonado-Lobón, J.A.; Luque, R.; Rodríguez, C.; Bañuelos, Ó.; López-Larramendi, J.L.; Olivares, M.; Blanco-Rojo, R. Effects of a Combination of Extracts from Olive Fruit and Almonds Skin on Oxidative and Inflammation Markers in Hypercholesterolemic Subjects: A Randomized Controlled Trial. *J. Med. Food* **2021**, *22*, 479–486. [CrossRef] [PubMed]
25. Caimari, A.; Puiggròs, F.; Suárez, M.; Crescenti, A.; Laos, S.; Ruiz, J.A.; Alonso, V.; Moragas, J.; del Bas, J.M.; Arola, L. The intake of a hazelnut skin extract improves the plasma lipid profile and reduces the lithocholic/deoxycholic bile acid faecal ratio, a risk factor for colon cancer, in hamsters fed a high-fat diet. *Food Chem.* **2015**, *167*, 138–144. [CrossRef]
26. Spagnuolo, L.; Della Posta, S.; Fanali, C.; Dugo, L.; De Gara, L. Antioxidant and Antiglycation Effects of Polyphenol Compounds Extracted from Hazelnut Skin on Advanced Glycation End-Products (AGEs) Formation. *Antioxidants* **2021**, *10*, 424. [CrossRef]
27. Ghasemynasabparizi, M.; Ahmadi, A.; Mazloomi, S.M. A review on pistachio: Its composition and benefits regarding the prevention or treatment of diseases. *J. Occup. Health Epidemiol.* **2015**, *4*, 57–69. [CrossRef]
28. Moreno-Rojas, J.M.; Velasco-Ruiz, I.; Lovera, M.; Ordoñez-Díaz, J.L.; Ortiz-Somovilla, V.; De Santiago, E.; Arquero, O.; Pereira-Caro, G. Valuation of Phenolic Profile and Antioxidant Activity of Eleven Pistachio Cultivars (*Pistacia vera* L.) Cultivated in Andalusia. *Antioxidants* **2022**, *11*, 609. [CrossRef]

29. Nuzzo, D.; Galizzi, G.; Amato, A.; Terzo, S.; Picone, P.; Cristaldi, L.; Mul, F.; Di Carlo, M. Regular Intake of Pistachio Mitigates the Deleterious Effects of a High Fat-Diet in the Brain of Obese Mice. *Antioxidants* **2020**, *9*, 317. [CrossRef]
30. Sauder, K.A.; McCrea, C.E.; Ulbrecht, J.S.; Kris-Etherton, P.M.; West, S.G. Pistachio nut consumption modifies systemic hemodynamics, increases heart rate variability, and reduces ambulatory blood pressure in well-controlled type 2 diabetes: A randomized trial. *J. Am. Heart Assoc.* **2014**, *3*, e000873. [CrossRef]
31. Fantino, M.; Bichard, C.; Mistretta, F.; Bellisle, F. Daily consumption of pistachios over 12 weeks improves dietary profile without increasing body weight in healthy women: A randomized controlled intervention. *Appetite* **2020**, *144*, 104483. [CrossRef]
32. Sari, I.; Baltaci, Y.; Bagci, C.; Davutoglu, V.; Erel, O.; Celik, H.; Ozer, O.; Aksoy, N.; Aksoy, M. Effect of pistachio diet on lipid parameters, endothelial function, inflammation, and oxidative status: A prospective study. *Nutrition* **2010**, *26*, 399–404. [CrossRef] [PubMed]
33. London, H.A.; Pawlak, R.; Colby, S.E.; Wall-Bassett, E.; Sira, N. The Impact of Pistachio Consumption on Blood Lipid Profile. *Am. J. Lifestyle Med.* **2013**, *7*, 274–277. [CrossRef]
34. Holligan, S.D.; West, S.G.; Gebauer, S.K.; Kay, C.D.; Kris-Etherton, P.M. A moderate-fat diet containing pistachios improves emerging markers of cardiometabolic syndrome in healthy adults with elevated LDL levels. *Br. J. Nutr.* **2014**, *112*, 744–752. [CrossRef] [PubMed]
35. Čolić, S.D.; Fotirić Akšić, M.M.; Lazarević, K.B.; Zec, G.N.; Gašić, U.M.; Dabić Zagorac, D.C.; Natić, M.M. Fatty acid and phenolic profiles of almond grown in Serbia. *Food Chem.* **2017**, *234*, 455–463. [CrossRef] [PubMed]
36. Xie, L.; Bolling, B.W. Characterisation of stilbenes in California almonds (*Prunus dulcis*) by UHPLC-MS. *Food Chem.* **2014**, *148*, 300–306. [CrossRef] [PubMed]
37. Jamshed, H.; Gilani, A.U.; Sultan, A.T.; Amin, F.; Arslan, J.; Ghani, S.; Masroor, M. Almond supplementation reduces serum uric acid in coronary artery disease patients: A randomized controlled trial. *Nutr. J.* **2015**, *15*, 77. [CrossRef] [PubMed]
38. Rajaram, S.; Connell, K.M.; Sabaté, J. Effect of almond-enriched high-monounsaturated fat diet on selected markers of inflammation: A randomised, controlled, crossover study. *Br. J. Nutr.* **2010**, *10*, 907–912. [CrossRef]
39. Soriano-Hernandez, A.D.; Madrigal-Perez, D.G.; Galvan-Salazar, H.R.; Arreola-Cruz, A.; Briseño-Gomez, L.; Guzmán-Esquivel, J.; Dobrovinskaya, O.; Lara-Esqueda, A.; Rodríguez-Sanchez, I.P.; Baltazar-Rodriguez, L.M.; et al. The protective effect of peanut, walnut, and almond consumption on the development of breast cancer. *Gynecol. Obstet. Investig.* **2015**, *80*, 89–92. [CrossRef]
40. Pelvan, E.; Olgun, E.Ö.; Karadağ, A.; Alasalvar, C. Phenolic profiles and antioxidant activity of Turkish Tombul hazelnut samples (natural, roasted, and roasted hazelnut skin). *Food Chem.* **2018**, *244*, 102–108. [CrossRef]
41. Pycia, K.; Kapusta, I.; Jaworska, G. Changes in Antioxidant Activity, Profile, and Content of Polyphenols and Tocopherols in Common Hazel Seed (*Corylus avellana* L.) Depending on Variety and Harvest Date. *Molecules* **2019**, *25*, 43. [CrossRef]
42. Guaraldi, F.; Deon, V.; Del Bo', C.; Vendrame, S.; Porrini, M.; Riso, P.; Guardamagna, O. Effect of short-term hazelnut consumption on DNA damage and oxidized LDL in children and adolescents with primary hyperlipidemia: A randomized controlled trial. *J. Nutr. Biochem.* **2018**, *57*, 206–211. [CrossRef] [PubMed]
43. Guiné, P.F.; Correia, M.R. Hazelnut: A Valuable Resource. *ETP Int. J. Food Eng.* **2020**, *6*, 67–72. [CrossRef]
44. Tey, L.S.; Brown, C.R.; Chisholm, W.A.; Delahunty, C.M.; Gray, R.A.; Williams, M.S. Effects of different forms of hazelnuts on blood lipids and α-tocopherol concentrations in mildly hypercholesterolemic individuals. *Eur. J. Clin. Nutr.* **2011**, *65*, 117–124. [CrossRef]
45. Perna, S.; Giacosa, A.; Bonitta, G.; Bologna, C.; Isu, A.; Guido, D.; Rondanelli, M. Effects of hazelnut consumption on blood lipids and body weight: A systematic review and Bayesian meta-analysis. *Nutrients* **2016**, *8*, 747. [CrossRef] [PubMed]
46. Seifaddinipour, M.; Farghadani, R.; Namvar, F.; Mohamad, J.; Abdul Kadir, H. Cytotoxic Effects and Anti-Angiogenesis Potential of Pistachio (*Pistacia vera* L.) Hulls against MCF-7 Human Breast Cancer Cells. *Molecules* **2018**, *23*, 110. [CrossRef]

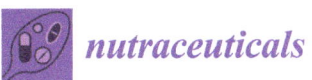

Review

Plant Seed Mucilage—Great Potential for Sticky Matter

Matúš Kučka [1], Katarína Ražná [1,*], Ľubomír Harenčár [1] and Terézia Kolarovičová [2]

1 Institute of Plant and Environmental Sciences, Faculty of Agrobiology and Food Resources, Slovak University of Agriculture, Tr. A. Hlinku 2, 94976 Nitra, Slovakia
2 Faculty of Agrobiology and Food Resources, Slovak University of Agriculture, Tr. A. Hlinku 2, 94976 Nitra, Slovakia
* Correspondence: katarina.razna@uniag.sk

Abstract: Some seeds of flowering plants can differentiate their seed coat epidermis into the specialized cell layer producing a hydrophilic mucilage with several ecological functions, such as seed hydration, protection, spatial fixation, stimulation of metabolic activity and development of seed. Due to the species- and genotype-dependent variabilities in the chemical composition of mucilage, mucilage does not display the same functional properties and its role depends on the respective species and environment. Mucilaginous substances, depending on their composition, exhibit many preventive and curative effects for human and animal health, which has significant potential in the agricultural, food, cosmetic and pharmaceutical industries. This paper summarizes the ecological, biological, and functional properties of mucilaginous plant substances and highlights their significant nutritional potential in terms of the development of functional foods, and nutraceuticals and dietary supplements. A paragraph describing the gene regulation of seed mucilage synthesis is included, and some recommendations for the direction of further research on mucilaginous substances are outlined.

Keywords: mucilages; ecological functions; human and animal health-promoting properties; application in agriculture; genes; nutritional components

1. Introduction

Some plants are characterized by producing a large quantity of various above- and below-ground secretions called mucilages or exudates. These can be secreted by roots, leaves, stems, or seeds, and perform different functions depending on the plant species [1]. Myxodiaspores are plants with the ability to initiate the differentiation of seed coat epidermis into the specialized cell layer upon fertilization, which synthesizes hydrophilic mucilage in the Golgi apparatus. Subsequently, the mucilage is secreted into the apoplastic compartment via secretory vesicles [2,3]. The mucilage forms a shell around the seed in the form of a gel-like transparent capsule, which represents a kind of modified cell wall with all typical polysaccharides, i.e., celluloses, pectins and hemicelluloses. Examples of plants with seeds that produce mucilage include *Arabidopsis thaliana* L., *Ocimum basilicum* L., *Lepidium sativum* L., *Salvia sclarea* L., *Artemisia annua* L., *Linum usitatissimum* L. and *Artemisia leucodes* Schrenk [4,5].

2. Methodology

We used the keywords (seed mucilage) to query the PubMed® database https://pubmed.ncbi.nlm.nih.gov/ (accessed on 24 May 2022), and the query returned a total of 528 search results. Since 1999, we have been observing a linear increase in the number of articles on this topic, with a few exceptions. The first article on seed mucilage was written in 1932, and the highest number of articles on seed mucilage was published in 2021 (70), which only confirms the current trend of increasing interest in this functional food ingredient. In our research, we tried to link the already established knowledge on plant seed mucilage with new information. In total, 92 articles related to plant seed mucilage were used, with 41 of these being less than 5 years old. Three articles were written in 2022, thirteen in 2021, five in 2020, nine in 2019 and eleven in 2018.

3. Ecological Functions of Mucilage

Mucilaginous substances have several ecological functions for plants (Figure 1), including seed hydration and protection from desiccation and spatial fixation in the soil, which affects their topochory, epizoochory, endozoochory and hydrochory. In addition, they maintain the metabolic activity of the seed and encourage its development. Mucilage contains substances that serve as a source of energy for the seeds and microorganisms in the soil. The exact role of mucilage seems to depend on the species and environmental context [3,6]. *Eragostris pilosa* (L.) BEAUV. seeds produce mucilage that allows them to survive in dry habitats. Their mucilage consists of pectins that form uniform layers on the inner surface of the cell walls, which are bounded by a thin layer of cellulose preventing them from being released into the cell lumen. In the presence of water, these pectins are hydrated and cause the mucilage cells to swell up. Subsequently, they start to detach. The aforementioned ability of Eragostris creates suitable conditions for germination [7]. Similarly, even the seeds of *Henophyton deserti* COSS. & DUR. are drought resistant. Mucilage represents 30% of the seed mass in this species. It can increase the weight of seeds by up to 550%. It has been shown that the mucilage of *H. deserti* works as a physical barrier in the regulation of the diffusion of water and oxygen into the inner seed coat. With this mechanism, it can prevent germination from occurring in unsuitable conditions. It was proved experimentally that higher concentrations of PEG inhibit mucilage hydration, but salt concentration has no effect on it. Mucilage reduces both the percentage and rate of seed germination, especially at 10 °C, and at high concentrations of NaCl and PEG [8]. The ability of mucilage to reduce germination under mild osmotic stress and subsequently to assist germination once this stress is relieved has also been confirmed in *Nepeta micrantha* BUNGE [9]. In addition to drought, plant survival on the desert dunes also depends on the burial depth in the sand. In the experiments conducted with the *Artemisia sphaerocephala* KRASCH. seeds, it was found that mucilage significantly increased seed emergence at a 0.5 and 10 mm burial depth under low irrigation, at a 0 and 5 mm burial depth under medium irrigation, and at a 0 and 10 mm burial depth under high irrigation. Seed mucilage also reduced seed mortality at shallow sand burial depths [10]. In addition, seed mucilage increased the surface dislocation force, allowing the seeds to anchor in highly erosive soils. When mucilage seeds from 52 plant species varying in their characteristics were tested, it was found that the largest effect on the resistance to water flow during erosion is due to the mucilage mass. Moreover, resistance to flow was largely dependent on the water flow speed and the rate of seed germination [11]. When mucilage is released from the seed, various particles of sand and dirt adhere to the seeds and remain on the seed surface after drying. This leads to the formation of a physical barrier that protects the seeds from predators (e.g., ants) [12]. Mucilaginous substances also affect seed germination. In optimal laboratory conditions, the difference between mucilaginous seeds (s1) and seeds with the mucilage removed (s2) was only in the germination rate (s1: 97% germination after 26 h; s2: 63% germination after 26 h). When exposed to salt stress, the s1 seeds germinated up to 48% more than the s2 seeds [13]. This may also be due to the presence of some enzymes in the mucilage that may assist in breaking the radicle envelope of the seeds, whereas demucilaged seeds do not contain such apoplast enzymes. Examples of such enzymes include pectinases, β-D-xylosidases and α-L-arabinofuranosidases, which are found in the mucilage of flaxseed [5,14].

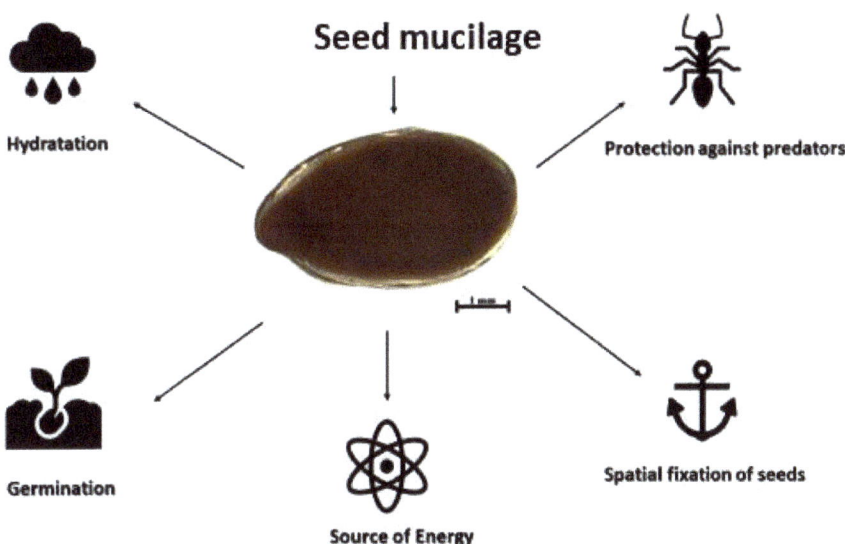

Figure 1. Ecological functions of mucilage (Kučka, elaborated based on [3–14].

4. Effects of Mucilage on Human and Animal Health

Depending on the composition, mucilaginous substances can exhibit antihypercholesterolemic, laxative and anticarcinogenic effects, and also have an effect on glucose metabolism. These effects help to prevent, or at least reduce, the risk of various major diseases such as diabetes, lupus nephritis, arteriosclerosis and hormone-dependent cancers [15–18]. *Cordia dichotoma* G. FORST. seed mucilage has been investigated for its antihypercholesterolemic effects. The study used rats, which were on a high-lipid diet, resulting in a significant increase in total cholesterol and low-density lipoprotein cholesterol, as well as in a significant decrease in antioxidant enzymes in the liver (glutathione reductase, glutathione peroxidase, glutathione-S-transferase, catalase and superoxide dismutase). Treatment with the *C. dichotoma* mucilage at a 0.5 and 1g per kg not only improved the lipid profile, but it also improved the liver and kidney function, even in the rats on a normal diet. Additionally, the antioxidant system in the liver was also improved [15]. The mucilage from *Abelmoschus esculentus* (L.) MOENCH, in addition to its antihypercholesterolemic effects, also had an effect on glucose levels when abnormal changes in body weight, water consumption, feed consumption and blood glucose levels occurred after 3 weeks of mucilage administration to alloxan-induced diabetic mice. At baseline, all mice had fasting blood glucose levels of approximately 4.1 mmol·L^{-1}. After the induction of alloxan, the blood glucose concentration increased to 12.3 ± 0.8 mmol·L^{-1} in one group and to 13.1 ± 0.8 mmol·L^{-1} in the other group. After the administration of 150 mg per kg of mucilage to the first group, the blood glucose level decreased to 7.1 ± 0.4 mmol·L^{-1} after three weeks, and in the second group the level decreased to 6.7 ± 0.4 mmol·L^{-1} [18] after the administration of 200 mg per kg of mucilage. The laxative activities of flaxseed mucilage and oil have also been investigated. Flaxseed mucilage had laxative effects at doses of 1 and 2.5 g·kg^{-1} with the resulting percentage increase of 65.06 ± 6.5% and 89.33 ± 4.04% in wet feces. The spasmogenic effect of flaxseed mucilage was completely blocked in the presence of atropine and partially blocked (63.9%) in the presence of pyrilamine. The laxative effect of both flaxseed mucilage and oil is probably mediated by the stimulation of cholinergic and histaminergic receptors, with a more pronounced cholinergic component in flaxseed mucilage [19]. Mucilage also exhibits anti-inflammatory and antioxidant effects, and the mucilage from fenugreek seeds showed a beneficial effect against rat arthritis when induced by intradermal injection of complete Freund's adjuvant. The maximum rate of edema inhibition was observed at a mucilage dose of 75 mg·kg^{-1} on the 21st day of adjuvant arthritis. After the treatment with mucilage from fenugreek seeds, the activity of inflammatory enzymes (cyclooxygenase-2 and myeloperoxidase) as well as the concentrations of thiobarbituric acid reactive substance decreased. On the other hand, there was an increase in the activity of antioxidant enzymes (catalase, superoxide dismutase, glutathione peroxidase), the levels of glutathione and vitamin C and lipid peroxidation. Additionally, the erythrocyte sedimentation rate and total white blood cell count increased significantly [20]. In addition, the prebiotic effect of chia mucilage, which is mainly due to the neutral mucilage polysaccharides, has been demonstrated. Compared to the low molecular weight prebiotics, the growth of some groups of intestinal bacteria, such as *Enterococcus* and *Lactobacillus*, is more delayed on mucilage but it lasts longer. The effects of chia mucilage at three different concentrations (0.3, 0.5 and 0.8%) on the growth and metabolic activity of human gut microbiota using the Simgi® dynamic gastrointestinal model have also been investigated. The researchers found that all mucilage concentrations significantly affected all bacterial groups of the gut microbiota, but the 0.3% concentration of chia mucilage had the most significant effect on the increase in total aerobes in the transverse colon and descending colon. Increases were also observed for lactic acid bacteria, *Enterococcus* spp. and *Staphylococcus* spp., and in contrast, no significant changes were observed for *Enterobacteriaceae*, *Clostridium* spp. and *Bifidobacterium* spp. By providing a substrate for the microorganisms, the chia mucilage also affects the resulting fermentation products, such as short-chain fatty acids (SCFAs). In the experiment, different values of SCFAs (acetic, propionic and butyric acid) were observed at different concentrations of chia mucilage, and the dependence of SCFA production on different parts of the gut was also observed. In the ascending colon, the greatest increase was observed on day 5 at a 0.5% concentration of chia mucilage, while in the transverse and descending colon, the increase was observed mainly on day 3 after the administration of chia mucilage. However, an increase was also observed in the transverse and descending colon on day 5 and day 8 at a 0.8% and 0.5% chia mucilage [21,22]. Recent studies suggest that flaxseed mucilage also exhibits antibacterial activity against several Gram-positive and Gram-negative bacteria using the agar well diffusion method and disk diffusion method. Mucilage showed strong antibacterial properties against all strains tested except *Listeria monocytogenes* [23]. There was also a potential to improve the course of chronic obstructive pulmonary diseases when the Pharmacopeial Unani formulation: linctus of flax mucilage [24] was used as the test drug. In Iranian traditional medicine, mucilage from quince seeds is used to treat skin wounds and burns. In a study on mucilage in rabbits, it was concluded that mucilage from quince seeds increases the level of growth factors in the wound fluids are involved in tissue repair, and therefore has good potential to promote wound healing at a 10–20% concentration [25]. The healing effects against the T-2 toxin-induced dermal toxicity in rabbits has also been demonstrated for mucilage obtained from quince seeds. This mucilage probably preserves the wound surface proteins whose synthesis is inhibited by the T-2 toxin. In addition, it is thought to act as a barrier against microorganisms and may also activate the growth factors and thereby facilitate skin healing [26]. In medicine, there is potential to use mucilage as a polymer capable of retaining water, for example, for wound dressings. An antibacterial wound dressing was prepared by the lyophilization of basil mucilage and with the addition of the antibacterial agent zinc oxide nanoparticles (ZnO-NPs). Hydrogen bonding and electrostatic interaction were confirmed between the slime and ZnO-NPs molecules. The resulting product was non-adhesive and non-toxic, with reasonable mechanical and thermal properties, which were further enhanced by the addition of ZnO to promote antibacterial capabilities. It was confirmed that the porosity, swelling and water retention of the product were suitable for use as a wound dressing. Due to its good porosity, basil mucilage gel is able to absorb a high volume of exudate from the wound surface. Water retention capacity is one of the most important properties of wound dressing because it allows the holding of water molecules within its structure.

The addition of ZnO-NPs slightly decreases porosity and swelling, but slightly increases water retention [27]. Mucilage has the potential to be used as a superdisintegrant in the production of pharmaceutical tablets by direct compression with other excipients and in wet granulation technology where the mucilage from basil seeds *(Ocimum basilicum* L.) was successfully used to produce the drug metoprolol tartarate [28]. Similarly, mucilage from plantain *(Plantago psyllium* L.) at a 3% *(w/w)* concentration can also be used as a drug binder. Studies indicate that paracetamol with this formulation is released more slowly than the traditional drug [29]. The *Ocimum basilicum* L. seed mucilage can also be used as a nasal gel containing paracetamol [30]. The mucilage from the seeds of *Lallemantia royleana* (BENTH.) itself exhibits analgesic effects, and was used to create a mixture of commercial 2% lidocaine gel and a mucilage-containing gel (0.01 g·ml^{-1}), which increased the efficacy of this local anesthetic [31].

5. Potential Uses of Mucilage in Agriculture and Industry

Mucilaginous substances have potential in agriculture, food, cosmetics and pharmaceutical industries (Table 1) [32]. In the food industry, chia mucilage can be used as a low-fat source of fiber. The addition of 7.5% chia seed mucilage to a yogurt recipe reduced the degree of syneresis during storage compared to full-fat yogurt and improved the nutritional value of the yogurt by increasing the fiber content. In addition, the resulting yogurt had a higher consistency, firmness, viscosity and better resistance to stress. The sensory acceptability of the resulting yogurts in terms of acidity, creaminess and viscosity was similar to full-fat yogurts [33]. Similarly, the addition of flaxseed mucilage increased the viscosity and decreased yogurt syneresis. In addition, it decreased the cohesiveness and increased the stickiness of the blended yogurt, while its addition in combination with carboxymethylcellulose resulted in decreased stickiness, increased cohesiveness and elasticity. The mucilage of flax with the addition of carboxymethylcellulose resulted in an increase in *Lactobacillus bulgaricus* in the blended yogurt, although the addition of mucilage alone had little effect on the growth of this lactic bacterium. On the other hand, the addition of mucilage itself had a considerable effect on the growth of *Streptococcus thermophilus* [34]. The mucilage from chia seeds can serve as a substitution for some oil in mayonnaise, thus increasing its stability, textural parameters and reducing the amount of fats [35]. Similarly, the addition of chia mucilage to pie dough reduces the fat content and increases fiber and protein contents [36], and some studies have shown that chia mucilage can replace emulsifiers and stabilizers in the preparation of ice cream [37]. Mucilage can also be used to encapsulate important substances, such as probiotics, which can improve the functional properties of food. It has been shown that quince seed mucilage is able to increase the survival rate of *Lactobacillus rhamnosus* up to 72 °C by encapsulation, and is also suitable as a transport matrix in the gastrointestinal environment when the bacteria are released at an appropriate time after reaching the intestinal tract [38]. The mucilage and soluble proteins from chia and flax seeds can be used as encapsulating material for two probiotic bacteria: *Bifidobacterium infantis* and *Lactobacillus plantarum* [39]. Using the electrospinning method, it was possible to incorporate the flavonoid hesperetin into basil mucilage nanofibers in conjunction with polyvinyl alcohol. After a successful encapsulation, there was an increase in resistance to high temperatures (from 182 °C to 314 °C) and a decrease in their release rate in acidic environments (pH 1.2) [40]. Vitamin A was also encapsulated by a similar principle using watercress seed mucilage and polyvinyl alcohol. Again, its stability in acidic environments and against high temperatures was enhanced [41]. Last but not least, mucilage can be used to produce biodegradable and antimicrobial edible films that increase the shelf life of food. Films made out of the psyllium seed mucilage, oregano extract and glycerol as a plasticizer had effective antimicrobial activities against *Staphylococcus aureus* and *Escherichia coli* and extended the postharvest shelf life of strawberries to 16 days [42].

Table 1. Application of mucilage in industry and agriculture.

Application Area	Plant Source	Applied Form	Achieved Properties	Reference
Food industry	*Salvia hispanica* L., *Linum usitatissimum* L.	Additive in yogurts	Improved nutritional properties, syneresis and viscosity	Refs. [33,34]
	Salvia hispanica L.	Additive in mayonnaise	Increased stability, reducing fat	Ref. [35]
	Salvia hispanica L.	Additive in cakes	Improved nutritional qualities	Ref. [36]
	Salvia hispanica L.	Additive in ice cream	Replacement for stabilizers and emulsifiers	Ref. [37]
	Salvia hispanica L. *Linum usitatissimum* L. *Cydonia oblonga* MILLER	Encapsulation of probiotics	Better resistance in the digestive tract	Refs. [38,39]
	Ocimum basilicum L. *Lepidium sativum* L.	Encapsulation of vitamins and flavonoids	Better resistance in the digestive tract	Refs. [40,41]
	Plantago psyllium L.	Production of edible films	Increased food shelf life	Ref. [42]
Pharmaceutical industry	*Lallemantia royleana* (BENTH.)	Formation of gels	Healing effects against dermal toxicity and burns	Ref. [31]
	Ocimum basilicum L.	Wound dressing formation	Antimicrobial effects	Ref. [27]
	Ocimum basilicum L. *Plantago psyllium* L.	Formation of medicinal tablets	Slower release, replacement of chemical preparations	Refs. [28,29]
	Ocimum basilicum L.	Formation of nasal gel	Analgesic effects	Ref. [30]
Cosmetics	*Salvia hispanica* L.	Gel formation	UV-protective effects	Ref. [43]
Agriculture	*Salvia hispanica* L.	Hydrogels in arid areas	Retention of water	Refs. [44,45]
Engineering industry	*Linum usitatissimum* L.	Biocomposite binder	Inexpensive and biocompound	Ref. [46]

In cosmetics, chia seed mucilage has promising potential due to its high photostability under UV light and muco-adhesion, which promotes the adhesion of the formulation to the mucosa [43]. In agriculture, mucilage can be used as a hydrogel that retains water in the rhizosphere, which, in addition, reduces surface tension and increases soil viscosity and the hysteresis index [44]. Therefore, it is potentially possible to use mucilage for plant growth in arid deserts [45]. In the industry, mucilage is used as a binder for biocomposite materials in which plant fibers serve as a reinforcing component [46].

6. Physical and Chemical Properties of Mucilage

As a natural product, the composition of mucilage can vary in space and time depending on a variety of external and internal conditions [47]. In addition, there are also significant variations in the chemical composition and functional properties of mucilage among different plant species and varieties (Table 2) [48]. In general, the seed mucilage of different plants is mainly composed of polysaccharides. Mucilaginous polysaccharides are a source of energy for microorganisms, absorb water, exchange cations and allow the plant to adhere to solid surfaces in the rhizosphere [49]. The composition of polysaccharides is mainly influenced by the enzymes secreted by the plant during water imbibition along with mucilage [5]. The mucilage coat of myxodiaspores seeds represents a modified cell wall. Chemically, it is mainly composed of the polysaccharide groups typical for the cell wall, mainly hemicelluloses (cellulose type of mucilage—e.g., *Neopallasia pectinata* (PALL.) POLJAKOV), but very often pectins are the main component (pectin type of mucilage—e.g., *Linum usitatissimum* L.) [50]. The flax mucilage of the Eden cultivar mainly consists of rhamnogalacturonan-I (52–62%), which is influenced by the enzymes rhamnogalacturonase and β-d-galactosidase, and arabinoxylan (27–36%), which is related to the activity of the enzymes α-l-arabinofuranosidase, β-d-xylosidase and β-xylanase. The highest value of xylanase activity was observed after 4 h of seed hydration, resulting in the low viscosity of the polysaccharides, which mainly contained pectic sugars. Maximum glycosidase activities were observed 24 to 48 hours after the application of water hydration, and mucilaginous substances, which were tightly bound to the cell walls, were released. The presence of β-d xylosidase and α-l-arabinofuranosidase activities was also confirmed [5]. By their high molecular weight, the polysaccharides of linseed mucilage represent about 3 to 9% of the total weight of the seed and are divided into two components: neutral and acidic. The neutral component is composed of D-xylose, L-arabinose and D-galactose in a ratio of 6.2:3.5:1, while the acidic component contains L-rhamnose, L-fucose, L-galactose and D-galacturonic acid in a ratio of 2.6:1:1.4:1.7 [48,51]. On average, flax varieties with yellow seeds were found to have a higher content of neutral polysaccharides (arabinoxylans) due to the presence of the s1 gene, while brown seeds had a higher content of acidic polysaccharides (pectins) [52]. In addition to polysaccharides, they also contain glycoproteins and various bioactive components, such as tannins, alkaloids and steroids to a lesser extent [32,49,53]. The main constituent of the mucilage of *Lepidium perfoliatum* L. species is the highly methyl esterified homogalacturonan (HG). In addition, a significant amount of callose and hemicellulose and a small amount of weakly methyl esterified HG were present in the seed coat mucilage of *L. perfoliatum* L. [2]. *Lallemantia royleana* (BENTH.) seed mucilage, similar to other mucilage, is mainly composed of carbohydrates (76.74%), of which the most abundant monosaccharides are galactose (36.28%) and arabinose (35.96%). The less abundant monosaccharides are rhamnose (15.18%), xylose (7.38%) and glucose (5.20%). In addition to carbohydrates, the mucilage of *L. royleana* (BENTH.) seeds is also composed of protein (3,86%), ash (9,92%) and moisture (9,48%). Overall, it contains 82.56 ± 1.6 µg GAE/mg of phenolic compounds [54]. A similar polysaccharide content of *Lallemantia royleana* (BENTH.) mucilage (Figure 2) was also determined by [55]. The researchers observed that *Lallemantia royleana* (BENTH.) mucilage consisted of arabinose (37.88%), galactose (33.54%), rhamnose (18.44%), xylose (6.02%) and glucose (4.11%) [55]. The mucilage from basil is mainly composed of high-molecular-weight polysaccharides (2320 kDa), which consist of glucose, galactose, mannose, arabinose, xylose and rhamnose. The polysaccharides of basil mucilage are slightly acidic due to the presence of uronic acid (6.51%) [56]. Chia seed mucilage contains 93.8% carbohydrates, which form the following monosaccharide units: xylose, glucose, arabinose, galactose, glucuronic acid and galacturonic acid [57]. These subsequently form D-xylosyl and D-glucosyl residues in a 2:1 ratio. Additionally, it contains 22 to 25% 4-0-methyl-D-glucuronopyranosyl residues. The acetates of xylitol, glucitol and 4-O-methylglucitol are present in a ratio of 8:4:3. Another component of the polymer is 4-O-methyl-D-glucuronic acid [58]. The mucilage from the seeds of *Hyptis suaveolens* L. contains acidic and neutral heteropolysaccharides in a ratio of approximately 1:1. The neutral polysaccharides are composed of galactose, glucose and mannose, which form the polysaccharides galactoglucan (30%) and galactoglucomannan (70%), while the acidic polysaccharides contain residues of fucose, xylose and 4-O-methylglucuronic acid [21,59]. The total carbohydrate content of watercress mucilage is 87.4%, of which the most abundant carbohydrates are mannose (38.9%), arabinose (19.4%), galacturonic acid (8.0%), fructose (6.8%), glucuronic acid (6.7%), galactose (4.7%), rhamnose (1.9%) and glucose (1.0%) [60].

Table 2. Carbohydrate composition of some seed mucilages.

Plant Source of Seed Mucilage	Carbohydrates	Reference
Linum usitatissimum L.	Rhamnogalacturonan and arabinoxylan	Ref. [5]
Linum usitatissimum L.	D-xylose, L-arabinose, D-galactose, L-ramnose, L-fucose, L-galactose, D-galacturonic acid	Ref. [51]
Lepidium perfoliatum L.	Methylesterified homogalacturonan, callose, hemicellulose	Ref. [2]
Lallemantia royleana BENTH.	Galactose, arabinose, rhamnose, xylose, glucose	Refs. [54,55]
Ocimum basilicum L.	Glucose, galactose, mannose, arabinose, xylose, rhamnose	Ref. [56]

Table 2. *Cont.*

Plant Source of Seed Mucilage	Carbohydrates	Reference
Salvia hispanica L.	Xylose, glucose, arabinose, galactose, glucuronic acid, galacturonic acid	Ref. [57]
Salvia hispanica L.	Residues of D-xylosyl, D-glucosyl, 4-0-methyl-D-glucuronopyranosyl	Ref. [58]
Hyptis suaveolens L.	Galactose, glucose, mannose, galactoglucan, galactoglucomannan, fucose, xylose, 4-O-methylglucuronic acid	Refs. [21,59]
Lepidium sativum L.	Mannose, arabinose, galacturonic acid, fructose, glucuronic acid, galactose, rhamnose, glucose	Ref. [60]

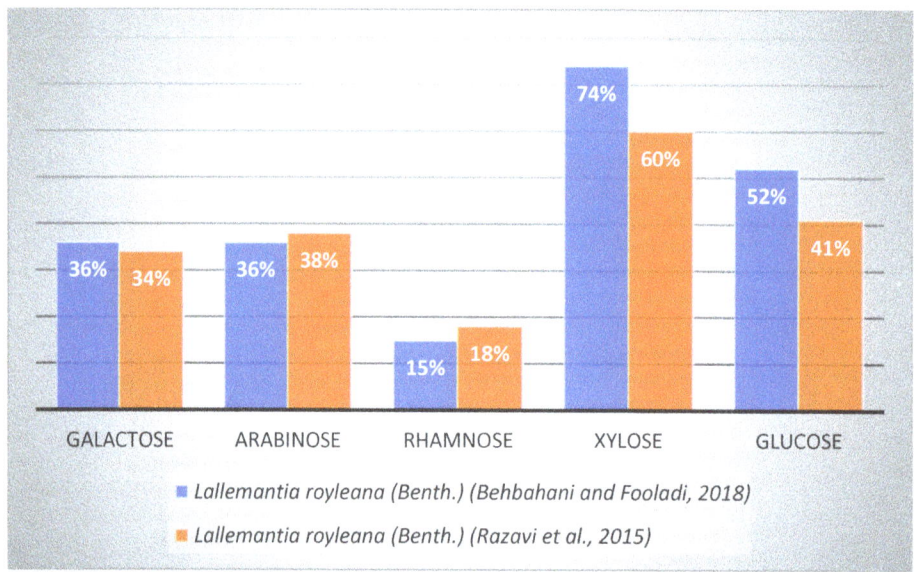

Figure 2. Difference in carbohydrate composition of *Lallemantia royleana* (BENTH.) seed mucilage between two studies [54,55].

When comparing the mucilage from several plants, it was observed that the lipid content of mucilage generally tended to be low. For example, the lipid content in the mucilage of yellow mustard was only 0.2%, 0.5 to 0.7% in flax, 4.76% in tamarind and 1.85% in watercress seeds. However, mucilage lipids provide important functions for the plant, improving their water uptake and desorbing the adsorbed phosphorus on the soil particles in the rhizosphere. The amount of protein varies considerably from plant to plant, with Indian plantain seed mucilage containing 0,94% protein, *Artemisia sphaerocephala* (KRASCH.) mucilage up to 24,1%, tamarind seed mucilage 14,78% and linseed mucilage having a protein content of between 4,4 and 15,1%. Mucilage proteins break down mucilage polysaccharides into the forms available to microorganisms, they respond to biotic and abiotic stresses, and mobilize nutrients in the rhizosphere [49,53,61]. An average mineral content of plant mucilage is 5.6% and they are also important in the exchange of cations between the plant and the rhizosphere and improve the coupling of the liquid phase of the soil with the water content [49]. Altogether, six chemical elements—copper, zinc, cobalt, lead, chromium, chromium and cadmium—have been detected in the mucilage of flaxseed [48]. The most abundant chemical element in cress mucilage is calcium (0.17%), but it also contains sodium, potassium and magnesium [60].

Although the chemical composition of mucilage is well known, its structural organization is unclear. The fibrillar character of the individual mucilage components is demonstrated by both the pectic and cellulosic types of mucilage. However, due to the presence of cellulose microfibrils, cellulose mucilage is much more organized [50]. Using critical point drying (CPD) and scanning electron microscopy (SEM), the structural details of mucilage were resolved down to the nanoscale. The mucilaginous fibrillar components generally form a network of cellulose fibers that serve as a scaffold for other polysaccharide fibers, which often branch out and are found between or on the surface of the cellulose fibers. The cellulose fibrils are long, thick, unbranched and, by being attached to the surface of the seeds, prevent the loss of the mucilage cover by mechanical impact. Interestingly, the structural organization of mucilage varies among plant species, which is important for water binding and storage [4]. Pectic mucilage, on the other hand, has a fibrous, convoluted and more homogeneous structure than the cellulosic type [50].

7. Functional Properties of Plant Seed Mucilage

The mucilaginous substances of the plants are odorless, colorless and tasteless. In addition, they are non-toxic and biodegradable [32]. Mucilage can also exhibit good photostability; for example, mucilage obtained from the seeds of *Salvia hispanica* L. showed a degradation percentage of 6.6% after 120 min under UV light [43]. Three parameters in the extraction of mucilage have a great influence on the functional properties of mucilage—temperature, pH and water/seed ratio. It has been observed that the maximum values of extraction, viscosity, emulsion stability, foam stability, solubility and water absorption capacity (9.3 g/g) of the *Eruca sativa* MILL. seed mucilage could be achieved at an extraction temperature of 65.5 °C, pH 4 and a water-to-seed ratio of 60:1 [62].

A very important indicator of the quality of mucilage is its molecular weight because the polymer chains interact when the mucilage dissolves, and mucilage with a high molecular weight can improve its viscosity. This property can be used to improve the texture of foods and it also affects the mouthfeel of the consumer [63]. The molecular weight of mucilage also affects the emulsifying and foaming properties [64]. The mucilage of different plants has different molecular weights, for example, the mucilage from the seeds of *Hyptis suaveolens* L. contains an anionic fraction responsible for swelling and viscous behavior with an average molar mass of 0.35×10^6 g·mol^{-1}, while the neutral polysaccharide fraction (in a 1:1 ratio) exhibits an average molar mass of 0.047×10^6 g·mol^{-1} [59]. The neutral component of flaxseed mucilage has a lower molecular weight (1.47×10^6 g·mol^{-1}) than the acidic part (1851×10^6 g·mol^{-1}) [65]. The molecular weight of the *Lallemantia royleana* BENTH. in WALL. seed mucilage is 1.19×10^6 g·mol^{-1}, *Salvia hispanica* L. 2.3×10^6 g·mol^{-1}, and the molecular weight of the *Ocimum basilicum* L. seed is 2.32×10^6 g·mol^{-1} [54,66]. Another study of *Lallemantia royleana* BENTH. in WALL. seed mucilage showed that the molecular weight was 1.294×10^6 g·mol^{-1} [55].

The solubility of mucilage improves with increasing temperatures, where the lowest solubility values for flax mucilage were observed at 20 °C (24.52% to 30.95%) and the highest at 80 °C (64.5% to 69.15%) [48]. It was observed that the mucilage from both white and black chia seeds showed similar solubility values between 30 and 60 °C. Black chia seed mucilage showed the greatest solubility at 70 °C (80.65%), while the solubility of white chia seed mucilage remained constant [67]. The solubility of *Eruca sativa* MILL. at 65.5 °C was 28.5% [61] and the solubility of *Lepidium perfoliatum* L. seed mucilage was approximately 20% at 60 °C [68].

Furthermore, mucilage exhibits thermostable properties with high degradation temperatures, for example, tamarind seed mucilage starts to lose weight at 175 °C and chia seed mucilage at 244 °C [49,53]. Black chia seed mucilage has a higher thermal decomposition temperature (286.8 °C) than white chia seed mucilage (269.4 °C) [67].

Another property of mucilage is its ability to retain water, which is dependent on pore size, capillary action and the amount of protein components present in the mucilage. Flax mucilage has a higher water retention capacity compared to microbial xanthan mucilage and lower water retention capacity compared to plant guar mucilage [69]. The mucilage from the seeds of *Lepidium perfoliatum* L. showed a similar trend; the water absorption capacity (around 20 g·g^{-1}) was lower than guar but almost identical to xanthan. It is suggested that the lower water absorption rate by *L. perfoliatum* L. seed mucilage compared to guar is due to the strong degree of interaction between the polysaccharide chains and hence the lower interaction with water [68]. In tamarind seed mucilage, the water holding and oil retention capacities have been shown to increase with temperature [61]. The water absorption capacity of basil seed mucilage is higher (35.16–38.96 g·g^{-1}) than its oil absorption capacity (5.40–17.38%) [70]. The water absorption capacity of chia seed mucilage is 54.24 ± 0.47 g·g^{-1} and the water holding capacity is greater (35.49 ± 0.24 g·g^{-1}) than its oil holding capacity (7.72 ± 0.36 g·g^{-1}) [67]. The water absorption capacity of *Eruca sativa* Mill. was 9.3 g·g^{-1} [62].

Mucilage proteins are characterized by their good foaming properties; foam stability increases with increasing the mucilage concentration. Chia seed mucilage has 96.5 ± 1.6% foam stability at a 0.1% concentration and 97.8 ± 1.2% at a 0.3% concentration [67]. Foam stabilization is also affected by the water/seed ratio (negatively) and temperature (positively) during mucilage extraction. Quince seed mucilage had a 94.89% emulsion stability and a 21.36% foam stability [71] and *Eruca sativa* MILL. mucilage had an emulsion stability of 87% and foam stability of 87.5% [62]. The foam stability of *Lepidium perfoliatum* L. seed gum also increased with increasing concentrations, but was lower compared to xanthan and guar gums at similar concentrations. This trend was probably due to the differences in viscosity of the continuation phase [68].

Mucilage can also form a cold-solidifying thermo-reversible gel. The strength of this gel is influenced by the dissolution temperature, pH and addition of minerals. With higher dissolution temperatures, the strength of the gel increases, and the addition of NaCl and complex phosphate salt decreases the strength. If we want to increase the strength, we can add CaCl$_2$ at a low concentration (<0.3 wt.%), and its strength decreases at higher concentrations [72]. The strength of *Hyptis suaveolens* (L.) Poit. seed mucilage gel also increased by the addition of sucrose (1, 3, 5, 10 and 20% w/v) to a 0.5% mucilage dispersion. This caused the gel to exhibit its shear-thinning behavior to a lesser extent, which had a stabilizing effect [73].

As the concentration of mucilage increases, its viscosity increases as well. The viscosity and elasticity are also influenced by chemical composition, with both variables increasing at a higher concentration of xylose and lower concentration of uronic acid. The viscosity of linseed mucilage ranges from 0.02 to 0.28 Pa·s, while the viscosity of basil seed mucilage ranges from 0.19 to 0.714 Pa·s. Depending on the variety and concentration, mucilage can behave as a viscous liquid, viscoelastic liquid or almost an elastic body [70,74]. The water/seed ratio during extraction had the highest effect on the viscosity of the quince seed mucilage, and increasing the extraction time at temperatures of up to 45 °C decreased the viscosity. Under optimum extraction conditions, the viscosity of the mucilage was 1.47396 Pa·s [71]. The viscosity of *Eruca sativa* MILL. in optimal conditions was 0.357 Pa·s [62]. The viscosity of the *Lepidium perfoliatum* L. seed gum decreased with the increasing shear rate. The highest viscosity (approximately 3 Pa·s) was noted at a shear rate of approximately 15 (1·s^{-1}). The comparison of the viscosity of *Lepidium perfoliatum* L. seed gum with other commercial gums with the same shear rate showed that the viscosity of this gum was higher than in locust beans, lower than in guar and almost identical to the viscosity of xanthan. As with other types of mucilage, increasing the concentration of the solution leads to an increase in the viscosity of *L. perfoliatum* seed mucilage, and increasing the temperature up to 65 °C leads to a decrease in viscosity. Interestingly, the addition of NaCl, KCl, CaCl$_2$ and MgCl$_2$ salts also influenced the viscosity of the mucilage, showing a rapid decrease in viscosity after the addition of 0.2% of any of the salts [68]. Although the mucilage from *Lallemantia royleana* Benth. exhibited a similar molecular weight to most seed mucilage, the intrinsic viscosity (23.06 dL·g^{-1}) was higher [55].

8. Gene Regulation of Seed Mucilage Synthesis

The epidermal cells of plants that secrete mucilage are influenced by several genes during the development phase, leading to changes in their extracellular matrices. Most research has focused on the epidermal cell genes of *Arabidopsis thaliana* L. Research on the *COBRA-LIKE 2* (*COBL2*) gene, a member of the COBRA-LIKE gene family, found that it has a specialized function in maintaining a proper cellulose deposition in the seed mucilage [75]. Additionally, the MUM 2 gene, a member of glycosyl hydrolase family 35, was identified. Its localization is in the cell wall of *A. thaliana*, with the MUM 2 protein entering the apoplast via the endoplasmic reticulum and the Golgi apparatus network. Overall, the MUM2 gene exhibits β-galactosidase activity and has a negligible effect on the amount of mucilage produced or the seed morphology; on the other hand, it is essential for the proper structure of the produced mucilage [76]. The β-galactosidase activity of the MUM2 gene may also be complemented by the TESTA-ABUNDANT2 (TBA2), PEROXIDASE36 (PER36) and MUCILAGE-MODIFIED4 (MUM4) genes, and thus may be involved in modifying the polysaccharide composition of seed mucilage [77]. It was possible to isolate a sequence of 308 base pairs of the MUM4 gene that controls the expression of the reporter gene in both *A. thaliana* L. and *Camelina sativa* (L.) Crantz seed coat cells and is regulated by the same cascade of transcription factors as endogenous MUM4 [78]. KNAT3 and KNAT7, members of the KNOX class II gene family, act as positive regulators of the biosynthetic gene RG-I MUCILAGE-MODIFIED 4 (MUM4, AT1G53500) and thus affect the production of mucilage in *A. thaliana* L. at early developmental stages [79]. The mucilage from *A. thaliana* L. is mainly composed of rhamnogalacturonan I, the size of which is influenced by the MUCILAGE-RELATED70 (MUCI70) gene with glycosyltransferase activity. Additionally, the CuAOα1 gene encoding a putative copper amine oxidase of clade 1a affects the production of pectin and influences the amount of rhamnogalacturonan I in the outer mucilage layer [80]. The MUM1 gene in *A. thaliana* L. encodes the transcription factor LEUNIG_HOMOLOG (LUH), which is localized in the nucleus. According to the research, the LUH/MUM1 transcriptional activator could be a positive regulator of the gene-encoding enzymes required for the extrusion of mucilage—MUM2, SUBSILIN PROTEASE1.7 and β-XYLOSIDASE1 [81]. The *A. thaliana* L. gene GALACTURONOSYLTRANSFERASE-LIKE5 (AtGATL5), which is localized in both the endoplasmic reticulum and Golgi system, could also be involved in the regulation of the final size of mucilage rhamnogalacturonan I [82]. The *A. thaliana* L. UUAT1 gene encodes a protein localized in the Golgi apparatus that transports the UDP-glucuronic acid and UDP-galacturonic acid in vitro. UDP-glucuronic acid is a precursor of many seed mucilage polysaccharides and, after synthesis in the cytosol, it is transported to the Golgi apparatus lumen where it is converted to UDP-galacturonic acid, UDP-arabinose and UDP-xylose. This suggests that the UUAT1 gene has a key role in the composition of seed mucilage [83]. CELLULOSE SYNTHASE 5 (CESA5)/MUCILAGE-MODIFIED 3 (MUM3), MUM5/MUCI21, SALT-OVERLY SENSITIVE 5 (SOS5) and FEI2 gene influences the adherence of A. thaliana mucilage. While MUM5 and CESA5 act as synergists by providing the adhesion of pectin to the seed through cellulose and xylan biosynthesis, SOS5 and FEI2 encode an arabinogalactan protein [84]. The PECTIN METHYLESTERASE INHIBITOR6 gene promotes mucilage release in *A. thaliana* L. by inhibiting the activities of endogenous pectin methylesterase that demethylate homogalacturonan [85]. The genes *A. thaliana* L. TRANSPARENT TESTA 8, SUBTILISIN-LIKE SERINE PROTEASE, GALACTUROSYL TRANSFERASE-LIKE 5, MUCILAGE-MODIFIED 4, AGAMOUS-LIKE MADS-BOX PROTEIN AGL62, GLYCOSYL HYDROLASE FAMILY 17 and UDP-GLUCOSE FLAVONOL 3-O-GLUCOSYLTRANSFERASE play a role in mucilage synthesis and release, seed coat development and anthocyanin biosynthesis, and are among the promising candidate genes of flaxseed [86]. The gene-encoding pectin methylesterases (PMEs), which control the level of pectin methylesterification, influence the structure and organization of *A. thaliana* mucilage. Of the PMEs observed, the PME58 gene showed the highest expression [87]. The direct activation of this gene is provided by two transcription factors in *A. thaliana* L., BLH2 and BLH4, which are significantly expressed in mucilage-secreting cells and thus positively regulate PMEs. In addition to PME58, they also affect the expression of the genes PECTIN METHYLESTERASE INHIBITOR6, SEEDSTICK, and MYB52 [88]. Conversely, the MUD1 gene, which encodes a nuclear RING domain protein and is highly expressed in the developing seed coat of *A. thaliana* L., negatively regulates the PME levels. MUD1 expression causes a reduction in the expression of PME-related genes, including MYB52, LUH, SBT1.7, PMEI6 and PMEI14 [89].

The production of mucilage at different developmental stages from the *Aechmea sphaerocephala* (GAUDICH.) Baker seeds is influenced by 21 key regulatory genes (AsNAM-1 to AsNAM-17, AsAP2-1, AsAP2-2, AsKNAT7 and AsTTG1) whose expressions were different at 10, 20, 30, 40, 50, 60 and 70 days after flowering. In the period of 10 to 30 days after flowering, both the AsNAM and AsAP2 genes stimulated the production of mucilage by their expression. In the period of 40 to 70 days after flowering, the expressions of AsNAM and AsAP2 were reduced, and conversely, the increase in AsKNAT7 expression inhibited the formation of mucilage [90]. The transcription factors MYB-bHLH-WD40 (MBW) and APETALA2 (AP2) had a key effect on the production of mucilage in the *A. sphaerocephala* (GAUDICH.) Baker seeds. The increased accumulation of UDP-glucose was mediated by an increased expression of phosphoglucomutase (pgm) and uridine glucose diphosphorylase (UGPase) and decreased expression of UDP-glucose 4-epimerase (GALE), UDP-glucose 6-dehydrogenase (UGDH) and UDP-glucose 4,6-dehydratase (RHM). The accumulation of UDP-xylose (UDP-Xyl) was influenced by an increased expression of UDP-apiose/xylose synthase (AXS) and decreased expression of UDP-arabinose 4-epimerase (UXE) [91]. The transparent testa glabra 1 (TTG1) gene encodes the transcription factor of *Lepidium perfoliatum* that plays a role in epidermal cell differentiation and the release of mucilage. This gene is 1032 bp long, it encodes 343 predicted amino acids and contains WD40 motifs [92]. An overview of the genes/transcription factors, their function in the mucilage process and spatial localization is shown in Tables 3 and 4.

Table 3. Function of genes/transcription factors in the mucilage process.

Function in the Process	Genes/Transcription Factors	Reference
Mucilage synthesis and release	Transparent testa 8; subtilisin-like serine protease; galacturosyl transferase-like 5; mucilage-modified 4; agamous-like MADS-box protein AGL62; glycosyl hydrolase family 17; pectin methylesterase inhibitor 6	Refs. [85,86]
Mucilage amount	Mucilage-modified 2 (MUM2)	Ref. [76]
Mucilage proper structure	Mucilage-modified 2 (MUM2)	Ref. [76]
Mucilage polysaccharide composition	Mucilage-modified 2 (MUM2) + testa-abundant 2 (TBA2); peroxidase 36 (PER36); mucilage-modified 4 (MUM4)	Ref. [77]
Mucilage production	Knotted arabidopsis thaliana 3 (KNAT3) and knotted arabidopsis thaliana 7 (KNAT7)	Ref. [79]
Mucilage cellulose deposition	Cobra-like 2 (COBL2)	Ref. [75]
Mucilage composition	UDP-uronic acid transporter1 (UUAT 1)	Ref. [83]
Mucilage extrusion	Leunig homolog (LUH)/mucilage-modified 1 (MUM 1); enzymes MUM 2; subsilin protease 1.7; beta-xylosidase 1	Ref. [81]
Mucilage adherence Mucilage structure and organization	Cellulose synthase 5 (CESA5)/mucilage-modified 3 (MUM3) Pectin methylesterase 8 (PME 8) + BLH 2 and BLH 4	Ref. [84] Refs. [87,88]
Mucilage rhamnogalacturonan I size	Mucilage-related 70 (MUCI 70); galacturonosyltransferase-like 5 (GATL 5)	Ref. [80]
Mucilage rhamnogalacturonan I amount	Copper amine oxidase 1 (CuAOX 1)	Ref. [80]

Notes: genes are shown in italics.

Table 4. Spatial localizations of some genes included in the mucilage process.

Spatial Localization	Genes/Transcription Factors	Reference
Epidermal cells	Cobra-like 2 (COBL2)	Ref. [75]
Cell wall	Mucilage-modified 2 (MUM2)	Ref. [76]
Seed coat cells	Mucilage-modified 4 (MUM4)	Ref. [77]
Mucilage-secreting cells	BLH 2 and BLH 4	Ref. [88]
Nucleus	Leunig homolog LUH	Ref. [81]
Endoplasmic reticulum; Golgi apparatus	Galacturonosyltransferase-like 5 (GATL5)	Ref. [82]
Golgi apparatus	UDP-uronic acid transporter1 (UUAT 1)	Ref. [83]
Developing seed coat	Mucilage defect 1 (MUD1)	Ref. [89]

Notes: genes are shown in italics.

9. Summary

Specific cells of some plants can produce hydrophilic mucilage in the Golgi apparatus and subsequently secrete it into the apoplastic space. This mucilage has several vital functions for the plant: it protects the seeds from desiccation, fixes the seeds in the soil, protects the seeds from predation, influences seed germination and serves as a source of energy for the seeds. In addition, it is priceless in agriculture and the food industry because it serves as an additive in various foods, and it is also used in the production of edible films and the encapsulation of probiotics. It is also used in human and veterinary medicines as it has antihypercholesterolemic, antibacterial, laxative, healing, anti-inflammatory and anticarcinogenic effects, and it influences glucose metabolism and acts as a prebiotic. It can be used in the manufacture of tablet medicines and for wound dressings.

Mucilage is mainly composed of polysaccharides, which vary between the species and varieties, but it also contains other components, such as proteins, lipids, ash, moisture, phenolics and minerals to a lesser extent. The mucilaginous substances of plants are odorless, colorless and tasteless; they have a high degradation temperature; good foaming properties and a high water retention capacity. In the future, mucilaginous substances have great potential to be used as potential nutraceuticals in disease prevention and treatment.

10. Future Perspectives

For the development of functional foods, food supplements or nutraceuticals, it is necessary to research more extensively the genotypic variability of the biochemical composition of mucilage and its biological and other properties (according to the purpose of use). The identification of the specific plant genotype reflecting the appropriate/required parameters of seed mucilage is crucial for advancing the usability of this potential nutraceutical. Therefore, detailed knowledge of the molecular mechanisms behind the regulation of mucilage biosynthesis mainly at the epigenetic level (microRNAs) should become the focus of future research.

Author Contributions: Conceptualization, M.K. and K.R.; methodology, M.K., K.R., Ľ.H. and T.K.; validation, K.R., M.K., Ľ.H. and T.K.; writing—original draft preparation, M.K. and K.R.; writing—review and editing, K.R., M.K., Ľ.H. and T.K.; visualization, M.K.; supervision, K.R.; project administration, K.R. All authors have read and agreed to the published version of the manuscript.

Funding: This research received no external funding.

Institutional Review Board Statement: Not applicable.

Informed Consent Statement: Not applicable.

Data Availability Statement: Not applicable.

Acknowledgments: This publication was created thanks to the support under the Operational Programme Integrated Infrastructure for the project: Long-term strategic research of prevention, intervention and mechanisms of obesity and its comorbidities, IMTS: 313011V344, co-financed by the European Regional Development Fund.

Conflicts of Interest: The authors declare no conflict of interest.

References

1. Galloway, A.F.; Knox, P.; Krause, K. Sticky mucilages and exudates of plants: Putative microenvironmental design elements with biotechnological value. *New Phytol.* **2020**, *225*, 1461–1469. [CrossRef]
2. Huang, D.; Wang, C.; Yuan, J.; Cao, J.; Lan, H. Differentiation of the seed coat and composition of the mucilage of *Lepidium perfoliatum* L.: A desert annual with typical myxospermy. *Acta Biochim. Biophys. Sin.* **2015**, *47*, 775–787. [CrossRef]
3. Western, T. The sticky tale of seed coat mucilages: Production, genetics, and role in seed germination and dispersal. *Seed Sci. Res.* **2012**, *22*, 1–25. [CrossRef]
4. Kreitschitz, A.; Gorb, S. The micro- and nanoscale spatial architecture of the seed mucilage—Comparative study of selected plant species. *PLoS ONE* **2018**, *13*, 0200522. [CrossRef]
5. Paynel, F.; Pavlov, A.; Ancelin, G.; Rihouey, C.; Picton, L.; Lebrun, L.; Morvan, C. Polysaccharide hydrolases are released with mucilages after water hydration of flax seeds. *Plant Physiol. Biochem.* **2012**, *62C*, 54–62. [CrossRef]
6. Yang, X.; Baskin, J.; Baskin, C.; Huang, Z.Y. More than just a coating: Ecological importance, taxonomic occurrence and phylogenetic relationships of seed coat mucilage. *Perspect. Plant Ecol. Evol. Syst.* **2012**, *14*, 434–442. [CrossRef]
7. Kreitschitz, A.; Tadele, Z.; Gola, E. Slime cells on the surface of *Eragrostis* seeds maintain a level of moisture around the grain to enhance germination. *Seed Sci. Res.* **2009**, *19*, 27–35. [CrossRef]
8. Gorai, M.; El Aloui, W.; Yang, X.; Neffati, M. Toward understanding the ecological role of mucilage in seed germination of a desert shrub *Henophyton deserti*: Interactive effects of temperature, salinity and osmotic stress. *Plant Soil* **2014**, *374*, 727–738. [CrossRef]
9. Zhao, C.; Jiang, L.; Shi, X.; Wang, L. Mucilage inhibits germination of desert ephemeral Nepeta micrantha under moderate osmotic stress and promotes recovery after release of this stress. *Seed Sci. Technol.* **2020**, *48*, 21–25. [CrossRef]
10. Yang, X.; Baskin, C.C.; Baskin, J.M.; Liu, G.; Huang, Z. Seed Mucilage Improves Seedling Emergence of a Sand Desert Shrub. *PLoS ONE* **2012**, *7*, e34597. [CrossRef]
11. Pan, V.S.; Girvin, C.; LoPresti, E.F. Anchorage by seed mucilage prevents seed dislodgement in high surface flow: A mechanistic investigation. *Ann. Bot.* **2022**, *129*, 30–37. [CrossRef] [PubMed]
12. LoPresti, E.; Pan, V.; Goidell, J.; Weber, M.; Karban, R. Mucilage-Bound Sand Reduces Seed Predation by Ants but Not by Reducing Apparency: A Field Test of 53 Plant Species. *Bull. Ecol. Soc. Am.* **2019**, *100*, e02809. [CrossRef]
13. Geneve, R.; Hildebrand, D.; Phillips, T.; AL-Amery, M.; Kester, S. Stress Influences Seed Germination in Mucilage-Producing Chia. *Crop Sci.* **2017**, *57*, 2160–2169. [CrossRef]
14. Zhou, Z.; Xing, J.; Zhao, J.; Liu, L.; Gu, L.; Lan, H. The ecological roles of seed mucilage on germination of *Lepidium perfoliatum*, a desert herb with typical myxospermy in Xinjiang. *Plant Growth Regul.* **2022**, *97*, 185–201. [CrossRef]
15. El-Newary, S.A. Mucilage of Cordia dichotoma seeds pulp: Isolation, purification and a new hypolipidemic agent in normal and hyperlipidemic rats. *Planta Med.* **2015**, *81*, 107. [CrossRef]
16. Kumar, D.; Pandey, J.; Kumar, P.; Raj, V. Psyllium Mucilage and Its Use in Pharmaceutical Field: An Overview. *Curr. Synth. Syst. Biotechnol.* **2017**, *5*, 1000134. [CrossRef]
17. Rubilar, M.; Gutiérrez, C.; Verdugo, M.; Shene, C.; Sineiro, J. Flaxseed as a source of functional ingredients. *J. Soil Sci. Plant Nutr.* **2010**, *10*, 373–377. [CrossRef]
18. Uddin Zim, A.F.M.I.; Khatun, J.; Khan, M.; Hossain, M.D.; Hauqe, M. Evaluation of in vitro antioxidant activity of okra mucilage and its antidiabetic and antihyperlipidemic effect in alloxan-induced diabetic mice. *Food Sci. Nutr.* **2021**, *9*, 6854–6865. [CrossRef]
19. Palla, A.H.; Gilani, A. Dual effectiveness of Flaxseed in constipation and diarrhea: Possible mechanism. *J. Ethnopharmacol.* **2015**, *169*, 60–68. [CrossRef]
20. Sindhu, G.; Ratheesh, M.; Shyni, G.L.; Nambisan, B.; Helen, A. Anti-inflammatory and antioxidative effects of mucilage of *Trigonella foenum graecum* (Fenugreek) on adjuvant induced arthritic rats. *Int. Immunopharmacol.* **2012**, *12*, 205–211. [CrossRef]
21. Mueller, M.; Čavarkapa, A.; Unger, F.M.; Viernstein, H.; Praznik, W. Prebiotic potential of neutral oligo- and polysaccharides from seed mucilage of *Hyptis suaveolens*. *Food Chem.* **2017**, *221*, 508–514. [CrossRef] [PubMed]
22. Muñoz, L.; Tamargo García, A.; Cueva, C.; Laguna, L.; Moreno Arribas, M.V. Understanding the impact of chia seed mucilage on human gut microbiota by using the dynamic gastrointestinal model simgi®. *J. Funct. Foods* **2018**, *50*, 104–111.
23. Mkedder, I.; Bouali, W.; Hassaine, H. Antibacterial Activity of Mucilage of *Linum usitatissimum* L. Seeds. *South Asian J. Exp. Biol.* **2021**, *11*, 305–310. [CrossRef]
24. Khan, A.A.; Alam, T.; Singh, S.; Wali, M.; Maaz, M.; Jabin, A. Efficacy Evaluation of *Linium usitatissimum* (Linctus of Flax Mucilage) in Chronic Obstructive Pulmonary Disease Patients. *Planta Med.* **2016**, *82*, PB20. [CrossRef]
25. Tamri, P.; Hemmati, A.A.; Ghafourian, M. Wound healing properties of quince seed mucilage: In vivo evaluation in rabbit full-thickness wound model. *Int. J. Surg.* **2014**, *12*, 843–847. [CrossRef]

26. Hemmati, A.A.; Kalantari, H.; Rezai, S.; Zadeh, H. Healing effect of quince seed mucilage on T-2 toxin-induced dermal toxicity in rabbit. *Exp. Toxicol. Pathol.* **2012**, *64*, 181–186. [CrossRef]
27. Tantiwatcharothai, S.; Prachayawarakorn, J. Characterization of an antibacterial wound dressing from basil seed (*Ocimum basilicum* L.) mucilage-ZnO nanocomposite. *Int. J. Biol. Macromol.* **2019**, *135*, 133–140. [CrossRef]
28. Sayyad, F.; Sakhare, S. Isolation, Characterization and Evaluation of *Ocimum basilicum* Seed Mucilage for Tableting Performance. *Indian J. Pharm. Sci.* **2018**, *80*, 282–290. [CrossRef]
29. Saeedi, M.; Morteza-Semnani, K.; Ansoroudi, F.; Fallah, S.; Amin, G. Evaluation of binding properties of *Plantago psyllium* seed mucilage. *Acta Pharm.* **2010**, *60*, 339–348. [CrossRef]
30. Avlani, D.; Ash, D.; Majee, S.; Roy Biswas, G. Sweet Basil Seed Mucilage as a Gelling agent in Nasal Drug Delivery. *Int. J. Pharmtech. Res.* **2019**, *12*, 42–49. [CrossRef]
31. Atabaki, R.; Hassanpour, M. Improvement of Lidocaine Local Anesthetic Action Using *Lallemantia royleana* Seed Mucilage as an Excipient. *Iran. J. Pharm. Sci.* **2014**, *13*, 1431–1436.
32. Tosif, M.M.; Najda, A.; Bains, A.; Kaushik, R.; Dhull, S.B.; Chawla, P.; Walasek-Janusz, M. A Comprehensive Review on Plant-Derived Mucilage: Characterization, Functional Properties, Applications, and Its Utilization for Nanocarrier Fabrication Polymers. *Polymers* **2021**, *13*, 1066. [CrossRef] [PubMed]
33. Ribes, S.; Gómez, N.; Fuentes, A.; Talens, P.; Barat, J. Chia (*Salvia hispanica* L.) seed mucilage as a fat replacer in yogurts: Effect on their nutritional, technological, and sensory properties. *J. Dairy Sci.* **2021**, *104*, 2822–2833. [CrossRef] [PubMed]
34. Basiri, S.; Haidary, N.; Shekarforoush, S.S.; Niakousari, M. Flaxseed mucilage: A natural stabilizer in stirred yogurt. *Carbohydr. Polym.* **2018**, *187*, 59–65. [CrossRef]
35. Fernandes, S.; Salas Mellado, M. Development of Mayonnaise with Substitution of Oil or Egg Yolk by the Addition of Chia (*Salvia hispânica* L.) Mucilage. *J. Food Sci.* **2017**, *83*, 74–83. [CrossRef]
36. Fernandes, S.; Filipini, G.; Salas Mellado, M. Development of cake mix with reduced fat and high practicality by adding chia mucilage. *Food Biosci.* **2021**, *42*, 101148. [CrossRef]
37. Campos, B.; Ruivo, T.; Scapim, M.; Madrona, G.; Bergamasco, R. Optimization of the Mucilage Extraction Process from Chia Seeds and Application in Ice Cream as a Stabilizer and Emulsifier. *Food Sci. Technol.* **2015**, *65*, 874–883. [CrossRef]
38. Dokoohaki, Z.; Sekhavatizadeh, S.; Hosseinzadeh, S. Dairy dessert containing microencapsulated *Lactobacillus rhamnosus* (ATCC 53103) with quince seed mucilage as a coating material. *LWT* **2019**, *115*, 108429. [CrossRef]
39. Bustamante, M.; Oomah, B.D.; Rubilar, M.; Shene, C. Effective Lactobacillus plantarum and Bifidobacterium infantis encapsulation with chia seed (*Salvia hispanica* L.) and flaxseed (*Linum usitatissimum* L.) mucilage and soluble protein by spray drying. *Food Chem.* **2016**, *216*, 97–105. [CrossRef]
40. Kurd, F.; Fathi, M.; Shekarchizadeh, H. Nanoencapsulation of hesperetin using basil seed mucilage nanofibers: Characterization and release modeling. *Food Biosci.* **2019**, *32*, 100475. [CrossRef]
41. Fahami, A.; Fathi, M. Development of cress seed mucilage/PVA nanofibers as a novel carrier for vitamin A delivery. *Food Hydrocoll.* **2018**, *81*, 31–38. [CrossRef]
42. Hajivand, P.; Aryanejad, S.; Akbari, I.; Hemmati, A. Fabrication and characterization of a promising oregano-extract/psyllium-seed mucilage edible film for food packaging. *J. Food Sci.* **2020**, *85*, 2481–2490. [CrossRef]
43. da Silveira Ramos, I.F.; Magalhães, L.M.; do OPessoa, C.; Ferreira, P.M.; dos Santos Rizzo, M.; Osajima, J.A.; Silva-Filho, E.C.; Nunes, C.; Raposo, F.; Coimbra, M.A.; et al. New properties of chia seed mucilage (*Salvia hispanica* L.) and potential application in cosmetic and pharmaceutical products. *Ind. Crops Prod.* **2021**, *171*, 113981. [CrossRef]
44. Naveed, M.; Ahmed, M.A.; Benard, P.; Brown, L.K.; George, T.S.; Bengough, A.G.; Roose, T.; Koebernick, N.; Hallett, P.D. Surface tension, rheology and hydrophobicity of rhizodeposits and seed mucilage influence soil water retention and hysteresis. *Plant Soil* **2019**, *437*, 65–81. [CrossRef] [PubMed]
45. Zhao, C.; Zheng, R.; Shi, X.; Wang, L. Soil microbes and seed mucilage promote growth of the desert ephemeral plant *Nepeta micrantha* under different water conditions. *Flora Morphol. Distrib. Funct. Ecol. Plants* **2021**, *280*, 151845. [CrossRef]
46. Paynel, F.; Morvan, C.; Marais, S.; Lebrun, L. Improvement of the hydrolytic stability of new flax-based biocomposite materials. *Polym. Degrad. Stab.* **2013**, *98*, 190–197. [CrossRef]
47. Ellerbrock, R.; Ahmed, M.; Gerke, H. Spectroscopic characterization of mucilage (Chia seed) and polygalacturonic acid. *J. Soil Sci. Plant Nutr.* **2019**, *182*, 888–895. [CrossRef]
48. Kaur, M.; Kaur, R.; Punia, S. Characterization of mucilages extracted from different flaxseed (*Linum usitatissiumum* L.) cultivars: A heteropolysaccharide with desirable functional and rheological properties. *Int. J. Biol. Macromol.* **2018**, *117*, 917–927. [CrossRef]
49. Nazari, M. Plant mucilage components and their functions in the rhizosphere. *Rhizosphere* **2021**, *18*, 100344. [CrossRef]
50. Kreitschitz, A.; Gorb, S. How does the cell wall 'stick' in the mucilage? A detailed microstructural analysis of the seed coat mucilaginous cell wall. *Flora* **2017**, *229*, 9–22. [CrossRef]
51. Oomah, B.D.; Kenaschuk, E.; Cui, S.; Mazza, G. Variation in the composition of water-soluble polysaccharides in flaxseed. *J. Agric. Food Chem.* **1995**, *43*, 1484–1488. [CrossRef]
52. Porokhovinova, E.; Pavlov, A.V.; Brutch, N.; Morvan, C. Carbohydrate composition of flax mucilage and its relation to morphological characters. *Agric. Biol.* **2017**, *52*, 161–171. [CrossRef]
53. Liu, Y.; Liu, Z.; Zhu, X.; Hu, X.; Zhang, H.; Guo, Q.; Yada, R.Y.; Cui, S.W. Seed coat mucilages: Structural, functional/bioactive properties, and genetic information. *Compr. Rev. Food Sci.* **2021**, *20*, 2534–2559. [CrossRef] [PubMed]

54. Alizadeh Behbahani, B.; Imani Fooladi, A.A. Shirazi balangu (*Lallemantia royleana*) seed mucilage: Chemical composition, molecular weight, biological activity and its evaluation as edible coating on beefs. *Int. J. Biol. Macromol.* **2018**, *114*, 882–889. [CrossRef]
55. Razavi, S.; Cui, S.; Ding, H. Structural and physicochemical characteristics of a novel water-soluble gum from *Lallemantia royleana* seed. *Int. J. Biol. Macromol.* **2016**, *83*, 142–151. [CrossRef]
56. Naji-Tabasi, S.; Razavi, S.M.A.; Mohebbi, M.; Malaekeh-Nikouei, B. New studies on basil (*Ocimum bacilicum* L.) seed gum: Part I—Fractionation, physicochemical and surface activity characterization. *Food Hydrocoll.* **2016**, *52*, 350–358. [CrossRef]
57. Timilsena, Y.; Adhikari, R.; Kasapis, S.; Adhikari, B. Molecular and functional characteristics of purified gum from Australian chia seeds. *Carbohydr. Polym.* **2016**, *136*, 128–136. [CrossRef]
58. Lin, K.Y.; Daniel, J.; Whistler, R. Structure of chia seed polysaccharide exudate. *Carbohyd. Polym.* **1994**, *23*, 13–18. [CrossRef]
59. Praznik, W.; Čavarkapa, A.; Unger, F.M.; Loeppert, R.; Holzer, W.; Viernstein, H.; Mueller, M. Molecular dimension and structural features of neutral polysaccharides from the seed mucilage of *Hyptis suaveolens* L. *Food Chem.* **2016**, *221*, 1997–2004. [CrossRef]
60. Karazhiyan, H.; Razavi, S.; Phillips, G.; Fang, Y.; Al-Assaf, S.; Nishinari, K. Rheological properties of Lepidium sativum seed extract as a function of concentration, temperature and time. *Food Hydrocoll.* **2009**, *23*, 2062–2068. [CrossRef]
61. Alpizar Reyes, E.; Carrillo Navas, H.; Gallardo Rivera, R.; Varela Guerrero, V.; Alvarez Ramirez, J.; Pérez Alonso, C. Functional properties and physicochemical characteristics of tamarind (*Tamarindus indica* L.) seed mucilage powder as a novel hydrocolloid. *J. Food Eng.* **2017**, *209*, 68–75. [CrossRef]
62. Koocheki, A.; Razavi, S.M.A.; Hesarinejad, M.A. Effect of Extraction Procedures on Functional Properties of Eruca sativa Seed Mucilage. *Food Biophys.* **2012**, *7*, 84–92. [CrossRef]
63. Yaseen, E.I.; Herald, T.J.; Aramouni, F.M.; Alavi, S. Rheological properties of selected gum solutions. *Food Res. Int.* **2005**, *38*, 111–119. [CrossRef]
64. Naji-Tabasi, S.; Razavi, S.M.A. New studies on basil (*Ocimum bacilicum* L.) seed gum: Part II—Emulsifying and foaming characterization. *Carbohydr. Polym.* **2016**, *149*, 140–150. [CrossRef] [PubMed]
65. Qian, K.; Cui, S.; Wu, Y.; Goff, H.D. Flaxseed gum from flaxseed hulls: Extraction, fractionation, and characterization. *Food Hydrocoll.* **2012**, *28*, 275–283. [CrossRef]
66. Naji-Tabasi, S.; Razavi, S. Functional properties and applications of basil seed gum: An overview. *Food Hydrocoll.* **2017**, *73*, 313–325. [CrossRef]
67. Muñoz, L.; Natalia, C.; Zúñiga-López, M.; Moncada-Basualto, M.; Haros, C.M. Physicochemical and functional properties of soluble fiber extracted from two phenotypes of chia (*Salvia hispanica* L.) seeds. *J. Food Compos. Anal.* **2021**, *104*, 104138. [CrossRef]
68. Koocheki, A.; Taherian, A.; Bostan, A. Studies on the steady shear flow behavior and functional properties of *Lepidium perfoliatum* seed gum. *Food Res. Int.* **2013**, *50*, 446–456. [CrossRef]
69. Rashid, F.; Ahmed, Z.; Hussain, S.; Huang, J.Y.; Ahmad, A. *Linum usitatissimum* L. seeds: Flax gum extraction, physicochemical and functional characterization. *Carbohydr. Polym.* **2019**, *215*, 29–38. [CrossRef]
70. Nazir, S.; Wani, I.A. Functional characterization of basil (*Ocimum basilicum* L.) seed mucilage. *Bioact. Carbohydr. Diet. Fibre.* **2021**, *25*, 100261. [CrossRef]
71. Jouki, M.; Mortazavi, S.; Tabatabaee, F.; Koocheki, A. Optimization of extraction, antioxidant activity and functional properties of quince seed mucilage by RSM. *Int. J. Biol. Macromol.* **2014**, *66*, 113–124. [CrossRef] [PubMed]
72. Chen, H.H.; Xu, S.Y.; Wang, Z. Gelation properties of flaxseed gum. *Int. J. Food Eng.* **2006**, *77*, 295–303. [CrossRef]
73. Pérez-Orozco, J.; Sanchez-Herrera, L.; Ortiz Basurto, R. Effect of concentration, temperature, pH, co-solutes on the rheological properties of *Hyptis suaveolens* L. mucilage dispersions. *Food Hydrocoll.* **2018**, *87*, 297–306. [CrossRef]
74. Wannerberger, K.; Nylander, T.; Nyman, M. Rheological and Chemical Properties of Mucilage in Different Varieties from Linseed (*Linum usitatissimum*). *Acta Agric. Scand.* **1991**, *41*, 311–319. [CrossRef]
75. Ben-Tov, D.; Idan-Molakandov, A.; Hugger, A.; Ben-Shlush, I.; Günl, M.; Yang, B.; Usadel, B.; Harpaz-Saad, S. The role of COBRA-LIKE 2 function, as part of the complex network of interacting pathways regulating Arabidopsis seed mucilage polysaccharide matrix organization. *Plant J.* **2018**, *94*, 497–512. [CrossRef]
76. Dean, G.; Zheng, H.; Tewari, J.; Huang, J.; Young, D.; Hwang, Y.; Western, T.; Carpita, N.; McCann, M.; Mansfield, S.; et al. The *Arabidopsis MUM2* Gene Encodes a β-Galactosidase Required for the Production of Seed Coat Mucilage with Correct Hydration Properties. *Plant Cell* **2018**, *19*, 4007–4021. [CrossRef]
77. McGee, R.; Dean, G.H.; Mansfield, S.D.; Haughn, G.W. Assessing the utility of seed coat-specific promoters to engineer cell wall polysaccharide composition of mucilage. *Plant Mol. Biol.* **2019**, *101*, 373–387. [CrossRef]
78. Dean, G.H.; Jin, Z.; Shi, L.; Esfandiari, E.; McGee, R.; Nabata, K.; Lee, T.; Kunst, L.; Western, T.L.; Haughn, G.W. Identification of a seed coat-specific promoter fragment from the Arabidopsis MUCILAGE-MODIFIED4 gene. *Plant Mol. Biol.* **2017**, *95*, 33–50. [CrossRef]
79. Zhang, Y.; Yin, Q.; Qin, W.; Gao, H.; Du, J.; Chen, J.; Li, H.; Zhou, G.; Wu, H.; Wu, A. The Class II KNOX family members KNAT3 and KNAT7 redundantly participate in Arabidopsis seed coat mucilage biosynthesis. *J. Exp. Bot.* **2022**, *73*, 3477–3495. [CrossRef]
80. Fabrissin, I.; Cueff, G.; Berger, A.; Granier, F.; Sallé, C.; Poulain, D.; Ralet, M.C.; North, H. Natural Variation Reveals a Key Role for Rhamnogalacturonan I in Seed Outer Mucilage and Underlying Genes. *Plant Physiol.* **2019**, *181*, 1498–1518. [CrossRef]
81. Huang, J.; DeBowles, D.; Esfandiari, E.; Dean, G.; Carpita, N.; Haughn, G. The Arabidopsis Transcription Factor LUH/MUM1 Is Required for Extrusion of Seed Coat Mucilage. *Plant Physiol.* **2011**, *156*, 491–502. [CrossRef] [PubMed]
82. Kong, Y.; Zhou, G.; Abdeen, A.; Schafhauser, J.; Richardson, B.; Atmodjo, M.; Jung, J.; Wicker, L.; Mohnen, D.; Western, T.L.; et al. AtGATL5 is Involved in the Production of Arabidopsis Seed Coat Mucilage. *Plant Physiol.* **2013**, *163*, 1203–1217. [CrossRef] [PubMed]

83. Saez-Aguayo, S.; Rautengarten, C.; Temple, H.; Sanhueza, D.; Ejsmentewicz, T.; Sandoval-Ibañez, O.; Doñas, D.; Parra-Rojas, J.P.; Ebert, B.; Lehner, A.; et al. UUAT1 Is a Golgi-Localized UDP-Uronic Acid Transporter That Modulates the Polysaccharide Composition of Arabidopsis Seed Mucilage. *Plant Cell* **2017**, *29*, 129–143. [CrossRef] [PubMed]
84. Griffiths, J.; Crepeau, M.-J.; Ralet, M.-C.; Seifert, G.; North, H. Dissecting seed mucilage adherence mediated by FEI2 and SOS5. *Front. Plant Sci.* **2016**, *7*, e0145092. [CrossRef] [PubMed]
85. Saez-Aguayo, S.; Ralet, M.C.; Berger, A.; Botran, L.; Ropartz, D.; Marion-Poll, A.; North, H. PECTIN METHYLESTERASE INHIBITOR6 promotes Arabidopsis mucilage release by limiting methylesterification of homogalacturonan in seed coat epidermal cells. *Plant Cell* **2013**, *25*, 308–323. [CrossRef]
86. Soto-Cerda, B.; Cloutier, S.; Quian Ulloa, R.; Gajardo Balboa, H.; Olivos, M.; You, F. Genome-Wide Association Analysis of Mucilage and Hull Content in Flax (*Linum usitatissimum* L.) Seeds. *Int. J. Mol. Sci.* **2018**, *19*, 2870. [CrossRef]
87. Turbant, A.; Fournet, F.; Lequart-Pillon, M.; Zabijak, L.; Pageau, K.; Bouton, S.; Van Wuytswinkel, O. PME58 plays a role in pectin distribution during seed coat mucilage extrusion through homogalacturonan modification. *J. Exp. Bot.* **2016**, *67*, 2177–2190. [CrossRef]
88. Xu, Y.; Wang, Y.; Wang, X.; Pei, S.; Kong, Y.; Hu, R.; Zhou, G. Transcription Factors BLH2 and BLH4 Regulate Demethylesterification of Homogalacturonan in Seed Mucilage. *Plant Physiol.* **2020**, *183*, 96–111. [CrossRef]
89. Sun, J.; Yuan, C.; Wang, M.; Ding, A.; Chai, G.; Sun, Y.; Zhou, G.; Yang, D.H.; Kong, Y. MUD1, a RING-v E3 ubiquitin ligase, has an important role in the regulation of pectin methylesterification in Arabidopsis seed coat mucilage. *Plant Physiol. Biochem.* **2021**, *168*, 230–238. [CrossRef]
90. Han, X.; Zhang, L.; Niu, D.; Shuzhen, N.; Miao, X.; Hu, X.; Li, C.; Fu, H. Transcriptome and co-expression network analysis reveal molecular mechanisms of mucilage formation during seed development in *Artemisia sphaerocephala*. *Carbohydr. Polym.* **2021**, *251*, 117044. [CrossRef]
91. Han, X.; Zhang, L.; Miao, X.; Hu, X.; Shuzhen, N.; Fu, H. Transcriptome analysis reveals the molecular mechanisms of mucilage biosynthesis during *Artemisia sphaerocephala* seed development. *Ind. Crops Prod.* **2020**, *145*, 111991. [CrossRef]
92. Cao, J.; Xu, D.; Huang, D.; Yuan, J.; Zhao, J.; Wang, W.; Lan, H. Cloning, characterization, and functional analysis of seed coat mucilage-related gene TTG1 from *Lepidium perfoliatum*. *Plant Sci. J.* **2014**, *32*, 371–382.

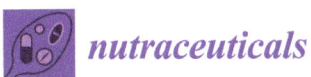

Review

Mushrooms as a Resource for Mibyou-Care Functional Food; The Role of Basidiomycetes-X (Shirayukidake) and Its Major Components

Seiichi Matsugo [1,2], Toshio Sakamoto [3], Koji Wakame [4], Yutaka Nakamura [1], Kenichi Watanabe [5] and Tetsuya Konishi [1,6,*]

[1] Faculty of Applied Life Sciences, Niigata University of Pharmacy and Applied Life Sciences, Higashi-jima, Akiha-ku, Niigata 956-8603, Japan; matsugoh@staff.kanazawa-u.ac.jp (S.M.); nakamura@nupals.ac.jp (Y.N.)
[2] Kanazawa University, Kakuma, Kanazawa 920-1192, Japan
[3] School of Biological Science and Technology, College of Science and Engineering, Kanazawa University, Kakuma, Kanazawa 920-1192, Japan; tsakamot@staff.kanazawa-u.ac.jp
[4] Faculty of Pharmaceutical Sciences, Hokkaido University of Science, Sapporo 006-8585, Japan; wakame-k@hus.ac.jp
[5] Department of Laboratory Medicine and Clinical Epidemiology for Prevention of Noncommunicable Diseases, Niigata University Graduate School of Medical and Dental Sciences, 757, Ichiban-cho, Asahimachi-dori, Chuo-ku, Niigata 951-8510, Japan; wataken@med.niigata-u.ac.jp
[6] Office HALD Food Function Research, Inc., Yuzawamachi Yuzawa, Niigata 949-6102, Japan
* Correspondence: konishi@nupals.ac.jp

Abstract: Mibyou has been defined in traditional oriental medicine as a certain physiological condition whereby an individual is not ill but not healthy; it is also often referred to as a sub-healthy condition. In a society focused on longevity, "Mibyou-care" becomes of primary importance for healthy lifespan expenditure. Functional foods can play crucial roles in Mibyou-care; thus, the search for novel resources of functional food is an important and attractive research field. Mushrooms are the target of such studies because of their wide variety of biological functions, such as immune modulation and anti-obesity and anticancer activities, in addition to their nutritional importance. Basidiomycetes-X (BDM-X; Shirayukidake in Japanese) is a mushroom which has several attractive beneficial health functions. A metabolome analysis revealed more than 470 components of both nutritional and functional interest in BDM-X. Further isolation and purification studies on its components using radical scavenging activity and UV absorbance identified ergosterol, (10E,12Z)-octadeca-10,12-dienoic acid (CLA), 2,3-dihydro-3,5-dihydroxy-6-methyl-4H-pyran-4-one (DDMP), formyl pyrrole analogues (FPA), including 4-[2-foemyl-5-(hydroxymethyl)-1H-pyrrole-1-yl] butanamide (FPAII), adenosine and uridine as major components. Biological activities attributed to these components were related to the observed biological functions of BDM-X, which suggest that this novel mushroom is a useful resource for Mibyou-care functional foods and medicines.

Keywords: Basidiomycetes-X (BDM-X); Shirayukidake; *Ceraceomyces tessulatus*; Mibyou; Mibyou-care functional food; healthy lifespan expenditure

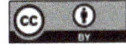

1. Introduction

As lifespans lengthen in developed countries, demands for a healthy lifespan are increasing, that is the life period, during which individuals are able to enjoy their health and well-being life without hospitalization or with the least amount of nursing care. Under these circumstances, "Mibyou"—a concept which originated in ancient oriental medicine—has been reevaluated, which refers to a certain physiological condition whereby an individual is not healthy but also not ill, leading to serious diagnosed endpoint diseases [1]. Mibyou-care is thus considered an important strategy for healthy life expenditure even in current preventive medicines.

According to the development of clinical examination technologies for diagnosing diseases, such as the biochemical assay of disease markers, and physical methods, including ultrasound and CT imaging, the definition of Mibyou has been updated in Western medicine as Mibyou I and II [2]. Mibyou I covers the condition in which individuals feel some unusual symptoms, such as malaise, anxiety, fatigue and pain, but clinical examinations do not show a significant abnormality. In Mibyou II, disease markers indicate certain disorders, but individuals can enjoy a normal life with the least amount of medical interventions (Figure 1).

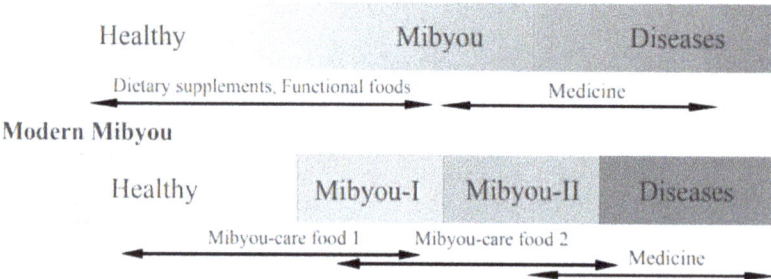

Figure 1. Traditional and modern Mibyou concept and Mibyou-care functional food.

The term "Mibyou-care" thus covers a wide range of practices, including daily routines such as self-medication, remedies, diet, exercise, brain storming, yoga and other activities with and without medical intervention for treating Mibyou; consequently, Mibyou-care is considered to be a basic strategy for maintaining health and well-being, both socially and individually. Functional foods and nutritional or dietary supplements obviously play important roles in Mibyou-care practices together with daily meals; thus, their roles are comprehensively discussed in the category of Mibyou-care functional food [3].

1.1. Mibyou-Care Functional Foods and Their Targets

Mibyou-care functional foods are broadly defined as any type of food used for Mibyou-care; that is, for disease prevention and the preservation of health and well-being. They therefore cover a wide range of food types, including nutrient-enriched fruits and vegetables and processed foods, as well as functional foods, such as food for special health use (FOSHU), nutraceuticals and medicinal food; all of these can be comprehensively grouped in the category of Mibyou-care functional foods. According to the purpose of their usage and application targets, they are currently classified into two categories: Mibyou-care functional foods 1 and 2 [3].

Mibyou-care functional food 1 is essentially used for disease prevention, health preservation and slowing the aging phenomena, and is used by healthy individuals as well as Mibyou I patients. Their major target is factors regulating metabolic homeostasis, such as immune, endocrine and neural systems, since distorted homeostatic potential is implicated as a primary condition of Mibyou in traditional oriental medicine. Foods and nutritional supplements with astringent and nourishing functions are included in this category. On the other hand, functional foods such as FOSHU and dietary supplements distributed in the current market are typical examples of Mibyou-care functional food 2. Their functions are characterized by food factors, with certain medicinal activity contributing to the treatment of Mibyou II conditions. As a result, disease markers are the target for managing respective conditions, such that levels of blood sugar, glycated proteins, blood pressure and LDL cholesterol are used to care for diabetic complications [4], and salivary AGE is suggested to be useful in the diagnosis of dementia [5]. Gsa (heterotrimeric G protein alpha) also could be a blood marker for diagnosing depression and evaluating anti-depressant drug effects [6].

Therefore, nutritional and pharmacological functions are both factors which are essential for Mibyou-care functional foods. In this context, edible mushrooms are an attractive target to be studied as a resource of Mibyou-care functional food, because they have been traditionally accepted as a food with health benefits and anti-aging functions [7].

1.2. Mushrooms as a Typical Resource for Mibyou-Care Functional Food

Mushrooms are not only a cuisine containing rich nutrients including vitamins and minerals [8], but they are also a medicinal resource with a variety of pharmacological functions [9,10], such as modulating immunity [11], being anticancer [12,13] and even preventing dementia [14]. Indeed, a recent meta-analysis on cohort studies indicates that mushroom consumption will reduce the risk of several diseases including cancer, and will therefore reduce the risk of mortality [15]. The social benefit of eating mushrooms has also been discussed in terms of reducing depression in the stressful conditions caused by the COVID-19 pandemic [16]. Large molecular components, such as polysaccharides including β-glucans, were primarily implicated as active principles in mushroom functions, and their anticancer function was discussed in the context of their immune modulation activity [17]. However, bioactive lower molecular weight components are also attracting significant attention, since phenylpropanoids isolated from *Inonotus obliquus (Chaga)*, for example, showed cancer cell cytotoxicity [18]. Now, a variety of components from low molecular weight compounds, such as simple phenolics, flavonoids and terpenoids, to large molecular weight components, such as polysaccharides, have been reported as the active principles of mushrooms [19–22], in addition to bioactive peptides and proteins such as ribotoxin-like protein [23,24]; their roles have been comprehensively discussed by Sanchez [25]. In addition to their nutrient composition, these bioactive ingredients characterize mushrooms as a promised resource for Mibyou-care functional food.

1.3. Basidiomycetes-X as a Mibyou-Care Functional Food Resource

Since mushrooms are part of the fungi family, which is a large biological kingdom [26], the search for new species of mushrooms with beneficial functions for human health is another important field of study. Basidiomycetes-X (BDM-X, Japanese name; Shirayuki-dake) is one such novel mushroom, which was originally isolated and cultivated in the mountainous district of Niigata, Japan. It was registered on the database for patented resources in Tsukuba, Ibaragi, Japan in 1999 (PCT/JP2004/006418) as a new mushroom species belonging to the Basidiomycota, which uniquely does not form mycelium. A more precise gene analysis identified BDM-X as one of the strains of *Ceraceomyces tessulatus*.

It is now artificially cultivated and provided as a cuisine, as well as a resource of functional food and medicine (Figure 2). Functional studies of BDM-X are currently progressing and have unveiled several physiological and pharmacological functions such as being anti-oxidative, anti-obesity and diabetic, and offering liver damage protection including NASH, as reviewed elsewhere [27]. The search for a functional component is also simultaneously being developed [28,29].

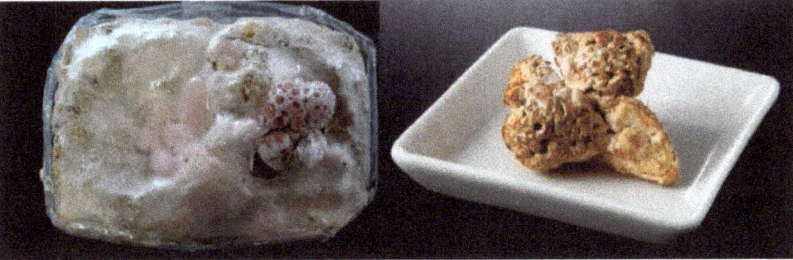

Figure 2. BDM-X culture and mycelium mass (provided by Mycology Techno Co. Ltd. in Niigata city, Japan).

1.4. Metabolome Analysis of BDM-X

To evaluate the potential of BDM-X as a functional food resource, profiling nutritionally and pharmacologically interesting components is of primary importance. Metabolomics is currently attracting attention as a method for profiling the comprehensive distribution of primary and secondary metabolites functioning in natural resources [30]. This method was applied to qualify lipophilic and hydrophilic low molecular weight organic components in BDM-X, to evaluate their nutritional and pharmacological significance. The Wide-Processed Metabolome (WPM) analysis, utilizing measurements via EC-MS and LC-MS, allowed us to detect at least 472 components (368 hydrophilic and 104 lipophilic compounds) in the BDM-X extract, which matched the migration time (MT) and mass-to-charge ratio (m/z) of the annotation list [31]. These include common nutrients such as amino acids, both saturated and unsaturated fatty acids, nucleotides, sugars, steroids such as ergosterol, testosterone and other secondary metabolites, including several unidentified components in addition to a variety of types of di- and tri-peptides. This wide variety of component distribution indicates the nutritional and pharmacological significance of this unique mushroom, as well as other edible mushrooms [19,23]. Notably, the metabolome analysis revealed the presence of several polyphenols, which were mainly flavonoids. The polyphenols qualitatively identified in BDM-X are as follows: 7,8-Dihydroxycoumarin, 7-Hydroxycoumarin, apigenin-7-*O*-glucoside, apigenin-8-*C*-glucoside, eriodictyol-7-*O*-neohesperidoside, eriocitrin, gallocatechin, chrysin, quercetin, delphinidin, baicalin and luteolin; their chemical structures are given in Figure 3. Polyphenols are a well-known food factor carrying anti-oxidant and anti-inflammatory functions, which play crucial roles in preventing oxidative stress-related disorders [32], and flavonoids such as apigenin and quercetin listed above are typical of them. It is generally known that the major polyphenols functioning as anti-oxidants in mushrooms are simple phenolic compounds such as phenolic acids, and flavonoids are minor since it is implicated that humans and fungi are not able to biosynthesize flavonoids [33,34]. The metabolome data suggest that the major polyphenolics in BDM-X are flavonoids, and not simple phenolic compounds. Moreover, antioxidant compounds such as ergothioneine and vitamin E, which are another group of antioxidant components found in edible mushrooms [35], were also not found in BDM-X by metabolomics and subsequent selective isolation studies [28,29]. Although the flavonoids listed above were not detected as a major ingredient in BDM-X through the isolation study, this wide variety of flavonoid distribution is unique and will significantly contribute not only to the antioxidant potential of BDM-X, but also to other physiological functions, which are both already cleared or yet to be uncovered. Further quantitative studies are required.

1.5. Selective Isolation and Quantification of Major Ingredients

Although the metabolome analysis identified more than 470 components of BDM-X, including a series of nutrients and the candidates of food factors, their quantitative information is limited. A further analysis of the specific components which may play significant roles in the beneficial health functions of BDM-X was carried out by solvent extraction following HPLC and TLC. The major components with UV absorption and/or DPPH radical scavenging activity were targeted for isolation, and the structures of purified compounds were assigned using mass spectrometry (MS) and nuclear magnetic resonance (NMR) [28,29]. From these studies, three types of formyl pyrrole alkaloids (FPA), ergosterol, (10*E*,12*Z*)-octadeca-10,12-dienoic acid ((10*E*,12*Z*)-CLA), 2,3-dihydro-3,5-dihydroxy-6-methyl-4*H*-pyran-4-one (DDMP), and two nucleosides, adenosine and uridine, were determined as the major ingredients existing at relatively high amounts and showing high or moderate DPPH radical scavenging activities in BDM-X. Their approximate contents determined in BDM-X are summarized in Table 1, and their chemical structures are given in Figure 4.

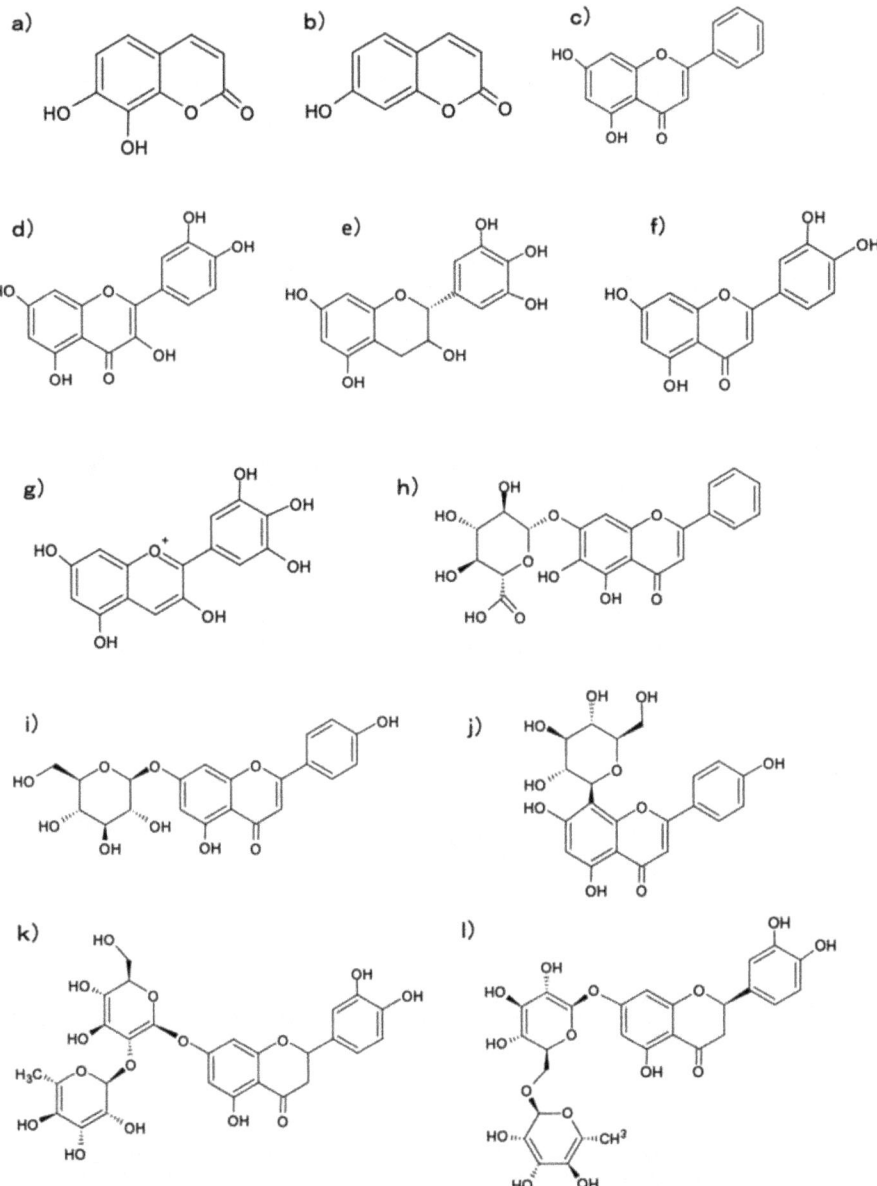

Figure 3. Polyphenols identified by a metabolome analysis. (**a**) 7,8-dihydroxycoumarin; (**b**) 7-hydroxycoumarin; (**c**) chrysin; (**d**) quercetin; (**e**) gallocatechin; (**f**) luteolin; (**g**) delphinidin; (**h**) baicalin; (**i**) apigenin-7-*O*-gucoside; (**j**) apigenin-8-*C*-glucoside; (**k**) eriocitrin; (**l**) eriodictyol-7-*O*-neohesperidoside.

Table 1. Approximate contents of major compounds identified in BDM-X.

Compound Identified	Structure Symbol in Figure 4	Contents (mg per 100 g BDM-X Dry Powder)	References
FPA-I	M	82.5	[28]
FPA-II	N	48.4	[28]
FPA-III	O	1.2	[28]
adenosine	P	42.4	[29]
uridine	Q	76.9	[29]
DDMP	R	350.0	[29]
ergosterol	S	16.7	[29]
(10E,12Z)-CLA	T	19.8	[29]

FPA-I; 4-[2-formyl-5-(hydroxymethyl)-1H-pyrrole-1-yl] butanoic acid, FPA-II; 4-[2-formyl-5-(hydroxymethyl)-1H-pyrrole-1-yl] butanamide, FPA-III; 5-(hydroxymethyl)-1H-pyrrole-2-carboxaldehyde.

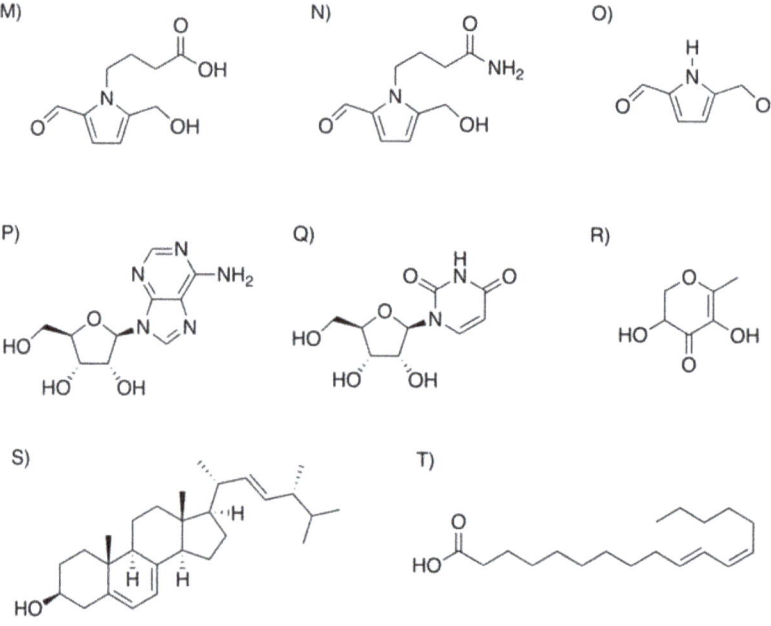

Figure 4. Structures of the major compounds identified in BDM-X (compound names are given in Table 1).

1.6. Role of the Major Components in Mibyou-Care Function of BDM-X

Among these identified components, formyl pyrrole analogue (FPA) carrying butyramide side chain (FPA-II) was the only new compound found in this mushroom, and is therefore a specific ingredient of BDM-X. Other compounds isolated and identified as major components of BDM-X are not new and commonly exist in many other food resources, including mushrooms. However, their nutritional and pharmacological functions suggest their pivotal role in the Mibyou-care function of BDM-X.

1.6.1. FPA

FPAs are commonly distributed in a wide variety of biological resources, and their structures are also varied [36]. FPA-I and -III are found in other sources such as *Morus alba* fruits (Bilberry fruit) [37], *Inonotus obliquus* (Chaga) [38], *Lycium chinense* fruits [39,40] and *Leccinum Extremiorientale* [41]; they show a range of bioactivities including being anti-oxidant and anti-inflammation, cancer chemoprevention, macrophage activation, hepatoprotective action, and anti-obesity and anti-diabetes functions.

Since the FPA-II-carrying *N*-butyramide structure was first found in BDM-X, the FPA-II was chemically synthesized in order to assign the precise structure and to obtain enough test samples for further functional studies, as shown in Figure 5. The structure of the isolated sample assigned by spectrometry, including NMR (^{1}H, ^{13}C 2D-NMR) and MS, was further confirmed by comparing all spectral patterns with this synthesized FPA-II. The biochemical and pharmacological functions of FPA-II therefore await clarification.

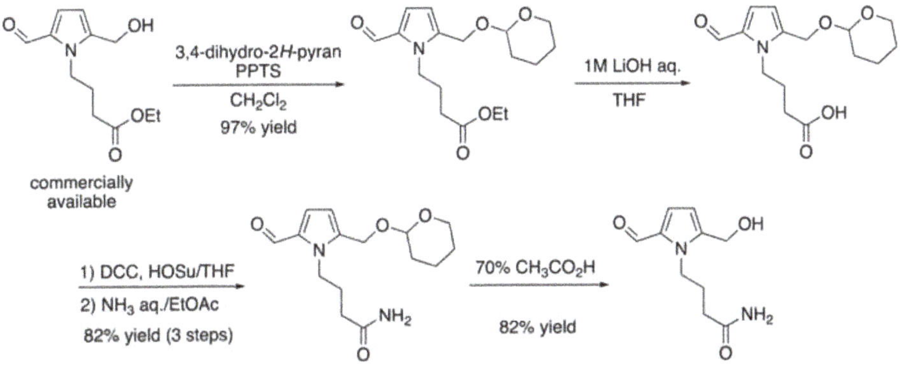

Figure 5. Synthetic route of newly found formyl pyrrole analogue in BDDM-X. Abbreviations: (PPTS; pyridinium *p*-toluenesulfonate, DCC; N,N'-dicyclohexylcarbodiimide, HOSu; N-hydroxysuccinimide, THF; tetrahydrofuran, EtOAc; ethyl acetate).

Since the formyl pyrrole structure (FPA-I) is chemically synthesized by the reaction of glucose and γ-butyric acid in strong acidic conditions in low yield [42], there are some discussions as to the origin of FPAs, and whether they are biosynthesized or artificially generated during the process of manufacturing dried powder. Since it is more difficult to consider the formation of FPA-bearing butyramide side chain (FPA-II) compared to FPA-I, the biosynthetic pathway of FPA-II is another target to be challenged for clarification.

1.6.2. DDMP

DDMP was identified as a major component with strong DPPH radical scavenging activity in the aqueous extract of BDM-X [29]. It is also isolated from several resources other than fungi, such as *lactobacterium* [43] and onion [44], and reported to have several physiological functions, such as being anti-inflammatory, anti-mutagenic and having cancer cell toxicity and affecting autonomic neurons. Tyrosinase inhibitory activity reported for DDMP is interesting because BDM-X has potential for cosmetic use [45]. DDMP, on the other hand, is implicated as a Maillard reaction product [46] which has mutagenic activity [47]. Further study is required for DDMP functioning as a food factor in BDM-X; the mechanism of biosynthetic production also awaits clarification.

1.6.3. Ergosterol

Ergosterol is a common component of fungal cytoplasmic membranes and plays a role in modulating membrane fluidity, similarly to the role of cholesterol in mammals; it is found in a variety of fungi or mushrooms [48]. Ergosterol is a well-known precursor of vitamin D. Ingested ergosterol is metabolized in the liver to ergocalciferol as provitamin D, and then converted to vitamins D3 with the assistance of a UV light [49]. Vitamin D is a source of hard skeletal structures such as bones and teeth, but it also contributes to the maintenance of muscle. Besides these essential roles as micronutrients, vitamin D plays a crucial role in many functions related to Mibyou-care, such as immune modulation [50], inflammation [51], hypertension and cardiovascular disease [52] and cancer [53]. A high ergosterol content in BDM-X as a vitamin D precursor suggests that BDM-X indirectly manipulates these functions.

1.6.4. CLA

CLA is known as one of the essential fatty acids which is a necessary nutrient, functioning both as energy fuel and as a component of cellular membranes, as well as a biosynthetic precursor of signaling molecules [54]. Moreover, pharmacological functions of CLA are currently attracting much attention [55,56] for their anti-obesity [57], anti-carcinogenic [58], anti-hypertensive [56] and immune modulating functions [59]. There are several isomers in which 9 c,11 t-18:2 and 10 t,12 c-18:2 isomers are the most representative. Although 9 c,11 t-18:2 is the most popular isomer found in dietary substances, the major CLA found in BDM-X is the 10 t,12 c isomer. The differential function of these isomers attracts additional attention, so that both isomers have high anti-inflammatory potential different from other fatty acids, but the activity is much higher in the 10 c,12 t isomer [60].

1.6.5. Adenosine and Uridine

Adenosine is a well-known nutrient molecule necessary for nucleic acids, DNA and RNA, as well as energy fuel molecule, ATP. Other phosphorylated derivatives, ADP and AMP, are metabolic intermediates acting as signaling molecules to regulate AMP kinase, which plays a pivotal role in energy homeostasis [61]. Moreover, free adenosine itself behaves as a signal molecule to modulate a variety of physiological functions related to pain, cancer and neurodegenerative, inflammatory and autoimmune diseases through interactions with adenosine receptors A1, A2A, A2B and A3 [62]. Therefore, adenosine externally taken might behave as a food factor contributing to physiological homeostasis, either directly or indirectly.

Uridine is a pyrimidine nucleoside and is a component of RNA. It is also the precursor for brain phosphatide biosynthesis, together with choline and DHA; the external administration of uridine together with DHA is therefore thought to increase synaptic proteins in the brain to protect brain aging [63].

1.6.6. β-Glucan

The presence of abundant polysaccharides besides low molecular functional ingredients is one of the characteristics of fungal resources, and the role of polysaccharides has been extensively discussed in the cancer preventive function of mushrooms [64]. BDM-X also contains polysaccharides in very high amounts—approximately 33 w/w%—and β-glucans (13% w/w) are one of the characteristic sugar components of BDM-X [27]. It is known that β-glucans play a critical role in the inert immune modulating activity of mushrooms as pathogen-associated molecular pattern molecules (PAMPs) to stimulate toll-like receptor 2 (TLR2) [65]. The possible application of BDM-X as a high β-glucan resource has previously been discussed in relation to the immune modulator used during the COVID-19 pandemic [66]. Preventing obesity is another important function of β-glucans as a source of dietary fiber [67].

1.7. Medicinal and Pharmacological Functions of BDM-X Contributing to Mibyou-Care

So far, several animal and human studies on the medicinal functions of BDM-X have been carried out and are summarized in Table 2; these include antioxidant protection [68], anti-obesity effects [69,70], hepatoprotective functions [69,71,72] and immune modulation, including the ameliorative effect on atopic dermatitis [73,74]. It is worth discussing the possible contribution of identified BDM-X components to those already known, as well as other unpublished functions.

Table 2. Reported biological and pharmacological functions of BDM-X.

	Medicinal Functions	Exp. System	Test Sample Form	Experimental and Results	Refs.
1	Antioxidant activity	in vitro, in situ	Aqueous extract	BDM-X prevented AAPH induced peroxidation in rat liver homogenate. Pre-administration of BDM-X to rat prevented nitrotyrosine formation followed LPS induced liver injury.	[68]
2	Anti-obesity, anti-diabetic and liver protective function	Male albino rat and OLETOF rat	BDM-X powder and extracts	BDM-X supplementation suppressed weight gain, visceral fat deposit and fatty liver injury caused by 15 weeks feeding on an HFHS diet, and ameliorated insulin sensitivity and adiponectin expression.	[69,70]
3	Amelioration of atopic dermatitis in humans	Human	BDM-X powder	Oral intake of BDM-X powder for two weeks ameliorated atopic dermatitis symptoms in volunteers.	[74]
4	Alleviation of atopic dermatitis in mice	Mouse	BDM-X powder	BDM-X administration to atopic dermatitis (AD) induced by house dust mite extract application in NC/Nga mouse attenuated ADlike clinical symptoms through modulating Th1/Th2 responses.	[73]
5	Prevention of nonalcoholic steatohepatitis (NASH)	Mouse	BDM-X powder	In NASH-HCC mice (C57BL/6J female pups) model produced by STZ-high fat diet treatment, BDM-X prevented pathogenesis of NASH by preventing inflammation and lipogenesis.	[71,72]
6	Hepatoprotective function	Human	BDM-X powder	The effect and safety of BDM-X on fatty liver were evaluated by a stratified randomized double-blind parallel group comparison.	[75]

Abbreviations: AAPH; 2,2′-azobis (2-amindino-propane) dihydrochloride, PS; lipopolysaccharide, HFHS diet; high fat, high sucrose diet, STZ; streptozotocin, HCC; hepatocellular carcinoma.

1.7.1. Protection against Oxidative Stress and Inflammation

Antioxidant and anti-inflammatory activities are a basic requirement of Mibyou-care functional foods, because they commonly occur in life processes to distort metabolic homeostasis, and are implicated as a causative factor of not only aging deterioration, but also pathogenesis and the progression of many diseases [33,76].

BDM-X has high potential for antioxidant or free radical scavenging activities, especially against the hydroxyl radical, which is the ultimate reactive species damaging cellular components including DNA by its hydrogen abstraction mechanism [77]. There are many antioxidant molecules which have been reported as quenching the hydroxyl radical effectively in vitro, but a few are also active in vivo. However, BDM-X has effective hydroxyl radical scavenging potential in vivo, too; it was previously shown that orally given BDM-X effectively prevented lipopolysaccharide induced liver damage in rodents, and nitrotyrosine formation, which is the marker of the hydroxyl radical induced damage, was also inhibited [68]. This early observation on the hydroxyl radical scavenging potential of BDM-X is rationalized by the action of major BDM-X ingredients listed in Table 2, especially FPAs, CLA, ergosterol and nucleotides, because they have the hydrogen atom as a target of hydroxyl radical attack. Indeed, the hydroxyl radical scavenging and cancer chemo preventive activity of Goji berry originated FPA-I has been reported [40].

Besides the hydroxyl radical scavenging activity, the high antioxidant potential of BDM-X has been proved by several other assay methods in vitro, such as DPPH radical scavenging activity, Fe^{3+}-reducing ability, Cu^{2+}-reducing ability and Fe^{2+}-chelating activity [78]. The total phenolic content in the aqueous extract determined elsewhere was as high as 8.1 mg gallic acid equivalent/g dry powder, and this value is comparable with the values reported for edible anti-oxidative mushrooms from Poland (3–12.8 mg gallic acid/g) [79]. This indicates that a series of polyphenols, mainly flavonoids, determined by the metabolome analysis (Figure 3) will also provide a significant contribution to the antioxidant potential of BDM-X. Since the oxidative damages are mediated by the reactive species with diverse reactivity and cellular localization in vivo, the synergistic functions of antioxidant components with different reactivity are also implicated in the high antioxidant potential of BDM-X.

1.7.2. Anti-Obesity and Anti-Metabolic Syndromes Function of BDM-X

Obesity is one of the major targets of Mibyou-care, because it is the major pathogenic condition of diabetes and related diseases including cardiac failure, stroke, dementia and cancer [80]. BDM-X has been shown to have a marked anti-obesity function in rodents, whereby male albino rats and genetically obese rats (OLETF) were fed a high-fat/high-sucrose (HFHS) diet with and without DBM-X supplementation for 90 days [69,70]. BDM-X supplementation markedly inhibited body weight gain, reduced visceral fat deposits and improved insulin tolerance acquired by the HFHS diet. Supporting this observation, anti-obesity and anti-diabetic functions have been studied for FPAs [36] and CLA [57], which were detected as the major components of BDM-X in addition to β-glucan as dietary fiber [67]. Polyphenols, typically catechins, have also been reported for their anti-obesity function through the manipulation of lipid metabolism [81]. Moreover, the high antioxidant and inflammation activities of BDM-X sustained by these antioxidant components including polyphenols [82] will obviously contribute to the regulation of insulin sensitivity, as was observed in HFHS feeding experiments [69,70].

1.7.3. Hepatoprotective Function of BDM-X

A strong hepatoprotective effect is one of the attractive pharmacological functions of BDM-X. Long-term feeding of an HFHS diet produced a fatty liver and increased the level of transaminases as the liver injury marker in rats, but BDM-X supplementation in the diet suppressed these changes [69], indicating their hepatoprotective function. The liver-protective function of BDM-X was further studied in the rodent model of non-alcoholic steatohepatitis (NASH), where NASH was induced by streptozotocin (STZ) in combination with feeding an HFHS diet [71,72]. NASH is the chronic liver disease regarded as Mibyou II, which can lead to liver cancer, and is closely associated with obesity and diabetes [83]. Gavage administration of BDM-X to mice in the nonalcoholic fatty liver stage (NAFLD) effectively prevented disease progression into NASH and inhibited fibrosis (Figure 6). The dietary supplemented BDM-X attenuated an enhanced expression of sterol regulatory element binding protein isoform (SREBP-I) and peroxisome proliferator-activated receptors (PPAR-alfa) during the development of NASH, indicating that BDM-X primarily manipulates lipogenesis in the liver [72]. The finding that BDM-X enhanced adiponectin expression in obese rats also suggests that BDM-X manipulates lipid metabolism, which leads to the prevention of obesity and fatty liver formation [70]. The ameliorative effect of BDM-X on fatty liver was also currently evaluated in humans by a randomized, double-blind, parallel-group comparison study, and a significant improvement of aminotransferase enzyme level was observed [75].

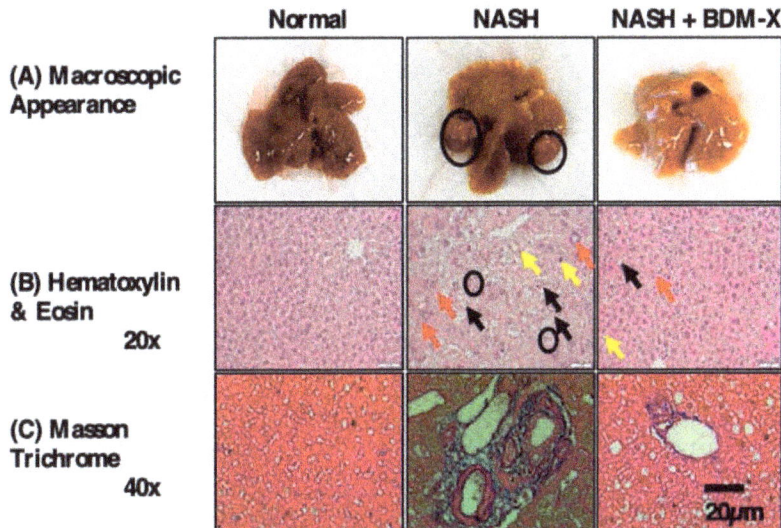

Figure 6. BDM-X attenuates clinicopathology in NASH-HCC mice. (**A**) Representative macroscopic appearance of livers (circles: liver tumors). (**B**) Hematoxylin/eosin staining (black arrow: macrovesicular steatosis, yellow arrow: microvesicular steatosis, red arrow: hypertrophy, circles: inflammatory cells). (**C**) Fibrosis deposition by Masson's trichrome staining (blue area). Normal, age-matched mice subjected to a normal diet; NASH, streptozotocin injected mice subjected to being fed a high-fat diet up to 16 weeks of age; NASH+BDM-X; streptozotocin injected mice subjected to the high-fat diet, treated with BDM-X (500 mg/Kg/day) from the age of 12 weeks to 16 weeks. Scale bar = 20 μm.

Liver disorders include NASH associated with oxidative stress and inflammation. The antioxidant components of BDM-X, including CLA, especially 10 c, 12 t CLA, ergosterol and adenosine, also convey anti-inflammatory activities and are therefore expected to contribute to the hepatoprotective function of BDM-X. FPA-I has the hepatoprotective function which reportedly carries anti-inflammatory and anti-oxidative stress activities [38,39]. It is also important to note that polyphenols, including flavonoids typically, display anti-inflammatory activities as well as anti-oxidant activities [84]. Indeed, the hepatoprotective function of flavonoids such as quercetin and naringin, for example, have been reported [85,86]. Therefore, the comprehensive and synergistic actions by these BDM-X components will be reflected in the effective prevention and amelioration of inflammation disorders, and typically liver damage diseases including NASH.

1.7.4. Immune Modulating Function

Regarding homeostasis regulation, the immune system is of primary importance [87] and is therefore the target of Mibyou-care, especially Mibyou I. Mushrooms have attracted attention as immune modulators because of their rich nutrients, encompassing both major and micro-nutrients, and also due to the presence of food factors, which modulate immune cell activity [88]. The immune activating function of polysaccharides, especially β-glucan, has been discussed mainly in relation to cancer therapy [89], and certain polysaccharide fractions such as Krestin are clinically used as medication to treat cancer [90].

BDM-X is also predicted to have immune modulation activity because of the high contents of β-glucan (13% w/w). Other components identified in BDM-X, especially FPAs and CLA, are reported to modulate immune cell activation [39,59]. Adenosine acts as an endogenous modulator of inert immunity, which plays a crucial role in Mibyou I care [91]. Ergosterol is another component, probably indirectly modulating the immune system through the formation of Vitamin D as an immunity modulator [50]. The effects associated with these major components may explain the observed functions of BDM-X, such as inhibition and amelioration of atopic dermatitis reported both in rodent [73] and human studies [74], where antioxidant and anti-inflammatory functions also have cooperative roles. Indeed, histochemical observation showed that BDM-X manipulated the accumulation of inflammatory must cells in the damaged skin of the atopic dermatitis model mice (Figure 7).

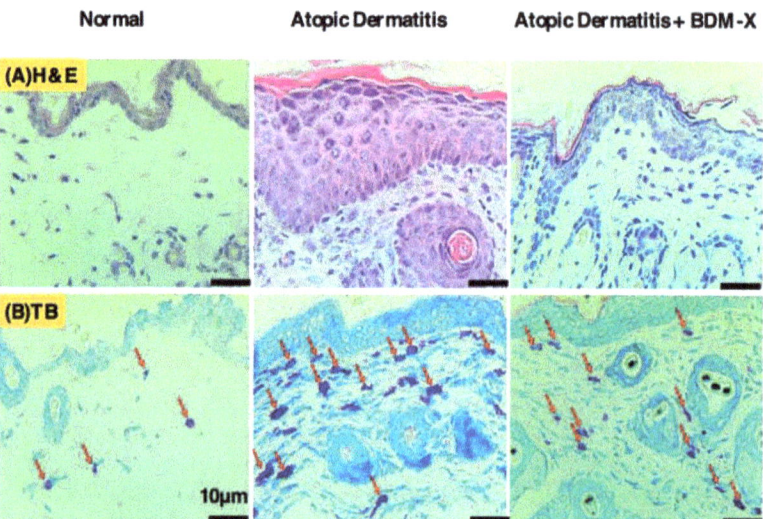

Figure 7. BDM-X treatment improves histopathological changes in atopic dermatitis in mice. (**A**) Hematoxylin/eosin (H&E) staining of the cross-sectional tissue slices of skin showing hyperkeratosis, parakeratosis, acanthosis and spongiosis. (**B**) Skin levels of mast cells (red arrow) by toluidine blue (TB) staining. Scale bar = 10 μm.

1.7.5. Cancer Preventive Function

The cancer immune activation is another aspect of the BDM-X function. There are a few preliminary unpublished observations, such that BDM-X administration stimulated lymphocyte formation in the spleen of rodents and increased cancer cell specific lymphocytes in the blood of a stage IV cancer patient. β-glucan is implicated as an active principle, but the contribution of lower molecular weight components determined in BDM-X is also plausible, since the chemo preventive function against cancer cells is reported for FPAs [36,40], CLA [58,92] and DDMP [44,93]. More precise studies are required before establishing the possible application of BDM-X in cancer prevention as a functional food to stimulate cancer immunity in Mibyou-care routines [88], as well as in the treatment of cancer in complimentary medicine as an adjuvant in chemo- and radio-therapies.

1.7.6. Other Prospective Functions

From the reported bioactivities of the respective components discussed above, BDM-X is an attractive research target for the study of functions such as blood pressure control, cardiovascular disease and the prevention of neuronal diseases, including dementia. For example, a BDM-X component, especially CLA, having high antioxidant and anti-inflammatory potential is reported to prevent neuroinflammatory conditions leading to brain damage [94].

There are currently many disorders including those described above, which are extensively discussed in relation to microbiome [95–97], and the β-glucans are the typical ingredient which can modulate intestinal bacterial flora [98]. However, the effect of other BDM-X components on intestinal bacteria also attracts attention besides their conventional pharmacological effects. We preliminarily observed that the long-term ingestion of BDM-X in rodents affected intestinal microbiome, so as to decrease certain bacterial families such as *Allobaculum*, which is associated with obesity, and to increase *Bacteroides* (not published). Therefore, further studies are warranted to clarify the effects of BDM-X and ingredients on gut bacteria.

1.8. Characteristic Feature of BDM-X as Mibyou-Care Functional Food

Among the major components of BDM-X, FPAs and DDMP are xenobiotics, but others are physiological substances. Pharmacologically interesting food factors are commonly xenobiotics such as polyphenols and dietary fibers, but it turns out that some cellular or physiological components show certain pharmacological functions, and are therefore called metabolic intermediate-type food factors, as exemplified by squalene [99]. Xenobiotics as a pharmacologically active substance obviously contribute to observed food functions, but latter-type food factors also play pivotal roles, especially in Mibyou-care, as shown by examples such as branched amino acids, especially leucine, which modulate skeletal muscle remodeling through attenuating inflammation [100] and Omega-3 fatty acids, especially EPA, which behave as an anti-inflammatory substance to prevent neuronal diseases [101]. Similarly, adenosine and uridine found in BDM-X as the major component make a significant contribution as metabolic intermediate-type food factors in the Mibyou-care functions of BDM-X.

Mibyou-care also involves medical intervention, especially in Mibyou II care. Although the mechanism of food factor action as a pharmacologically active molecule is rationalized by ligand–receptor interaction, the specificity and binding strength of food factors are generally weak compared to medicine, and strong pharmacological activity is therefore not the primary requirement of food factors [102]. Metabolic intermediate-type food factors, including adenosine and uridine as signaling molecules [103], might play a pivotal role in the homeostatic regulation of physiological reactions, which is one of the basic targets of Mibyou-care. In this context, the biological response modifier (BRM) effect that was primarily implicated for the anticancer function of mushrooms [104] might be important as an underlying mechanism of the Mibyou-care function of BDM-X.

Although the pharmacological contributions of respective components have not been precisely studied yet, comprehensive action, including synergism among the components, is considered to play a pivotal role in the beneficial health functions of BDM-X as an edible mushroom, and characterizing the potential of BDM-X as a Mibyou-care functional food.

2. Conclusions

The major components identified in BDM-X strongly indicate that BDM-X has attractive properties, which may play significant roles in Mibyou-care practice as a cuisine and also as functional food resources. Its medicinal application should also be further discussed elsewhere.

Further mechanistic studies are needed at a molecular level to understand how the isolated components, especially FPA-II, are involved in the observed functions of BDM-X. However, the discussion above indicates that BDM-X itself is a promising food applicable to Mibyou-care, especially Mibyou I care.

Author Contributions: Conceptualization, T.K.; validation, S.M., T.S., K.W. (Koji Wakame), K.W. (Kenichi Watanabe), and Y.N.; resources, T.K., S.M., T.S., K.W. (Koji Wakame), K.W. (Kenichi Watanabe). and Y.N.; data curation, T.S., K.W. (Koji Wakame), K.W. (Kenichi Watanabe). and Y.N.; writing—original draft preparation, T.K.; writing—review and editing, T.K., S.M., T.S., K.W. (Koji Wakame). and Y.N.; visualization, K.W. (Koji Wakame), K.W. (Kenichi Watanabe). and Y.N.; project administration, T.K.; funding acquisition, T.K. All authors have read and agreed to the published version of the manuscript.

Funding: This review paper is not funded by any profit or organization. Original studies by coauthors sited here were funded by several sources of grant including the grant from the Ministry of Education, Culture, Sports, Science and Technology of Japan for K. Watanabe (23602012), and from the Promotion and Mutual Aid Corporation for Private Schools, Japan for K. Watanabe (26460239) and also T.K., and from the Joint research contract with Kanazawa University and Mycology Techno Co., Ltd. (Niigata, Japan) for T. S. These are described in their original papers published.

Institutional Review Board Statement: None of the data presented in this study required approval from any institution or board.

Informed Consent Statement: There are no descriptions in this study which need informed consent agreement.

Data Availability Statement: None.

Conflicts of Interest: The authors declare no conflict of interest.

Abbreviations

CT	Computed Tomography
HPLC	High-Performance Liquid Chromatography
GC	Gas Chromatography
GC-MS	Gas Chromatography-Mass Spectroscopy
EC-MS	Electrochemical Mass Spectroscopy
LC-MS	Liquid Chromatography Mass Spectroscopy
NMR	Nuclear Magnetic Resonance
UV	Ultraviolet
DPPH	2,2-Diphenyl-1-Dipicryl Hydrazyl Radical

References

1. *Yellow Emperor's Classic of Internal Medicine*; Veithy, L., Translator; 1975, Foreword by Barnes L.L.; University of California Press: Orkland, CA, USA, 2016.
2. Fukuo, Y. Destructive creation in the Reiwa Era Utilization of "The concept of Modern Mibyou" as Presymptomatic Medicine. *J. Int. Soc. Inf. Sci.* **2020**, *38*, 15.
3. Konishi, T. Mibyou Care is A Key for Healthy Life Elongation: The Role of Mibyou-Care Functional Foods. In *Complementary Therapies*; Bernardo-Filho, M., Ed.; IntechOpen: London, UK, 2021. [CrossRef]
4. Hussain, N. Implications of using HBA1c as a diagnostic marker for diabetes. *Diabetol. Int.* **2016**, *7*, 18–24. [CrossRef] [PubMed]
5. Choromanska, M.; Klimiuk, A.; Kostecka-Sochon, P.; Wilczynska, K.; Kwiatkowski, M.; Okuniewska, N.; Waszkiewicz, N.; Zalewska, A.; Maciejczyk, M. Antioxidant Defense, Oxidative Stress and Oxidative Damage in Saliva, Plasma and Erythrocytes of Dementia Patients. Can Salivary AGE be a Marker of Dementia? *Int. J. Mol. Sci.* **2017**, *18*, 2205. [CrossRef]
6. Targum, S.D.; Schappi, J.; Koutsouris, A.; Bhaumik, R.; Rapaport, M.H.; Rasgon, N.; Rasenick, M.M. A novel peripheral biomarker for depression and antidepressant response. *Mol. Psych.* **2022**, *27*, 1640–1646. [CrossRef]
7. Mattila, P.; Suonpää, K.; Piironen, V. Functional properties of edible mushrooms. *Nutrition* **2000**, *16*, 694–696. [CrossRef]
8. Rathore, H.; Prasad, S.; Sharma, S. Mushroom nutraceuticals for improved nutrition and better human health: A review. *Pharma Nutr.* **2017**, *5*, 35–46. [CrossRef]
9. Lindequist, U.; Niedermeyer, T.H.J.; Jülich, W.-D. The Pharmacological Potential of Mushrooms. *Evid. Based Complement. Altern. Med.* **2005**, *2*, 285–299. [CrossRef] [PubMed]
10. Anusiya, G.; Prabu, U.G.; Yamini, N.V.; Sivarajasekar, N.; Rambabu, K.; Bhaeraath, G.; Fawzi, B. A review of the therapeutic and biological effects of edible and wild mushrooms. *Bioengineered* **2021**, *12*, 11239–11268. [CrossRef]
11. Lull, C.; Wichers, H.J.; Savelkoul, H.F.J. Anitiinflammatory and Immunomodulating Properties of Fungal Metabolites. *Mediat. Inflamm.* **2005**, *2*, 63–80. [CrossRef]
12. Smith, J.E.; Rowan, N.J.; Sullivan, R. Medicinal mushrooms: A rapidly developing area of biotechnology for cancer therapy and other bioactivities. *Biotechnol. Lett.* **2002**, *24*, 1839–1845. [CrossRef]
13. Ferreira, J.C.F.R.; Vaz, J.A.; Vasconcelos, M.H.; Martins, A. Compounds from Wild Mushrooms with Antitumor Potential. *Anticancer. Agents Med. Chem.* **2010**, *10*, 424–436. [CrossRef] [PubMed]
14. Zhang, S.; Tomata, Y.; Sugiyama, K.; Tsuji, I. Mushroom consumption and Incident Dementia in Elderly Japanese: The Ohsaki Cohort 2006 Study. *J. Am. Geriatr. Soc.* **2017**, *65*, 1462–1469. [CrossRef] [PubMed]
15. Ba, D.M.; Gao, X.; Muscat, J.; Al-Shaar, L.; Chinchilli, V.; Zhang, X.; Ssentongo, P.; Beelman, R.B.; Richie, J.P., Jr. Association of mushroom consumption with all-cause and cause-specific mortality among American adults: Prospective cohort study findings from NHANES III. *Nutr. J.* **2021**, *20*, 38. [CrossRef]
16. Ba, D.M.; Gao, X.; Al-Shaar, L.; Muscat, J.E.; Chinchilli, V.M.; Beelman, R.B.; Richie, J.P. Mushroom intake and depression: A population-based study using data from the US National Health and Nutrition Examination Survey (NHANES), 2005–2016. *J. Affect. Disord.* **2021**, *294*, 686–692. [CrossRef] [PubMed]
17. Guggenheim, A.G.; Wright, K.M.; Zwickey, H.L. Immune modulation From five Major Mushrooms: Application to Integrative Oncology. *Intgr. Med.* **2014**, *13*, 32–44.

18. Nakajima, Y.; Sato, Y.; Konishi, T. Antioxidant small phenolic ingredients in *Inonotus obliquus* (Persoon) pilat (Chaga). *Chem. Pharm. Bull.* **2007**, *55*, 1222–1226. [CrossRef]
19. Venturella, G.; Ferraro, V.; Cierlincione, F.; Gargano, M.L. Medicinal Mushrooms: Bioactive Compounds, Use, and Clinical Trials. *Int. J. Mol. Sci.* **2021**, *11*, 634. [CrossRef]
20. Kumar, K.; Mehra, R.; Guine, R.P.F.; Lima, M.J.; Kumar, N.; Kaushik, R.; Ahmed, N.; Yadav, A.N.; Kumar, H. Edible Mushrooms: A Comprehensive Reciew on Bioactive Compounds with Health Benefits and Processing Aspects. *Foods* **2021**, *10*, 2996. [CrossRef]
21. Rahi, D.K.; Malik, D. Diversity of mushrooms and their metabolites of nutraceutical and therapeutic significance. *J. Mycol.* **2016**, *2016*, 7654123. [CrossRef]
22. Shama, D.; Singh, V.P.; Singh, N.K. A Review on Phytochemistry and Pharmacology of Medicinal as well as Poisonous Mushrooms. *Mini Rev. Med. Chem.* **2018**, *18*, 1095–1109. [CrossRef]
23. Ragucci, S.; Landi, N.; Russo, R.; Valletta, M.; Pedone, P.V.; Chambery, A.; Maro, A.D. Ageritin from Pioppino Mushroom: The Prototype of Ribotoxin-Like Proteins, a Novel Family of Specific Ribonucleases in Edible Mushrooms. *Toxins* **2021**, *13*, 263. [CrossRef]
24. Landi, N.; Clemente, A.; Pedone, P.V.; Ragucci, S.; Maro, A.D. An Updated Review of Bioactive Peptides from Mushrooms in a Well-Defined Molecular Weight Range. *Toxins* **2022**, *14*, 84. [CrossRef] [PubMed]
25. Sanchez, C. Bioactives from Mushroom and Their Application. In *Food Bioactive*; Puri, M., Ed.; Springer International Publishing: Cham, Switzerland, 2017; Chapter 2; pp. 23–57.
26. Feeney, M.J.; Miller, A.M.; Roupas, P. Mushrooms-biologically distinct and nutritionally unique: Exploring a "third food kingdom". *Nutr. Today* **2014**, *49*, 301–307. [CrossRef] [PubMed]
27. Konishi, T.; Watanabe, K.; Arummugam, S.; Sakurai, M.; Sato, S.; Matsugo, S.; Watanabe, T.; Wakame, K. Nutraceutical and therapeutic significance of Echigoshirayukidake (*Bashikiomycetes-X*), a novel mushroom found in Niigata, Japan. *Glycative Stress Res.* **2019**, *6*, 248–257.
28. Sakamoto, T.; Nishida, A.; Wada, N.; Nakamura, Y.; Sato, S.; Konishi, T.; Matsugo, S. Identification of a novel alkaloid from the Edible Mushroom *Basidiomycetes-X* (Echigoshirayukidake). *Molecules* **2020**, *25*, 4879. [CrossRef]
29. Sakamoto, T.; Li, Z.; Nishida, A.; Kadokawa, A.; Yoshida, T.; Wada, N.; Matsugo, S.; Nakamura, Y.; Sato, S.; Konishi, T. Identification of Major antioxidant Compounds from the Edible Mushroom *Basidiomycetes-X* (Echigoshirayukidake). *Front. Biosci.* **2022**, *14*, 10. [CrossRef]
30. Soga, T.; Ueno, Y.; Naraoka, H.; Ohashi, Y.; Tomita, M.; Nishioka, T. Simultaneous determination of anionic intermediates for Bacillus subtilis metabolic pathways by capillary electrophoresis electrospray ionization mass spectrometry. *Anal. Chem.* **2002**, *74*, 2233–2239. [CrossRef]
31. Wakame, K. Shirayuki-Dake Mushroom (BDM-X) Powder and Extract Metabolomic Analysis by CE-TOFMS and LC-TOFMS. Mendeley Data, V1. 2021. Available online: https://doi.org/10.17632/sdx9g4dwmp.1 (accessed on 6 June 2022).
32. Topmás-Barberán, F.A.; Andrés-Lacueva, C. Polyphenols and Health: Current State and Progress. *J. Agric. Food Chem.* **2012**, *36*, 8773–9775. [CrossRef]
33. Kozarski, M.; Klaus, A.; Jaqkovljevic, D.; Todorovic, N.; Vunduk, J.; Petrovic, P.; Niksic, M.; Vrvic, M.M.; Griensven, L.V. Antioxidant s of Edible Mushrooms. *Molecules* **2015**, *20*, 19489–19525. [CrossRef]
34. Ferreira, I.C.F.R.; Borros, L.; Abreu, R.M.V. Antioxidants in wild mushrooms. *Curr. Med. Chem.* **2014**, *68*, 305–320. [CrossRef]
35. Martinez-Medina, G.A.; Chávez-González, M.L.; Verma, D.K.; Prado-Barragagán, L.A.; Martínez-Hernández, J.L.; Flores-Gallegos, A.C.; Thakur, M.; Srivastav, P.P.; Aguilar, C.N. Bio-functional components in mushrooms, a health opportunity: Ergothionine and huitlacohe as recent trends. *J. Funct. Foods* **2021**, *77*, 104326. [CrossRef]
36. Wood, J.M.; Furkert, D.P.; Brimble, M.A. 2-Formylpyrrole natural products: Origin, structural diversity, bioactivity and synthesis. *Nat. Prod. Rep.* **2019**, *36*, 289–306. [CrossRef] [PubMed]
37. Kim, S.B.; Chang, B.Y.; Jo, Y.H.; Lee, S.H.; Han, S.-B.; Hwang, B.Y.; Kim, S.Y.; Lee, M.K. Macrophage activating activity of pyrrole alkaloids from *Morus alba* fruits. *J. Ethnopharmacol.* **2013**, *145*, 393–396. [CrossRef] [PubMed]
38. Shan, W.G.; Wang, Y.; Ma, L.-F.; Zhan, Z.-J. A New pyrrole alkaloid form mycelium of *Inonotus obliquus*. *J. Chem. Res.* **2017**, *41*, 392–393. [CrossRef]
39. Chin, Y.-W.; Lim, S.-W.; Kim, S.-H.; Shin, D.-Y.; Suh, Y.-G.; Kim, Y.-B.; Kim, Y.C.; Kim, J. Hepatoprotective pyrrole derivatives of *Lycium chinense* fruits. *Bioorg. Med. Chem. Lett.* **2003**, *13*, 79–81. [CrossRef]
40. Li, J.; Pan, L.; Naman, C.B.; Deng, Y.; Chai, H.; Keller, W.J.; Kinghorn, A.D. Pyrrole Alkaloids with Potential Cancer Chemopreventive Activity Isolated from a Goji Berry-contaminated Commercial Sample of African Mango. *J. Agric. Food Chem.* **2014**, *62*, 5054–5060. [CrossRef]
41. Yang, N.-N.; Huang, S.-Z.; Ma, Q.-Y.; Dai, H.-F.; Guo, Z.-K.; Yu, Z.-F.; Zhao, Y.-X. A New Pyrrole Alkaloid from *Leccinum Extremiorientale*. *Chem. Nat. Compd.* **2015**, *51*, 730–732. [CrossRef]
42. Li, H.; Yu, S.-J. Review of pentosidine and pyrraline in food and chemical models: Formation, potential risks and determination. *J. Sci. Food Agric.* **2018**, *98*, 3225–3233. [CrossRef]
43. Beppu, Y.; Komura, H.; Izumo, T.; Horii, Y.; Shen, J.; Tanida, M.; Nakashima, T.; Tsuruoka, N.; Nagai, K. Identification of 2,3-dihydro-3,5-dihydroxy-6-methyl-4H-pyran-4-one isolated from *Lactobacillus pentosus* strain S-PT84 culture supernatants as a compound that stimulates autonomic nerve activities in rats. *J. Agric. Food Chem.* **2012**, *60*, 11044–11049. [CrossRef]

44. Ban, J.O.; Hwang, I.G.; Kim, T.M.; Hwang, B.Y.; Lee, U.S.; Jeong, H.S.; Yoon, Y.W.; Kimz, D.J.; Hong, J.T. Anti-proliferate and pro-apoptotic effects of 2, 3-dihydro-3, 5-dihydroxy-6-methyl-4*H*-pyranone through inactivation of NF-κB in human colon cancer cells. *Arch. Pharm. Res.* **2007**, *30*, 1455–1463. [CrossRef]
45. Takara, K.; Otsuka, K.; Wada, K.; Iwasaki, H.; Yamashita, M. 1,1-Diphenyl-2-picrylhydrazyl Radical Scavenging Activity and Tyrosinase Inhibitory Effects of Constituents of Sugarcane Molasses. *Biosci. Biotechnol. Biochem.* **2007**, *71*, 183–191. [CrossRef] [PubMed]
46. Chen, Z.; Xi, G.; Fu, Y.; Wang, Q.; Cai, L.; Zhao, Z.; Liu, Q.; Bai, B.; Ma, Y. Synthesis of 2,3- dihydro-3,5-dihydroxy-6-methyl-4*H*-pyran-4-one from maltol and its taste identification. *Food Chem.* **2021**, *361*, 130052. [CrossRef] [PubMed]
47. Hiramoto, K.; Nasuhara, A.; Michikoshi, K.; Kikugawa, K. DNA strand-breaking activity and mutagenicity of 2,3-dihydro-3,5-dihydroxy-6-methyl-4*H*-pyran-4-one (DDMP), a Maillard reaction product of glucose and glycine. *Mutat. Res.* **1997**, *395*, 47–56. [CrossRef]
48. Villares, A.; Mateo-Vivaracho, L.; García-Lafuente, A.; Guillamón, E. Storage temperature and UV-irradiation influence on the ergosterol content in edible mushrooms. *Food Chem.* **2014**, *147*, 252–256. [CrossRef] [PubMed]
49. Wimalawansa, S.J. Non-musculoskeletal benefits of vitamin D. *J. Steroid Biochem. Mol. Biol.* **2018**, *175*, 60–81. [CrossRef] [PubMed]
50. Baeke, F.; Takiishi, T.; Korf, H.; Gysemans, C.; Mathieu, C. Vitaminn D: Modulator of the immune system. *Curr. Opin. Pharmacol.* **2010**, *10*, 482–496. [CrossRef] [PubMed]
51. Guillot., X.; Semerano, L.; Saidenberg-Kermanac'h, N.; Falgarone, G.; Boissier, M.-C. Vitamin D and inflammation. *Joint Bone Spine* **2010**, *77*, 552–557. [CrossRef]
52. Danik, J.S.; Manson, J.E. Vitamin D and Cardiovascular Disease. *Curr. Treat. Options Cardiovasc. Med.* **2012**, *14*, 414–424. [CrossRef]
53. Jeon, S.M.; Shin, E.A. Exploring vitamin D metabolism and function in cancer. *Exp. Mol. Med.* **2018**, *50*, 1–14. [CrossRef]
54. Hashimoto, M.; Hossain, S. Fatty Acids: From Membrane Ingredients to Signaling Molecules. In *Biochemistry and Health Benefits of Fatty Acids*; Waisundara, V., Ed.; IntechOpen: London, UK, 2018. [CrossRef]
55. Whigham, L.D.; Cook, M.E.; Atkinson, R.L. Conjugated linoleic acid: Implications for human health. *Pharmacol. Res.* **2000**, *42*, 503–510. [CrossRef]
56. den Hartigh, L.J. Conjugated Linoleic Acid Effects on Cancer, Obesity, and Atherosclerosis: A Review of Pre-Clinical and Human Trials with Current Perspectives. *Nutrients* **2019**, *11*, 370. [CrossRef] [PubMed]
57. Siolveira, M.B.; Carraro, R.; Monereo, S.; Tébar, J. Conjugated linoleic acid (CLA) and obesity. *Public Health Nutr.* **2007**, *10*, 1181–1186. [CrossRef] [PubMed]
58. Tanaka, T.; Hosokawa, M.; Yaui, Y.; Ishigamori, R.; Miyashita, K. Cancer chemopreventive ability of conjugated linoleic acids. *Int. J. Mol. Sci.* **2011**, *12*, 7495–7509. [CrossRef] [PubMed]
59. Viladomiu, M.; Hontecillas, R.; Bassaganya-Riera, J. Modulation of inflammation and immunity by dietary conjugated linoleic acid. *Eur. J. Pharmacol.* **2016**, *785*, 87–95. [CrossRef]
60. Masso-Welch, P.A.; Zangani, D.; Ip, C.; Vaughan, M.M.; Shoemaker, S.F.; McGee, S.O.; Ip, M.M. Isomers of Conjugated Linoleic Acid Differ in Their Effects on Angiogenesis and Survival of Mouse Mammary Adipose Vasculature. *J. Nutr.* **2004**, *134*, 299–307. [CrossRef]
61. Hardie, D.G. AMP-activated protein kinase- an energy sensor that regulates all aspects of cell function. *Genes Dev.* **2011**, *25*, 1895–1908. [CrossRef]
62. Borea, P.A.; Gessi, S.; Merighi, S.; Vincenzi, F.; Varani, K. Pharmacology of Adenosine Receptors; The State of the Art. *Physiol. Rev.* **2018**, *98*, 1591–1625. [CrossRef]
63. Wurtman, R.J.; Cansev, M.; Sakamoto, T.; Ulus, I. Nutritional modifiers of aging brain function: Use of uridine and other phosphatide precursors to increase formation of brain synapses. *Nutr. Rev.* **2010**, *68*, S88–S101. [CrossRef]
64. Zong, A.; Gao, H.; Wang, F. Anticancer polysaccharides from natural resources: A review of recent research. *Carbohydr. Polym.* **2012**, *90*, 1395–1410. [CrossRef]
65. Zhang, J.; Tyler, H.L.; Haron, M.H.; Jackson, C.R.; Pasco, D.S.; Pugh, N.D. Macrophage activation by edible mushrooms is due to the collaborative interaction of toll-like receptor agonists and dectin-1b activating beta glucans derived from colonizing microorganisms. *Food Funct.* **2019**, *10*, 8208–8217. [CrossRef]
66. Khatun, M.A.; Matsugo, S.; Konishi, T. Novel Edible Mushroom BDM-X as an Immune Modulator: Possible Role in Dietary Self-Protection Against COVID-19 Pandemic. *Am. J. Biomed. Sci. Res.* **2021**, *12*, 611–616.
67. Khoury, E.D.; Cuda, C.; Luthovyy, B.L.; Anderson, G.H. Beta Glucan: Health Benefits in Obesity and Metabolic Syndrome. *J. Nutr. Metab.* **2012**, *2012*, 851362. [CrossRef] [PubMed]
68. Watanabe, T.; Nakajima, K.; Konishi, T. In vitro and in vivo anti-oxidant activity of hot water extract of basidiomycetes-X, newly identified edible fungus. *Biol. Pharm. Bull.* **2008**, *31*, 111–117. [CrossRef] [PubMed]
69. Sato, S.; Sakurai, M.; Konishi, T.; Nishikawa, K.; Tsuno, Y. Anti-obesity effect of Echigoshirayukidake (*Basidiomytetes-X*) in rats. *Glycative Stress Res.* **2019**, *6*, 198–211.
70. Khatun, M.A.; Sato, S.; Konishi, T. Obesity Preventive function of novel edible mushroom, *Basidiomycetes-X* (Echigoshirayukidake): Manipulations of insulin resistance and lipid metabolism. *J. Traad. Compl. Med.* **2020**, *10*, 245–251. [CrossRef] [PubMed]
71. Watanabe, K.; Afrin, R.; Sreedhar, R.; Karuppagounder, V.; Harima, M.; Alexander, X.; Velayutham, R.; Arumugam, S. Pharmacological Investigation of *Ceraceomyces tessulatus* (Agaricomycetes) in Mice with Nonalcoholic Steatohepatitis. *Int. J. Med. Mushrooms* **2020**, *22*, 683–692. [CrossRef]

72. Suzuki, H.; Watababe, K.; Arumugum, S.; Yellurkar, M.L.; Sreedhar, R.; Afrin, R.; Sone, H. Meal Ingestion of *Ceraceomyces tessulatus* Strain BDM-X (Agaricomycetes) Protects against Nonalcoholic steatohepatitis in Mice. *Int. J. Med. Mushrooms* **2022**, *24*, 41–52. [CrossRef]
73. Watanabe, K.; Karuppagounder, V.; Sreedhar, R.; Kandasamy, G.; Harima, M.; Velayutham, R.; Arumugam, S. *Basidiomycetes-X*, an edible mushroom, alleviates the development of atopic dermatitis in NC/Nga mouse model. *Exp. Mol. Pathol.* **2018**, *105*, 322–327. [CrossRef]
74. Minami, K.; Watanabe, T.; Yukami, S.; Nomoto, K. Clinical trials of Basidiomycetes-X (FERMP-19241) on the patients with atopic dermatitis. *Med. Biol.* **2007**, *151*, 306–311, (In Japanese with Abstract in English).
75. Yonei, Y.; Yagi, M.; Takabe, A.; Nishikawa, K.; Tsuno, Y. Effect and safety of Echigoshirayukidake (*Basidiomycetes-X*) on fatty liver: Stratified randomized, double-blind, parallel-group comparison study and safety evaluation study. *Glycative Stress Res.* **2019**, *6*, 258–269.
76. Liguori, I.; Russo, G.; Curcio, F.; Bulli, G.; Aran, L.; Della-Morta, D.; Gargiulo, G.; Testa, G.; Cacciatore, F.; Bonaduce, D.; et al. Oxidative stress, aging and diseases. *Clin. Interv. Aging* **2018**, *13*, 757–772. [CrossRef] [PubMed]
77. Lipinski, B. Hydroxyl Radical and Its Scavengers in Health and Disease. *Oxid. Med. Cell. Longev.* **2011**, *2011*, 809696. [CrossRef] [PubMed]
78. Matsugo, S.; Sakamoto, T.; Nishida, A.; Wada, N.; Konishi, T. Pyrrole Compound. JP Patent No. 6859566, 26 November 2021.
79. Radzki, W.; Staswinska, A.; Jabtoriska-Rys, E. Antioxidant capacity and polyphenolic content of dried wild edible mushrooms from Poland. *Int. J. Med. Mushrooms* **2014**, *16*, 65–75. [CrossRef]
80. Field, A.E.; Coakley, E.H.; Must, A.; Spadano, J.L.; Laird, N.; Dietz, W.H.; Rimm, E.; Colditz, G.A. Impact of Overweight on the Risk of Developing Common Chronic Diseases During a 10-Year Period. *Arch. Intern. Med.* **2001**, *161*, 1581–1586. [CrossRef]
81. Li, F.; Gao, C.; Yan, P.; Zhang, M.; Wang, Y.; Hu, Y.; Wu, X.; Wang, X.; Sheng, J. EGCG Reduces Obesity and White Adipose Tissue Gain Partly Through AMPK Activation in Mice. *Front. Pharmacol.* **2018**, *9*, 1366. [CrossRef]
82. Martín, M.Á.; Ramos, S. Dietary Flavonoids and Insulin Signaling in Diabetes and Obesity. *Cells* **2021**, *10*, 1474. [CrossRef]
83. Postic, C.; Girard, J. Contribution of de novo fatty acid synthesis to hepatic steatosis and insulin resistance: Lessons from genetically engineered mice. *J. Clin. Investig.* **2008**, *118*, 829–838. [CrossRef]
84. Tripoli, E.; Guardia, M.L.; Giammanco, S.; Di Majo, D.; Giammonco, M. Citrus flavonoids. Molecular structures, biological activity and nutritional properties: A review. *Food Chem.* **2007**, *104*, 466–479. [CrossRef]
85. Miltonprabu, S.; Tomczyk, M.; Skalicka-Woźniak, K.; Ractrelli, L.; Daglia, M.; Nabavi, F.; Alavian, S.M.; Nabavi, S.M. Hepatoprotective effect of quercetin: From chemistry to medicine. *Food Chem. Toxicol.* **2017**, *108*, 365–374. [CrossRef]
86. Yadav, M.; Sehrawat, N.; Singh, M.; Upadhyay, S.K.; Aggarwal, D.; Sharma, A.K. Cardioprotective and Hepatoprotective Potential of Citrus Flavonoid Naringin: Current Status and Future Perspectives for Health Benefits. *Asian J. Biol. Life Sci.* **2020**, *9*, 1–5. [CrossRef]
87. Maggini, S.; Fierre, A.; Calder, P.G. Immune Function ad Micronutrient Requirements Change over the Life Course. *Nutrients* **2018**, *10*, 1531. [CrossRef] [PubMed]
88. Ayeka, P.A. Potential of Mushroom Compounds as Immunomodulators in Cancer Immunotherapy: A Review. *Evid. Based Complement. Alternat. Med.* **2018**, *2018*, 7271509. [CrossRef]
89. Vetvicka, V.; Teplyakova, T.V.; Shintyapina, A.B.; Korolenko, T.A. Effects of Medicinal Fungi-Derived β-Glucan on Tumor Progression. *J. Fungi* **2021**, *7*, 250. [CrossRef] [PubMed]
90. Tsukagoshi, S.; Hashimoto, Y.; Fujii, G.; Nomoto, K.; Orita, K. Krestin (PSK). *Cancer Treat. Rev.* **1984**, *11*, 131–155. [CrossRef]
91. Kumar, V.; Sharma, A. Adenosine: An endogenous modulator of innate immune system with therapeutic potential. *Eur. J. Pharmacol.* **2009**, *616*, 7–15. [CrossRef]
92. Kim, K.-J.; Lee, J.; Park, Y.; Lee, S.H. ATF3 Mediates Anti-Cancer Activity of *Trans*-10, *cis*-12-Conjugated Linoleic Acid in human Colon Cancer Cells. *Biomol. Ther.* **2015**, *23*, 134–140. [CrossRef]
93. Sharma, N.; Samarakoon, K.W.; Gyawail, R.; Park, Y.-H.; Lee, S.-J.; Oh, S.J.; Lee, T.-H.; Jeong, D.K. Evaluation of the Antioxidant, Anti-Inflammatory, and Anticancer Activities of *Euphorbia hirta* Ethanolic Extract. *Molecules* **2014**, *19*, 14567–14581. [CrossRef]
94. Murru, E.; Carta, G.; Manca, C.; Sogos, V.; Pistis, M.; Melis, M.; Banni, S. Conjugated Linoleic Acid and Brain Metabolism: A Possible Anti-Neuroinflammatory Role Mediated by PPARα Activation. *Front. Pharmacol.* **2020**, *11*, 587410. [CrossRef]
95. Trøseid, M.; Andersen, G.Ø.; Broch, K.; Hov, J.R. The gut microbiome in coronary artery disease and heart failure: Current knowledge and future directions. *eBioMedicine* **2020**, *52*, 102649. [CrossRef]
96. Davis, C.D. The Gut Microbiome and Its Role in Obesity. *Nutr. Today* **2016**, *51*, 167–174. [CrossRef] [PubMed]
97. Foley, S.E.; Tuohy, C.; Dunford, M.; Grey, M.J.; De Luca, H.; Cawley, C.; Szabady, R.L.; Maldonado-Contreras, A.; Houghton, J.M.; Ward, D.V.; et al. Gut microbiota regulation of P-glycoprotein in the intestinal epithelium in maintenance of homeostasis. *Microbiome* **2021**, *9*, 183. [CrossRef] [PubMed]
98. Golisch, B.; Lei, Z.; Tamura, K.; Brumer, H. Configured for the Human Gut Microbiota: Molecular Mechanisms of Dietary β-Glucan Utilization. *ACS Chem. Biol.* **2021**, *16*, 2087–2102. [CrossRef]
99. Bhilwade, H.N.; Tatewaki, N.; Konishi, T.; Nishida, M.; Eitsuka, T.; Yasui, H.; Inanami, O.; Honda, O.; Naito, Y.; Ikekawa, N.; et al. The Adjuvant Effect of Squalene, an Active Ingredient of Functional Foods, on Doxorubicin-Treated Allograft Mice. *Nutr. Cancer* **2019**, *71*, 1153–1164. [CrossRef] [PubMed]

100. Nicastro, H.; de Luz, C.R.; Chaves, D.F.S.; Bechara, L.R.G.; Voltarelli, V.A.; Rogero, M.M.; Lancha, A.H., Jr. Does Branched-chain Amino Acids Supplementation Modulate Skeletal Muscle Remodeling through Inflammation Modulation? Possible Mechanism. *J. Nut. Metab.* **2021**, *2021*, 136937. [CrossRef] [PubMed]
101. Giacobbe, J.; Benoiton, B.; Zuriszain, P.; Pariante, C.M.; Borsini, A. The Anti-Inflammatory Role of Omega-3 Polyunsaturated Fatty Acids Metabolites in Pre-Clinical Models of Psychiatoric, Neurodegenerative, and Neurological Disorders. *Front. Psychiatry* **2020**, *11*, 122. [CrossRef]
102. Konishi, T. Weak direct and strong indirect interactions are the mode of action of food factors. *Funct. Food. Health Dis.* **2014**, *4*, 254–263. [CrossRef]
103. Chen, Z.P.; Levy, A.; Lightman, S.L. Nucleotides as extracellular signalling molecules. *J. Neuroendocr.* **1995**, *7*, 83–96. [CrossRef]
104. Kuroki, M.; Miyamoto, S.; Morisaki, T.; Yotsumoto, F.; Shirasu, N.; Taniguchi, Y.; Soma, G. Biological Response Modifiers Used in Cancer Biotherapy. *Anticancer Res.* **2012**, *32*, 2229–2233.

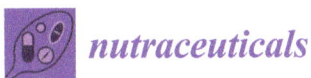

Review

Potential of Microalgae as Functional Foods Applied to Mitochondria Protection and Healthy Aging Promotion

Lorenzo Zanella and Fabio Vianello *

Department of Comparative Biomedicine and Food Science, University of Padua, Viale dell'Università 16, 35020 Legnaro, Italy
* Correspondence: fabio.vianello@unipd.it

Abstract: The rapid aging of the Western countries' populations makes increasingly necessary the promotion of healthy lifestyles in order to prevent/delay the onset of age-related diseases. The use of functional foods can significantly help to achieve this aim, thanks to the contribution of biologically active compounds suitable to protect cellular and metabolic homeostasis from damage caused by stress factors. Indeed, the excessive production of reactive oxygen species (ROS), favored by incorrect eating and behavioral habits, are considered causal elements of oxidative stress, which in turn favors tissue and organism aging. Microalgae represent a convenient and suitable functional food because of their extraordinary ability to concentrate various active compounds, comprising omega-3 polyunsaturated fatty acids, sterols, phenolic compounds, carotenoids and others. Within cells, mitochondria are the cellular organelles most affected by the accumulation of molecular damage produced by oxidative stress. Since, in addition to producing the chemical energy for cellular metabolism, mitochondria control numerous cell cycle regulation processes, including intrinsic apoptosis, responses to inflammatory signals and other biochemical pathways, their dysfunction is considered decisive for many pathologies. Among these, some degenerative diseases of the nervous system, cardiovascular system, kidney function and even cancer are found. From this viewpoint, bioactive compounds of microalgae, in addition to possessing high antioxidant properties, can enhance mitochondrial functionality by modulating the expression of numerous protective factors and enzymes, which in turn regulate some essential biochemical pathways for the preservation of the functional integrity of the cell. Here, we summarize the current knowledge on the role played by microalgal compounds in the regulation of the mitochondrial life cycle, expression of protective and reparative enzymes, regulation of intrinsic apoptosis and modulation of some key biochemical pathways. Special attention was paid to the composition of some cultivable microalgae strains selected for their high content of active compounds suitable to protect and improve mitochondrial functions.

Keywords: microalgae; mitochondria; oxidative stress; antioxidants; PUFA; carotenoids; sterols; polyphenols; chronic diseases

Citation: Zanella, L.; Vianello, F. Potential of Microalgae as Functional Foods Applied to Mitochondria Protection and Healthy Aging Promotion. *Nutraceuticals* **2023**, *3*, 119–152. https://doi.org/10.3390/nutraceuticals3010010

Academic Editor: Ivan Cruz-Chamorro

Received: 23 December 2022
Revised: 21 January 2023
Accepted: 1 February 2023
Published: 6 February 2023

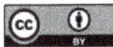

Copyright: © 2023 by the authors. Licensee MDPI, Basel, Switzerland. This article is an open access article distributed under the terms and conditions of the Creative Commons Attribution (CC BY) license (https://creativecommons.org/licenses/by/4.0/).

1. Introduction

In the last 70 years, the world population has grown from 2.5 billion to over 7 billion, but a general aging process has been occurring since 1980, albeit geographically uneven, which will lead to the number of people aged between 15 and 59 in developed countries halving by 2100 [1]. Among the consequent impacts, healthcare costs represent a problem deserving special attention, both for the present situation and, in perspective, for the future evolution of the world population [2–5]. In particular, long-term chronic-degenerative diseases increase with the fraction of the elderly population [2], and the adoption of policies aimed at delaying the onset and severity of these diseases represents the best strategy for managing their social and economic impact [3–5].

There is a general scientific consensus considering the diet as one of the main factors promoting and maintaining human health status, especially aiming at the prevention of diseases due to aging [6,7]. Unfortunately, the Western diet constitutes a primary risk factor, together with insufficient physical activity, being characterized by an excessive intake of calories, ultra-processed foods, saturated fats, carbohydrates with a high glycemic index and salt [8]. At the same time, it is often deficient in healthy compounds which are abundant in plants, i.e., antioxidants, minerals, vitamins and fibers [9], and which can significantly contribute to the reduction of certain diseases and extend lifespan [7].

As part of a synergistic effort of scientific research and sustainable economic development aimed at promoting healthy aging, the identification and characterization of functional foods assume great relevance. These, even taken in modest amounts, can effectively contribute to favor the improvement of the diet of populations with a high aging rate while, at the same time, supporting economic policies oriented towards a sustainable development model [10–12]. In this context, many microalgae are now considered innovative functional foods which could play an important role in delaying aging and also in reducing the impact of many age-related diseases [13–16]. The literature reports on a huge variety of studies highlighting the value of microalgae as a source of healthful substances, especially antioxidant compounds [14,16–21]. Indeed, oxidative stress represents one of the main mechanisms of alteration of cellular and tissue homeostasis at the basis of aging and many important diseases, including various types of cancer and neurological diseases [22,23].

Mitochondria represent the cellular components in which the highest number of redox reactions take place and are, therefore, the organelles most exposed to oxidative damage. The significant endowment of enzymes aimed at preventing oxidative damage and the related functional implications confers a primary role to the mitochondrion in the protection of the cell from oxidative stress and related pathologies [24–26]. Notwithstanding, the importance of proper nutrition for preserving the mitochondrion's functional integrity is still an insufficiently understood topic, despite being increasingly at the center of clinical research. In this short review, the potential benefits of microalgal compounds in the prevention of functional mitochondrial disorders are specifically discussed. In particular, we tried to summarize some mechanisms of action of the main active compounds present in microalgae, highlighting how their action is not only due to mere chemical protection from oxidant compounds but also to their ability to modulate the life cycle of mitochondria and their main biochemical pathways.

This contribution is dedicated to the memory of Prof. Mario Roberto Tredici (University of Florence) in recognition of his irreplaceable contribution to the development of microalgae biotechnology and of his passionate dedication, which he passed to those who had the fortune to collaborate with him.

2. Functions of Mitochondria

Mitochondria are involved in many other essential metabolic activities, including the control of cellular apoptosis, in addition to being responsible for the processes of cellular respiration and ATP synthesis.

Their outer membrane delimits a space further compartmentalized by the inner membrane, very developed and folded into ridges, where numerous enzymes are integrated, such as those constituting the respiratory chain, also known as the electron transport chain. The inner membrane delimits an internal matrix in which a specific DNA strand and ribosomes can be found, allowing the synthesis of part of mitochondrial structural and enzymatic proteins. However, most of them must be synthesized in the cytoplasm and then imported by specific transporters. Mitochondria follow a complex life cycle within the cell, the main phases of which are defined as biogenesis, fusion, fission and mitophagy (Figure 1). These phases, also called mitochondrial dynamics, are characterized by interactive processes among the organelles, which behave as an integrated mitochondrial reticulum [27]. During the biogenesis phase, mitochondria modulate their mass, function, size and morphology through processes controlled by a network of transcription factors and coregulators (cf. Table 1) which, in addition to the fewer but essential genes of the mtDNA, also require the coordinated transcription of a large number of genes in the nucleus [28–30]. Furthermore, mitochondria can mix their content and generate extended organelle networks through a process named fusion [27]. This phase implies the fusion of the outer membrane controlled by mitofusins, i.e., large Mfn1 and Mfn2 GTPases, whereas OPA1 Mitochondrial Dynamin Like GTPase (OPA1) intermembrane protein is required for inner membrane fusion [31,32].

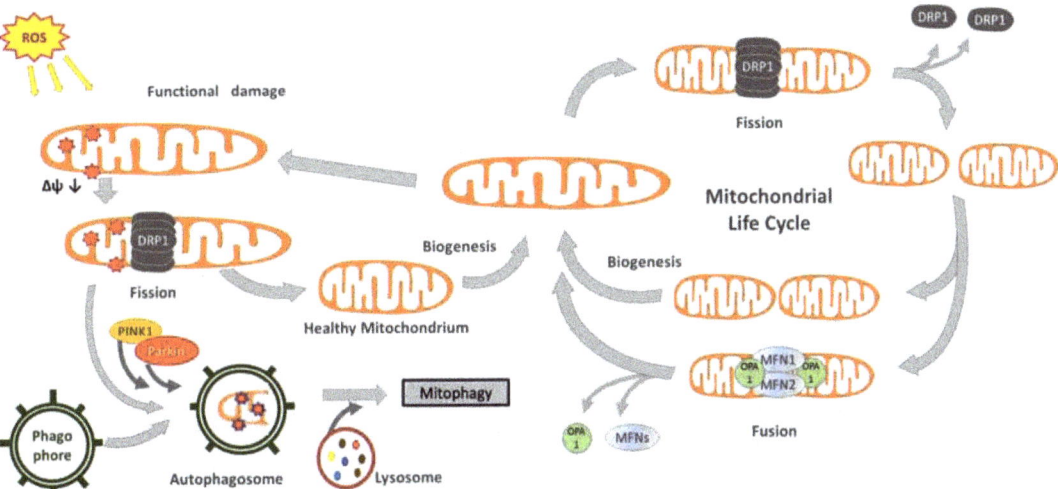

Figure 1. Conceptual illustration of the mitochondrial life cycle and the contribution of mitochondrial dynamics and mitophagy to maintain organelle shape, size and functionality. Abbreviations: Drp1, dynamin-related-protein 1; Mfn, mitofusin; OPA1, mitochondrial dynamin like GTPase; parkin, E3 ubiquitin-protein ligase parkin; Pink1, PTEN-induced putative kinase protein 1.

Following the replication of their single chromosome, mitochondria can proceed to the division phase, called fission [33]. This allows for the replacement of dysfunctional mitochondria or, in the case of cell replication, provides an adequate number of organelles to be segregated between daughter cells. Fission requires the intervention of dynamin-related protein 1 (Drp1), a cytosolic GTPase that translocates to the outer mitochondrial membrane for assembling multimeric rings, which induce mitochondrial division [27,34–36]. Importantly, fission also allows the separation of dysfunctional parts of the mitochondrion [37]. The degradation of dysfunctional parts, or entire damaged mitochondria, occurs through a special autophagy clearance phase known as mitophagy. This phase is controlled by the PTEN-induced putative kinase protein 1 (PINK1), a protein kinase activated by the depolarization of the organelle membrane and which recruits the E3 ubiquitin-protein ligase parkin (parkin) to the outer mitochondrial membrane, which in turn promotes mitophagy by binding ubiquitin moieties as degradation signal (ubiquitination) [38–40]. An alternative pathway is regulated by the mitophagic receptors BCL-2 interacting protein 3 Like (Bnip3L alias Nix) and BCL-2 interacting protein 3 (Bnip3) [40]. Mitophagy, however, is a complex phase involving selective autophagic events, in which mitochondrial and other cytoplasmic materials are sequestered in double-membrane-delimited vesicles, called autophagosomes, then fused to lysosomes to form autolysosomes where materials are degraded. Several enzymes, membrane transporters and receptors are involved, among which a pivotal function is attributed to processing regulators, such as autophagy related 5 (Atg5) and beclin-1 (BECN1) [40].

Table 1. Compounds known for their modulatory activities on the main mitochondrial cycle phases and on their main regulatory enzymes/pathways (the compounds found in microalgae are underlined). Abbreviations: Atg5, autophagy related 5; BCN1, beclin-1; Bnip3, BCL-2 interacting protein 3; DHA, docosahexaenoic acid; Drp1, dynamin-related-protein 1; EPA, eicosapentaenoic acid; Fis1, mitochondrial fission 1 protein; Mfns, mitofusins; MT, mitochondrion; NRF1, nuclear respiratory factor-1; parkin, E3 ubiquitin-protein ligase parkin; Nrf2, nuclear factor erythroid 2-related factor 2; OPA1, mitochondrial dynamin like GTPase; PGC-1α, peroxisome proliferator-activated receptor-γ coactivator-1α; Pink1, PTEN-induced kinase 1; Prk2, protein kinase C-related kinase 2; SIRT1, silent information regulator-1; TFAM, transcription factor A mitochondrial; TFBM, transcription factor B mitochondrial.

Modulatory Active Compound	Ref.	Key Regulatory Enzymes or Pathways	Cycle Phase	Description
Astaxanthin	[41,42]	PGC-1α, Tfam		
EPA	[43]	NRF-1, TFAM, COXIV, SIRT1, PGC-1α		
EPA/DHA, curcumin	[44–46]	PGC-1α, NRF1	Biogenesis	MTs increase by organelle division. The organelles undergo mtDNA replication and subsequent division.
Fucoxanthin	[47]	NRF1, NRF2		
Quercetin, resveratrol	[45]	Nrf2		
Salidroside (Rhodiola)	[48]	SIRT1		
Fucoxanthin, curcumin	[45,47,49]	PGC1α, Tfam		
Fucoxanthin	[47]	Mfns; Opa1		Coordinated fusion of the inner and outer membranes between two organelles aimed to merge intact and slightly dysfunctional MTs. It is particularly useful in case of damaged mtDNA.
Omega-3 fatty acids	[46]	Mfns; Opa1	Fusion	
Resveratrol	[32]	Mfn2		
Omega-3 fatty acids	[46]	Drp1, Fis1		Separation of the MT into two smaller units. Fission allows the isolation of damaged MT parts for elimination, but it becomes massive in the case of apoptosis.
1H-pyrrole-2-carboxamide compounds (synthetic)	[34]	Drp1	Fission	
Astaxanthin	[42,50]	Drp1		
Curcumin, astaxanthin, resveratrol, hydroxytyrosol, oleuropein, spermidine	[51]	Modulation of several mitophagy mediators		Autophagic degradation of irreversibly damaged MTs or part of them.
Astaxanthin	[42]	PINK, parkin	Mitophagy	
Fucoxanthin	[49]	Pink1, Prk2, Bnip3, BECN1, Atg5		

The regulation of mitochondrial dynamics can directly affect the mass and functionality of the mitochondrial reticulum. Many compounds, some reported in Table 1, modulate mitochondrial dynamics by acting on key enzymes or regulating the expression of relevant cytosolic and mitochondrial factors. Among these, central functions are performed by peroxisome proliferator-activated receptor-γ coactivator-1α (PGC-1α), nuclear respiratory factor-1 (NRF1), nuclear factor erythroid 2-related factor 2 (Nrf2), transcription factor A mitochondrial (TFAM) and transcription factor B mitochondrial (TFBM), which are all positive regulators of the mitochondrial biogenesis.

PGC-1α interacts with many cell functions and is regulated at both transcription and post-translation levels, e.g., activated by deacetylation by silent information regulator-1 (SIRT1). Among other effects, it modulates mitochondrial biogenesis by interacting with both NRF1 and Nrf2 nuclear respiratory factors [29]. In turn, NRF1 and Nrf2 regulate the expression of subunits of the electron transfer chain and promote mtDNA transcription [29]. NRF1 is also a promoter factor of the expression of TFAM and of other promoters required for the basal transcription of mitochondrial DNA, in particular of TFB1M and TFB2M (transcription factor B1 and B2, mitochondrial, respectively) [29,52]. In the activated form, Nrf2 translocates to the nucleus, where it regulates the expression of several genes by binding to the antioxidant response elements (AREs) included in their promoter regions, four of which are also in the NRF1 promoter [29].

As the powerhouse of the cell, the mitochondrial enzymatic machinery carries out the redox processes by which the chemical energy of organic compounds is transferred to ATP molecules (glycolysis, Krebs cycle and beta-oxidation of fatty acids), then directly used as an energy source for the cell. The transfer of electrons through the respiratory chain implies the production of a high amount of reactive oxygen species (ROS), i.e., the main actors involved in the oxidative stress, which in turn is believed to be the main cause of the molecular damage at the base of cellular aging processes [24,53–55]. Oxidative damage produced by ROS is kept under control by several enzymes (Table 2), which perform two essential functions: the prevention of the excessive concentration or persistence of ROS and the repair of molecular damage produced by these reactive compounds.

The biochemical network of protection mechanisms against oxidative damage and related signaling pathways is indicated by the term "mitohormesis" [30]. Despite defense mechanisms, the progressive accumulation of oxidative damage leads to dysfunctionalities of the mitochondrial reticulum, which is considered to be among the main causes of aging [56,57] and of numerous chronic degenerative noncommunicable diseases (NCDs), such as nonalcoholic steatohepatitis (NASH) [58–61], muscle insulin resistance related to obesity [62,63], kidney pathologies [64], cardiovascular pathologies [25,65,66], Parkinson's disease [67], Huntington's disease [68], and Alzheimer's disease [54,69]. The study of the correlation among the morpho-functional alteration of mitochondria, the aging processes and the onset of numerous chronic and degenerative diseases made it possible to highlight the importance of diet in the preservation of mitohormesis. In particular, the intake of foods containing compounds suitable to enhance the protective mechanisms of mitochondrial functionality is now considered a primary factor for delaying aging and for preventing related diseases [51]. Tables 1 and 2 list some compounds which have been shown to modulate protective enzymes or specific processes of the mitochondrial life cycle. Notably, most of these molecules present antioxidant properties in vitro, therefore, they are able to inactivate ROS by direct chemical interaction, and this has often led to the belief that their primary biological activity is due to this mechanism. However, even if it is evident that antioxidant activity is, to varying degrees, involved in the effects produced by antioxidants, it was demonstrated that these compounds often trigger much more complex interactions and show biological properties different from those just attributable to antioxidant activity. As an illustrative example, the highly studied case of resveratrol can be considered referring to the so-called "French paradox" [70]. This consists in the low incidence of coronary heart disease observed in French people, while having a diet relatively rich in saturated fats. According to authors' hypothesis, this was attributed to the protective effect of resveratrol, taken through a moderate consumption of red wine. Resveratrol is a polyphenol with antioxidant properties modulating various cellular and even mitochondrial processes (cf. Tables 1 and 2), producing a protective action against cardiovascular pathologies. However, this protection occurs even assuming very small amounts of this compound, which would not justify a significant effect in terms of chemical antioxidant action.

Table 2. Factors/proteins/compounds known as regulators of activity or gene expression of mitochondrial enzymes involved in the prevention and repair of damage due to ROS. Abbreviations: AP-1, activator protein 1; AP-2, adaptor protein complex 2; ARE, antioxidant response element; C/EPB, CCAAT/enhancer-binding protein; CREB, cAMP response element-binding protein; DHA, docosahexaenoic acid; Egr1, Early growth response protein 1; FOXO3a, forkhead box O3a; HIF-1, hypoxia-inducible factor 1; NF-κB, nuclear factor kappa-light-chain-enhancer of activated B cells; NRF-1, nuclear respiratory factor-1; Nrf2, nuclear factor erythroid 2-related factor 2; Oct-1, POU domain, class 2, transcription factor 1; p53, cellular tumor antigen p53; PIG3, p53 inducible gene 3; PPARγ, peroxisome proliferator activated receptor γ; SIRT, sirtuin; Sp1, specificity protein 1.

Factor/Protein/Compound Able to Regulate Target Enzyme or Its Gene Expression	Effect	Ref.	Target Enzyme	Target Enzyme Function
PPARγ	Up	[71]		
Oct-1	Up	[71]		
Astaxanthin	Up	[72]	Catalase	Hydrogen peroxide (H_2O_2) decomposition to oxygen (O_2) and water (H_2O).
DHA (via Nrf2)	Up	[73]		
p53, PIG3	Down	[74]		
MicroRNA-30b	Up	[75]		
NF-κB, (Sp1), C/EBP, SIRT, FOXO3a, CREB	Up	[73,76–78]		
AP-1	Up	[79]		Manganese enzyme expressed in the inner matrix catalyzes the dismutation of the superoxide radical ($O_2 \bullet^-$) into ordinary molecular oxygen (O_2) and hydrogen peroxide (H_2O_2).
AP-2	Down	[76]		
p53, p50	Down	[78,80]	Mn-Superoxide dismutase (SOD2)	
miR-146a	Down	[81]		
Quercetin	Down	[82]		
Curcumin	Up	[83]		
Astaxanthin	Up	[72]		
Sp1, C/EBP, Egr1, Nrf2, NF-κB, ELAV-like proteins, resveratrol	Up	[84–87]	Cu,Zn-Superoxide dismutase (SOD1)	Copper-zinc enzyme with the same function as SOD-2 but expressed in the inter-membrane space [77,88].
AP-1	Down	[78,89]		
Quercetin	Down	[82]		
ARE/EpRE	Up	[90]	Peroxiredoxins (Prx3)	Enzymes are able to catalyze the oxidation of the redox-active cysteine (i.e., peroxidatic cysteine) to a sulfenic acid by the peroxide substrate.
Angiotensin II	Down	[91]		
SOD2	Up	[92]	Thioredoxin (TNX2)	Enzymes are expressed by a nuclear gene and imported into the mitochondrion, which carries out ROS scavenging activity with the concomitant anti-apoptotic effect [93].
Curcumin	Up	[83]		
Resveratrol	Up	[85]	Glutathione peroxidase-1(GPx-1)	A selenocysteine-containing enzyme involved in the reductive detoxification of peroxides. Its expression seems stimulated by the epidermal growth factor (EGF).
Genistein	Up	[94]		
Quercetin	Down	[82]		
Resveratrol	Up	[85]	Glutathione (GSH)	It protects the cell from respiration-induced reactive oxygen species and detoxifies lipid hydroperoxides and electrophiles.
Quercetin	Down	[45]		
Nrf2/Nrf1 via ARE, AP-1 and NF-kB	Up	[95]		
Procyanidin B2 (upregulation of P1 isoform via nuclear translocation of Nrf2)	Up	[96]	Glutathione-S-transferases (GSTs)	Mitochondrial GSTs display both GSH transferase and peroxidase activities for the detoxification of harmful byproducts [97].
Obtusilactone A (OA) and (−)-sesamin	Down	[98]	Lon proteases	They decompose damaged and misfolded proteins tagged for degradation at their –COOH or –NH3 terminus [57]. Mitochondrial biogenesis in mammalian cells is partly regulated by the matrix Lon protease [99].
Acute stressors, such as heat shock, serum starvation, and oxidative stress (Nrf-2, HIF-1)	Up	[100]		
Only synthetic molecules are known: β-lactones (A2-32-01); Phenyl esters (AV167, TG42, TG53); α-aminoboronic acid	Down	[101]	Clp proteases	Variants of chaperon ATPase subunits (ClpA, ClpC, ClpE etc.) combined with a proteolytic subunit (ClpP) [57].
Only synthetic molecules are known: Acyldepsipeptide analogs (ADEP-41); imipridones (ONC201, ONC212, TR57)	Up	[101]		

Mitochondrial Apoptosis and the Role of BCL-2 Family Proteins

Many compounds found in microalgae show to affect the regulation of apoptosis, a cell death process in which mitochondria are key players. Apoptosis is a complex and still not fully understood process, the discussion of which is beyond the scope of the present review. However, some essential mechanisms of action are summarized here since they will be frequently mentioned in the following discussion of the bioactivities of microalgal compounds.

In healthy subjects, apoptosis is a physiological mechanism by which the transformation of cells into cancerous cells is prevented; therefore, its regulation assumes relevant therapeutic applications. Mitochondrial activation of apoptosis is controlled by proteins of the BCL-2 family, i.e., proteins sharing the BCL-2 homology (BH) domains, numbered from 1 to 4, and playing both pro- and anti-apoptotic roles. The antiapoptotic proteins which contain four BH domains (BH1-BH4) include B-cell lymphoma 2 (BCL-2), B-cell lymphoma-extra-large (BCL-xL), BCL-2-like protein 2 (BCL2L2 alias BCL-w), BCL-2 family protein myeloid cell leukemia-1 (Mcl-1), and BCL-2-related protein A1 (A1) [102]. Proapoptotic BH1-BH4 effectors, which directly promote the mitochondrial outer membrane permeabilization, consist of BCL-2-associated X protein (Bax) and BCL-2 homologous antagonist killer (Bak) [102]. The BCL-2 family also includes pro-apoptotic BH-3 only proteins: BH3 interacting-domain death agonist (Bid), BCL-2-like protein 11 (Bim), BCL-2-interacting killer (Bik), BCL-2-associated death promoter (Bad), BCL-2-modifying factor (Bmf), harakiri BCL-2 interacting protein (Hrk), phorbol-12-myristate-13-acetate-induced protein 1 (PMAIP1, generally mentioned with the alias Noxa), and p53-upregulated modulator of apoptosis (Puma) [103,104].

The interaction among these apoptosis actors and regulators is complicated and not completely elucidated, but some recent reviews with complementary insights were published by Peña-Blanco and García-Sáez [102], Kale et al. [105], and Roufayel et al. [103], from which some of the following concepts were here synthesized.

As a very schematic model, Bak and Bax represent the apoptotic effectors, which translocate from cytosol to the mitochondrial outer membrane following their activation, where they can accumulate. There, they induce the formation of pores though which activators of the caspase cascade, such as SMAC/DIABLO protein and cytochrome c (Cyt-c), are released to the cytosol, triggering cell death in a short time. Concerning the apoptotic event, Bak/Bax can be activated by the interaction with BH3-only proteins or by dephosphorylation as an effect of specific direct activators. On the contrary, their inhibition occurs by dimerization binding with antiapoptotic BCL-2 proteins. On the other side, BH3-only proteins can antagonize Bak/Bax to bind antiapoptotic BCL-2 proteins and form heterodimers, thus releasing the apoptotic proteins, which can accumulate on the mitochondrial membrane.

Various models describe how BCL-2 family proteins competitively interact with each other to control apoptosis [103]. It is interesting to note that activation/inhibition of different BCL-2 proteins is triggered by some biochemical pathways, with which compounds found in microalgae can interact and by oxidative stress itself. For instance, the regulation of the activity of BCL-2 proteins, which can occur at the gene expression level and/or by phosphorylation/de-phosphorylation, is strongly affected by the ERK1/2 MAP kinase signaling (ERK, extracellular signal-regulated kinase; MAP, mitogen-activated protein) through several and alternative biochemical routes [106].

3. Conceptualization of the Functionality of Foods and Implications of Their Active Compounds

Many compounds with an activity on the protection of mitochondria, and other cellular components, are normally present in the human diet, but only in very small amounts. The recent awareness of their relevance has progressively pushed the research to look for functional foods, i.e., foods particularly rich in suitable molecules for significant diet supplementation. There is no internationally agreed definition of functional food, but the regulations issued by several countries share the assumption that it *"has the ability to promote well-being and health beyond basic nutritional properties"* [107]. The definition introduced by the European Food Safety Authority (EFSA) specifies that the effects of functional foods must be: *"...relevant to either an improved state of health and well-being and/or reduction of risk of disease. [...] and it must demonstrate their effects in amounts that can normally be expected to be consumed in the diet"*, while experts of the Functional Food Center (USA) specified that active food compounds must *"...provide a clinically proven and documented health benefit utilizing specific biomarkers for the prevention, management, or treatment of chronic disease or its symptoms"* [10]. Beyond the above definitions, a shared concept is that a functional food must contain compounds considered not essential for human nutrition and yet able to positively modulate metabolic processes and cellular functions as well as to protect from detrimental alterations of the well-being state. The latter can be intended as consistent with the functional decay due to aging or even related to actual pathological conditions. Furthermore, some compounds found in functional foods could be included in a further functional category of relatively recent and fairly uncertain definition, namely nutraceutical compounds. This term implies an intermediate biological activity between that of a nutrient and that of a drug, but the proposed definitions are, once again, grounded on the effectiveness of preventing or treating pathologies or metabolic disorders [108,109]. The significant overlap with the definition of functional food is evident, even if nutraceuticals do not necessarily have to be foods or part of them. Generally, nutraceuticals are provided as one or more natural nutrients in powder or tablet form, therefore similar to typical drug preparations, without however falling into this category [110]. It is worth noting here that the concepts underlying these definitions, often influenced by commercial needs, are not really new, having already been implicitly introduced by various forms of traditional or alternative medicine, such as traditional Chinese medicine, Indian Ayurvedic medicine or, for some aspects, homeopathic medicine [111,112].

The most interesting point of this heritage of concepts, beyond the implicit interpretations of many definitions, relies on a novel approach for the interaction among diet, metabolism and health state. The ever deeper understanding of the mechanisms of action of biologically active substances, such as polyphenols, carotenoids, omega-3 polyunsaturated fatty acids (PUFAs), polysaccharides, alkaloids, etc., has encouraged the research for novel sources of compounds suitable to support a thriving industry focused on the development of food supplements.

In the last two decades, microalgae have been particularly studied for their ability to concentrate in a unique cell, several actives suitable to promote well-being and health, which are often rare in foods from terrestrial ecosystems [13,14,16,113–116]. Even if some microalgal species can be considered for their relevant contribution to macronutrients, in general, the nutritional interest of these microorganisms is closely related to their supply of active compounds. For instance, the food use of *Haematococcus* derivatives provides a high amount of astaxanthin (a very active carotenoid) which cannot be compared with any traditional food [19]. Furthermore, an ethical issue concerning the preservation of natural resources should be considered. In a previous review, we showed that a daily intake of 6 g dry weight (DW) of *Nannochloropsis* can guarantee the intake of 240 mg/day of eicosapentaenoic acid (EPA), as recommended by EFSA, comparable to a weekly consumption of about 236 g fresh weight of seabream or seabass [117]. Fish oil required to produce these prized fishes can be obtained from 800–1200 g of wild forage fish, which appears ecologically unsustainable.

Generally, microalgae are cultivated for the content of their most represented active compound, justifying the claim of their nutritional "functionality". However, if also all minor active compounds comprised in the same biomass are considered, microalgae should be regarded as "multifunctional" foods, as will become evident in the following part of the present review. Indeed, it is opportune here to mention that microalgae and cyanobacteria are rich in several compounds, not treated in the following discussion, but very useful for human health and even for therapeutic applications. For instance, the cyanobacteria

Arthrospira can contain up to 60% DW of proteins rich in essential amino acids [118]. Microalgal polysaccharides of the cell wall can contribute approximately 10% of the DW [119] and comprise different heteropolysaccharides and monosaccharides, with potential and still unexplored bioactivities, whereas some microalgae are known sources of extracellular sulfated polysaccharides with relevant effects on the human metabolism [120]. Moreover, microalgae are a valuable source of vitamins such as tocopherols and important vitamins of the B group (e.g., B_6, B_9, B_{12}), also comprising some of them poorly found in terrestrial plants, such as vitamins D and K [15]. The high content of minerals is consistent with the composition of ash, which can vary between 13–18% in marine microalgae and 4.5–6.7% in some freshwater species, such as *Chlorella* and *Arthrospira* [119]. Some minerals of high interest for nutritional scopes can be abundant: for instance, *Phaeodactylum tricornutum* contains about 5% DW of Ca and 0.24% DW of Fe [119].

Importantly, fish farmers exploited for decades the exceptional nutritional properties of some microalgae for weaning larvae of fish and shrimps [117]. This provided strong evidence of their potential and safety as a source of bioactive compounds for human nutritional applications, also because microalgae do not share common pathogens with humans. Interestingly, their rigid cell wall can be exploited as a natural encapsulation to protect new-generation therapeutics from the aggressive environment of the stomach, as recently proposed for an edible preparation of S-glycoprotein and soluble angiotensin-converting enzyme 2 (ACE2) for the treatment/inhibition of SARS-CoV-2 [121]. Despite this, still few microalgal strains are Generally Recognized As Safe (GRAS) in the USA or are authorized for human food use in other relevant markets. In this regard, the situation is quite confusing since some microalgae were already approved as raw biomass ingredients, but in other cases, only as a source of edible extracts (generally oils). However, there are inconsistencies among the consulted references, whereas databases of national authorities are not easily searchable. Consequently, some inaccuracies or deficiencies could also be reported in the present work. To the best of our knowledge, only the following species were authorized for human consumption [117,122,123]: *Arthrospira platensis* in the USA, Canada, the EU, India, Japan and China; *Haematococcus pluvialis*, and *Chlamydomonas reinhardtii* in the USA and China; *Auxenochlorella pyrenoidosa* in the EU and China; *A. prototheocoides* in the USA, the EU and Japan; *Chlorella vulgaris* in the EU and Japan; *C. sorokiniana* in Canada and the EU; *C. regularis* in Canada; *Dunaliella bardawil* in the USA; *Dunaliella salina* in Canada and China; *Euglena gracilis* in Canada, the EU, China and Japan; *Schizochytrium* sp. as a fermented ingredient in the USA; *Aphanizomenon flos-aquae*, *Parachlorella kessleri*, *Jaagichlorella luteoviridis*, *Tetraselmis chui* and *Odontella aurita* in the EU; *Nostoc sphaeroides* and *Microchloropsis gaditana* in China. Furthermore, the following algal derivatives (not the algal biomass) were authorized as food ingredients:

- In the EU [117]: β-carotene and a mixture of carotenoids from *Dunaliella salina*; oil rich in PUFAs from *Ulkenia* sp.; DHA and EPA ethyl esters oil from *Schizochytrium* sp.; astaxanthin-rich oleoresin from *Haematococcus pluvialis*; oil rich in EPA from *Phaeodactylum tricornutum*;
- In the USA (data by Food and Drug Administration or cited reference): DHA Algal Oil from *Schizochytrium* sp.; EPA oil from *Microchloropsis gaditana* [124]; Astaxanthin extracted from *Haematococcus pluvialis*; algal fat from *Prototheca zopfii* (syn. *moriformis*) [125]; oil from *Ulkenia* sp.;
- National Health Commission (People's Republic of China): DHA oil from *Schizochytrium* sp., *Ulkenia amoeboida*, *Crypthecodinium cohnii*.

Surprisingly, moreover, the analysis of these microorganisms as potential sources of compounds useful for the maintenance of mitohormesis was still insufficiently investigated.

3.1. Protective Features of Crude Extracts of Microalgae

Studies focused on the use of microalgae as food for their protective action on mitochondria are still very scarce, and most of the information, therefore, comes from the study of individual compounds present in their composition. In this section, the few works to our knowledge were considered, including experimental results obtained on cultivated cells.

An ethanol/water extract obtained from *Tetraselmis suecica* (phylum: Chlorophyta, class: Chlorodendrophyceae [126]) was tested on a human lung cancer cell line challenged with H_2O_2 and showed enhanced oxidative stress resilience and cell survival by the upregulation of several enzymes, including mitochondrial SOD2 and GPx1 [127]. Interestingly, the extract treatment also upregulated the expression of SIRT2, a cytosolic deacetylase, which promotes mitochondrial biogenesis, whereas it inhibited Drp1 and the related fission activity [128]. A 10% dietary supplementation with *Nannochloropsis gaditana* (phylum: Ochrophyta, class: Eustigmatophyceae, currently accepted name: *Microchloropsis gaditana* [126]) was able to reduce the peroxidation on some mitochondrial components of the liver of diabetic rats, using malondialdehyde and carbonyl proteins as damage markers [129]. These effects mitigated the decreased activities of catalase (CAT) and superoxide dismutase (SOD), as well as the concentration of reduced glutathione (GSH) observed in untreated diabetic rats in comparison to healthy controls. A 70% methanolic extract of *Euglena tuba* (phylum: Euglenozoa, class: Euglenophyceae [126]) showed antitumoral activity against Dalton's lymphoma cells in inbred populations of a BALB/c (H2d) mice strain [130]. This result was consistent with the detected alteration of the mitochondrial membrane potential, upregulation of proapoptotic proteins Bax and cellular tumor antigen p53 (p53), while the anti-apoptotic protein regulator BCL-2 was downregulated. Mitochondria-mediated apoptosis in non-small cell lung cancer lines was also demonstrated for hot water extracts of *Chlorella sorokiniana* (phylum: Chlorophyta, class: Trebouxiophyceae [126]). This conclusion was supported by the downregulation of the anti-apoptotic BCL-2, E3 ubiquitin-protein ligase XIAP (XIAP) and survivin, whereas the proapoptotic caspase-3, caspase-9, and poly [ADP-ribose] polymerase (PARP) were activated by peptide bond cleavage [131]. An anticancer effect due to mitochondrial apoptosis was also proposed for methanol and ethyl acetate extracts of *Picochlorum* sp. RCC486 [132] (phylum: Chlorophyta, class: Trebouxiophyceae [126]), ethanol extracts of an unclassified Antarctic freshwater of the Botryidiopsidaceae family [133] (phylum: Ochrophyta, class: Xanthophyceae [126]), and ethanol extracts of *Chaetoceros calcitrans* [134] (phylum: Bacillariophyta, class: Mediophyceae [126]). Most of these anticarcinogenic activities can be explained by the high content of polyphenols and carotenoids in microalgae, suitable to modulate mitochondrial metabolism, reported below. However, it should be kept in mind that part of these results was obtained only on tumor-derived cell lines, and their verification in vivo is recommended for robust confirmation.

Other activities of interest mainly concerned disorders related to aging and chronic diseases. The attenuation of hepatic steatosis was shown in a murine model following the treatment with ethanol extracts of *Nitzschia laevis* (phylum: Bacillariophyta, class: Bacillariophyceae, accepted name: *Nitzschia amabilis* [126]) prepared using a Super High Pressure-Low Temperature Flowing Cell Cracker. The disease improvement was due to the enhancement of hepatic mitochondrial function and the repression of fatty acid synthesis by the phosphorylation of acetyl-CoA carboxylase [135]. In another study carried out in vitro, both on primary skin cells and on ex vivo full-thickness skin, an aqueous extract of *Scenedesmus rubescens* (phylum: Chlorophyta, class: Chlorophyceae, accepted name: *Halochlorella rubescens* [126]) showed protective effects against UV radiation damage by an increase of both mitochondrial efficiency and of cell proliferation [136].

An interesting finding was obtained using *Spirulina platensis* (phylum: Cyanobacteria, class: Cyanophyceae, currently accepted name: *Arthrospira platensis* [126]) treating a horse's endocrine disorder named Equine Metabolic Syndrome, a severe pathology linked to insulin resistance, oxidative stress, and systemic inflammation [137]. In vivo trials carried out with pelleted *Spirulina*, as well as in vitro tests on cell line models with a water extract of *Spirulina*, have shown that this cyanobacterium improved the mitochondrial functionality, downregulated the proapoptotic proteins p21, p53 and Bax, as well as the pro-mitophagic proteins PINK1 and parkin.

3.2. Activity of Long-Chain Polyunsaturated Fatty Acids (PUFAs)

Microalgae are known for their ability to synthesize and concentrate long-chain PUFAs, and in particular EPA and docosahexaenoic acid (DHA), especially if culture conditions aimed at maximizing the accumulation of these compounds are adopted. For instance, DHA can reach up to 40% of the total fatty acids in some Dinophytes, 30% of the total fatty acids in some Haptophytes and even up to 60% of total fatty acids in the form of triacylglycerols in Thraustochytrids belonging to the genus *Aurantiochytrium* and *Schizochytrium* [115]. The content of EPA, on the other hand, can reach up to 20% of the fatty acids in Diatoms, e.g., *Phaeodactylum tricornutum*, while among the Eustigmatophytes, EPA can range between 15 and 30% of the lipo-acidic profile of *Nannochloropsis oculata* [115].

In addition to presenting an antioxidant effect, PUFAs provide benefits to human health through various mechanisms of action and metabolic pathways. Clinical trials involving PUFAs are generally based on the intake of fish oil, whose EPA and DHA content, in any case, derives from microalgae through the fish food chain. When focusing on the biology of mitochondria, it has been shown that omega-3-rich diets improved mitochondrial dynamics and morphology, increasing the expression of mitofusins (Mfns) and OPA1, while a downregulation of Drp1 and mitochondrial fission 1 protein (Fis1) was observed [46]. The overall effect was to promote mitochondrial fusion and inhibit fission processes, thus increasing the mitochondrial reticulum and enhancing its functionality.

It is worth mentioning that a diet rich in EPA and DHA modifies the composition of the mitochondrial membrane phospholipids by partially replacing arachidonic acid [138], so improving stress tolerance and reducing the incidence of heart attack [65,139]. Among the lipids almost exclusively synthesized in mitochondria, cardiolipins constitute approximately 15–20% of the total mitochondrial phospholipids. Among many functions, they regulate mitochondrial dynamics stabilizing the interaction of key enzymes with the organelle membrane, especially Drp1 and OPA1 [65]. Cardiolipins anchor Cyt-c to the internal mitochondrial membrane, and their integrity seems to be fundamental for the prevention of the "mitochondrial permeability transition pore" opening, which triggers the release of Cyt-c into the cytosol and cell apoptosis [65]. However, cardiolipins' integrity is threatened by oxidative reactions, to which they are particularly exposed due to their position with respect to oxidative phosphorylation enzymes. Several studies have shown that PUFAs play an important role in the functionality and protection of cardiolipins (see the review by Paradies et al. [65]). Dietary supplementation with DHA and EPA can increase the total cardiolipin content in cardiac mitochondria [139]. In hearts subjected to prolonged ischemic conditions, DHA has been shown to counteract the decline of tetralinoleyl cardiolipin, i.e., the primary moiety of cardiolipin, preventing cardiomyocyte death by the formation of the mitochondrial permeability transition pore [65,139].

Studies focused on overweight subjects show that EPA-treated adipocytes improved their mitochondrial reticulum and its functionality through the upregulation of mRNA expression of NRF-1, MTFA and Cyt-c oxidase [43]. These effects were accompanied by the upregulation of genes involved in mitochondrial biogenesis, such as sirtuin 1, PGC1-α and 5'-AMP-activated protein kinase (AMPK). Moreover, mitochondrial biogenesis was stimulated via upregulation of PGC1-α and NRF-1 also by treating C57BL/6J mice with a high-fat diet comprising an EPA and DHA concentrate (6% EPA, 51% DHA) [44]. At the same time, a tissue-specific modulation of lipid metabolism was observed. Indeed, the expression of carnitine palmitoyltransferase 1A and fatty acid catabolism were increased in epididymal, but not subcutaneous, fat cells.

Interestingly, it has long been known that EPA can be found in low amounts in the fatty liver of diabetic patients [140]. A study carried out on myotubes prepared using cells obtained from obese type 2 diabetic patients have shown an impaired mitochondrial capacity for fatty acid and glucose oxidation. The treatment with EPA (100 µmol/L) enhanced glucose oxidation, whereas positive effects on lipid metabolism were also observed, but with less clear results [141]. Furthermore, in rats, EPA significantly increased the expression of thermogenic genes, such as uncoupling protein 1-3 (UCP1-3), cell death-inducing DFFAlike effector A (CIDEA) and vascular endothelial growth factor A (VEGFα) [142], consistent with the promotion of the beige-like adipocytes differentiation observed in humans [43].

3.3. Sterols

These compounds are synthesized in microalgae mainly as components of the cell membrane, in quantities that can vary in response to environmental conditions, such as salinity, temperature and light intensity [143]. Several microalgal sterol compounds have been described, including campesterol, stigmasterol, beta-sitosterol, monomethylsterol, brassicasterol, ergosterol and cholesterol [143,144]. Some molecules of this group are quite uncommon if compared to those occurring among higher plants, such as poriferasterol and clionasterol, identified in *Chlorella pringsheimii* (phylum: Chlorophyta, class: Trebouxiophyceae, currently accepted name: *Pseudochlorella pringsheimii* [126]), or ergosterol and chondrillasterol in *Chlorella fusca* (phylum: Chlorophyta, class: Chlorophyceae, currently accepted name: *Desmodesmus abundans* [126]) [18]. Interestingly, appreciable contents of β-sitosterol and stigmasterol were detected in *Nannochloropsis* sp. [145].

The interactions of sterols with the biology of mitochondria have been studied mainly as modulators of the apoptotic process and, in general, for the related effects on cancer prevention. Stigmasterol, a sterol extracted from *Navicula incerta* (phylum: Bacillariophyta, class: Bacillariophyceae [126]), promoted the apoptosis of hepatocarcinoma cells (HepG2) by upregulating the expression of BAX and P53, both powerful pro-apoptotic genes, and by downregulating the anti-apoptotic BCL2 gene [146]. The activation of cellular apoptosis via the mitochondrial route suggests possible applications of microalgal sterols for the treatment of cancer, but also potential uses aimed at promoting the clearance of dysfunctional cells, which could be candidates to transform into neoplastic cells, thus favoring the renewal of tissue composition.

In a cellular model of colon cancer, the effect of different phytosterols, pure substances or mixtures, was also studied in combination with a carotenoid, i.e., β-cryptoxanthin, by treatments at concentrations comparable to values present in human serum after the intake of functional drinks. Various effects were detected at the mitochondrial level with consequent apoptosis activation and inhibition of cell proliferation, according to the following efficacy scale: phytosterols-mix > stigmasterol > β-cryptoxanthin + phytosterols-mix > campesterol > β-cryptoxanthin [147].

3.4. Phenolic Compounds

Phenolic compounds are secondary metabolites with antioxidant properties and several biological activities. They are abundant in plants and comprise phenolic acids and polyphenols (i.e., flavonoids and tannins), stilbenes, lignans and lignins [148]. Considering the data reported in the literature for this group of compounds, it should be kept in mind that the quantification of phenolic compounds is a challenging topic since they generally show limited solubility in water, and the extraction efficiency varies significantly with the method and solvent used. The commonest methodologies are based on the extraction using hydrophilic solvents, or their mixtures, such as ethanol, methanol, or water (in the latter case, preferably with a microwave-assisted process), but various other techniques are currently also available [149,150]. The composition of phenolic compounds in different microalgal species, however, should be critically considered for representing their actual total amount. In general, results obtained by a specific extraction process, even if deemed sufficiently efficient, still represent an underestimate of the actual content of phenolic compounds, as will be evident in some examples below. Importantly, the quantification is generally expressed in terms of standard antioxidant capacity, conventionally established in µmol or, more frequently, in mg of gallic acid equivalents (mg GAE) per gram of sample. However, the latter conventional concentration unit can be applied just for the antioxidant capacity, and it is not suitable for representing the impact of these substances on biological functions, such as the regulation of enzymes and nuclear factors.

Goiris et al. [151] studied the fractional extraction of phenolic compounds from microalgae, obtaining the highest quantities with an ethanol–water mixture, followed by hot water, and only modest amounts with hexane or ethyl acetate. This is consistent with the abundance of polar hydroxyl groups in the molecules of phenolic compounds, which therefore confer a prevailingly hydrophilic behavior, as also demonstrated by studies on the partitioning between aqueous and olive oil phases of phenolic compounds of olive fruits [152]. In work carried out on biomasses of *Nannochlorospis* sp. and of *Spirulina* sp., Scaglioni et al. [153] quantified the insoluble part of phenolic compounds, believed to be bound to cell walls after extraction of the soluble fraction using methanol and/or ethanol. Extractions of *Spirulina* using the two alcohols produced quantitatively similar extracts, while the ethanolic fraction obtained from *Nannochloropsis* was higher than the methanolic fraction by about 40%. Finally, the insoluble polyphenol fraction was quantitatively lower than 4% and 8% of the phenols extracted by ethanol (i.e., the most effective solvent) in *Spirulina* and *Nannochloropsis*, respectively.

The few data presented here point out that phenolic composition varies significantly with the adopted extraction technique and the species-specific composition of the microalgal cell wall. This should suggest a reflection on the criticalities inherent in the available literature, but also on the bioavailability of phenolic compounds of microalgae for nutritional purposes. Their effectiveness, in fact, does not only depend on their content and composition in the considered microalga, but also on their relative bioavailability and their uncertain stability throughout the digestive processes of the human intestine. From a biochemical point of view, there are well-founded reasons to consider that the in vitro antioxidant activity of microalgal polyphenols is less relevant than other, more specific, effects of microalgal compounds.

Goh et al. [154] quantified the phenolic compounds obtained by different solvents from *Chaetoceros* and *Nannochloropsis*, two algal genera widely used in aquaculture, and then compared their antioxidant activity by means of widely used assays. Surprisingly, this study showed that the extracts with the highest antioxidant activity were not those richest in phenolic compounds. Therefore, antioxidant capacity must have been mainly attributable to different antioxidant compounds, of which many microalgae are rich. It is noteworthy that the antioxidant activity of polyphenols is strongly dependent on their chemical structure, beyond their abundance, and influenced by the arrangements of hydroxyl groups and double bounds in their molecule [155]. Considering the abovementioned results, literature data on microalgae indicate highly variable total contents of phenolic compounds among genera (Table 3). Andriopoulos et al. [156] revised the total phenolic content (TPC) in 35 genera of microalgae and cyanobacteria, showing that these compounds range on average between 0.9 and 38.5 mg GAE/g DW, with few exceptions below the minimum value and most of the data ranging between 2 and 7 mg GAE/g DW. The same authors cultivated and analyzed five species of microalgae (*Chlorella minutissima* (phylum: Chlorophyta, class: Chlorophyceae, currently accepted name: *Mychonastes homosphaera* [126]), *Dunaliella salina*, *Nannochloropsis oculata*, *Tisochrysis lutea* and *Isochrysis galbana*) detecting values of TPC (calculated as the sum of aqueous and methanolic extracts) between 6 and 12 mg GAE/g DW. An example of TPC occurring in some microalgae is shown in Table 3.

Table 3. Total phenolic content in some microalgae biomasses (mgGAE/g DW).

Species	Total Phenolic Content mg GAE/g Biomass DW	Reference
Euglena cantabrica	0.6–12.6	[157]
Demodesmus sp.	7.7	[158]
Tetraselmis suecica	4.3	[151]
Dunaliella salina	4.5	[158]
Haematococcus pluvialis	1.9	[151]
Nannochloropsis limnetica	5.8	[158]
Nannochloropsis salina	6.5	[158]
Galdieria sulphuraria	1.6–5.3	[159]
Nannochloropsis sp.	2.2	[151]
Isochrysis sp.	7.8	[151]
Chaetoceros calcitrans	2.3	[151]
Porphyridium cruentum	1	[151]
Phaeodactylum tricornutum	3.2–6.1	[151,158]
Chlorella sorokiniana	5.8–5.9	[158]
Auxenochlorella pyrenoidosa	13.2–25.8	[160]
Arthrospira platensis	17–43.2	[160]
Arthrospira fusiformis	47.3–88.5	[161]
Nostoc commune	0.9	[162]

Many phenolic acids and polyphenols can have strong positive effects on human metabolism, and their importance as micronutrients for preserving health is now well documented [163]. The specific activities of these substances on the regulation of mitochondrial functions have been investigated: Chodari et al. [164] reviewed the activities of polyphenols on biogenesis, Sandoval-Acuna et al. [165] their activities not explained by antioxidant effects, and Naoi et al. [166] their modulatory effects on the mitochondrial apoptosis machinery. However, studies relating polyphenols obtained from microalgal extraction on mitochondria are lacking. Note that the mechanisms of action of this group of compounds are far from being well understood and can vary in relation to cell type and metabolic conditions.

Some polyphenols have been shown to modulate the biochemical pathways involved in mitochondrial biogenesis. The disclosed activity of resveratrol as an upregulator of SIRT1, which in turn inactivates the proapoptotic p53 by deacetylation, shined a light on the importance of polyphenols for cell cycle regulation [167]. It was shown that this activity was not explained by the mere antioxidant property and was also observed with quercetin and with other polyphenols, which are not known in microalgae (fisetin, piceatannol, butein, and soliquiritigenin) [167]. As already said, SIRT1 is an activator of PGC-1α, which in turn is a strong enhancer of mitochondrial biogenesis. According to Chodari et al. [164], the activation of AMPK by resveratrol represents a collateral effect of biogenesis activation via PGC-1α. A significant increase of SIRT1, PGC-1α, mtDNA, Cyt-c, and mitochondrial biogenesis was detected in the muscle and brain of mice following dietary administration of quercetin [168]. It should be noted, however, that the treated groups received 12.5 mg/kg or 25 mg/kg, which are considered quite high dosages. Moreover, polyphenols have been shown to increase mitochondrial biogenesis and activation of AREs by upregulating Nrf2, possibly by displacing this factor from the inhibition binding to Kelch ECH associating protein 1 (Keap1) [165]. Apocynin, epicatechin, cyanidin, cyanidin-3-glucoside and curcumin (not all identified in microalgae) have been shown to inhibit or repress some superoxide anion generators, among which are xanthine oxidase and monoamine oxidase (MAO) [165]. In this regard, the inhibition of MAO-B can have relevant neuroprotective effects [166]. Apigenin, biapigenin, curcumin, oroxylin A, ferulic acid, quercetin, resveratrol, and hesperidin were reported to interact with the mitochondrial membrane in complex ways, promoting or inhibiting the opening of the mitochondrial permeability transition pore [166], above discussed considering the role of cardiolipins. Even if it is not possible to explain in detail here the structure and regulation of the mitochondrial permeability transition pore, the overall results of these effects lead to a neuroprotective activity against important neurodegenerative pathologies [166].

As examples of biological activities of polyphenols, hydroxytyrosol, an abundant polyphenol in olives that is not yet identified in microalgae, was reported to stimulate the mitochondrial functionality and biogenesis via PCG-1α and to increase the activity and protein expression of respiratory complexes I, II, III and V in 3T3-L1 adipocytes [169]. The same compound produced a similar upregulation of the respiratory chain in human fibroblast cultures, explained by the activation of protein kinase A (PKA), cAMP response element-binding protein (CREB) and PGC-1α [170]. Moreover, a trial conducted on high-fat, high-sucrose (HFHS) diet-fed rats showed that a polyphenol extract from red wine could significantly enhance the mitochondrial respiratory chain and NADPH oxidase system, reducing oxidative stress in liver and heart tissues, with a strong preventive effect on steatosis development in the liver [171].

Considering some polyphenols found in microalgae (Table 4), ellagic acid, a compound found at a concentration of 860 µg/g DW in *Galdieria sulphuraria* cultivated under specific conditions [172], regulated ROS production in hepatocytes under oxidative stress, preventing cell damage and consequent apoptosis [173]. Moreover, this substance showed protective activities toward inflammations induced by arsenic on nerve cells via mitochondrial regulation [174] and against BCL-2 protein Bnip3-mediated oxidative stress in cardiomyocytes [175]. In apparent contrast with these cytoprotective activities, the same compound has shown proapoptotic mitochondrial effects in different types of cancer cells, such as human colon adenocarcinoma Caco-2 cells [176], in cancerous B-lymphocytes [177], in bladder cancer cells [178], in pancreatic cancer cells [179] and in lung cancer [180]. A very scholarly review discussing the anticancer mechanisms of action of selected polyphenols was published by Gorlach et al. [181]. Furthermore, apigenin, luteolin, kaempferol, and quercetin inhibited the growth of HepG2 cells and induced morphological changes associated with apoptosis in a dosage- and time-dependent manner by upregulating the expression of the proapoptotic p53-inducible gene 3 (PIG3) [182]. Therefore, even if polyphenols were reported to improve several mitochondrial functions, especially the electron transport chain activity, by modulating the redox state and inhibiting the apoptotic process, they can also promote this last phenomenon depending on their concentration and cell environmental conditions [166,183]. Indeed, the fine-tuning of biochemical mechanisms need to be elucidated in detail, in consideration that many of the reported results, although not all, have been obtained using cell models. In this last case, even if the demonstrated interactions are surely well founded, there are no certainties about the reproducibility in vivo.

Table 4. Phenolic compounds detected in microalgae species. For each strain, any compound reported in at least one of the cited references was included. Synonyms: *Porphyridium purpureum* = *Porphyridium cruentum*; *Microchloropsis salina* = *Nannochloropsis salina*; *Auxenochlorella pyrenoidosa* = *Chlorella pyrenoidosa*; *Arthrospira platensis* = *Spirulina platensis* [126].

Phenolic Compound	*Euglena cantabrica*	*Desmodesmus* sp.	*Tetraselmis suecica*	*Dunaliella salina*	*Haematoc. pluvialis*	*Nannochl. limnetica*	*Microchl. salina*	*Galdieria sulphuraria*	*Nannochloropsis* sp.	*Diacronema lutheri*	*Porph. purpureum*	*Phaeod. tricornutum*	*Chlorella sorokiniana*	*Auxenoc. pyrenoidosa*	*Arthrospira platensis*	*Arthrospira* sp.	*Nostoc commune*
Phloroglucinol			+		+					+	+	+			+	+	+
Pyrocatechol															+		
Pyrogallol															+		
Gallic ac.	+	+			+	+			+			+		+	+	+	+
4-Hydroxy benzoic ac.								+						+	+	+	
3,4-Dihydroxy benzoic ac.							+					+			+		
Protocatechuic ac.	+								+						+		
Quinic ac.															+		
Salicylic ac.						+	+	+			+				+		
Syringic ac.	+								+						+	+	
Vanillic ac.												+			+		
Vanillin											+				+	+	
4-Aminobenzoic ac.								+									
Caffeic ac.		+	+	+	+				+			+	+		+		
Cinnamic ac.		+			+								+				
Ferulic ac.		+	+	+	+	+			+	+	+	+	+		+		
2/3/4-Hydroxy-cinnamic ac.															+		
P-Coumaric ac.		+	+	+		+			+	+	+	+			+		
Chlorogenic ac.	+									+					+	+	+
Phloretin										+							
Rosmarinic ac.															+		
Apigenin		+			+					+	+	+			+		
Catechin hydrate	+							+							+		
Daidzein					+						+	+					
Dihydrokaempferol					+												
Dihydroquercetin					+												
Epicatechin	+														+		
Epigallocatechin														+			
Genistein					+						+	+					
Kaempferol					+												
Luteolin					+			+									
Naringenin					+			+									
Quercetin					+			+				+			+		
Ellagic ac.								+							+		
Rutin															+		
Resveratrol															+		
References	[150]	[158]	[150,184]	[158]	[184]	[158]	[158]	[172]	[153]	[184]	[184]	[142,150,176]	[158]	[160]	[160,184–186]	[153]	[150]

3.5. Carotenoids

Carotenoids are excellent antioxidants, which can contribute to preventing dysfunctions due to oxidative stress and appear to be particularly active on membranes and the enzymatic machinery of the mitochondria, nuclei and microsomes [120]. It is widely accepted that their intake is able to modulate the metabolism of cancer cells and significantly reduce the incidence of various types of cancer [187]. However, the activity of carotenoids depends on their bioavailability, which appears to be variable; e.g., fucoxanthin was described to be better absorbed than lutein or astaxanthin in mice [120].

Over 1100 naturally occurring carotenoids were estimated [125], among which more than 750 have been identified, whereas only 40 are commonly consumed, mainly represented by β-carotene, lycopene, lutein, β-cryptoxanthin, α-carotene and zeaxanthin [188].

Each microalgal species is generally characterized by a few prevailing carotenoids. For instance, β-carotene is the main metabolite in algae of the genus *Dunaliella*, astaxanthin in *Haematococcus pluvialis* (phylum: Chlorophyta; class: Chlorophyceae [126]), violaxanthin and vaucheriaxanthin in *Nannochloropsis*, accompanied by other compounds of the violaxanthin cycle, i.e., antheraxanthin and zeaxanthin [189] (Table 5).

However, the synthetic pathways of carotenoids lead to the production of several intermediate metabolites. Thus, many of them are detected in the microalgal composition in addition to the main metabolite, albeit at lower concentrations.

The beneficial activity of carotenoids on human health has been studied for only a few of them, and often with insufficient detail. Among these, the most studied are probably: β-carotene, astaxanthin and fucoxanthin. Specifically, β-carotene belongs to the carotene family, i.e., carotenoids which do not contain oxygen, and, possibly, it represents the molecule studied for the longest time as a supplement in the human diet, always being considered an excellent provitamin A.

Some clinical studies associated the intake of β-carotene with several beneficial outcomes, such as a reduced risk of cardiovascular disease, the prevention of several age-related cancers and the improvement of endogenous cellular antioxidants via modulation of Nrf2/ARE pathway in response to oxidative stress conditions [190]. Moreover, β-carotene has been shown to protect mitochondrial membranes from the impairment of mitochondrial import receptor subunit TOM20 homolog (Tom20) due to oxidative stress [190]. Notably, Tom20 is an import receptor of the outer-membrane translocator TOM40 complex and plays an essential role in the import of mitochondrial proteins [191]. Low-doses of β-carotene were shown to modulate autophagy and to downregulate the NF-κB inflammatory factor, whereas mitochondrial biogenesis was stimulated via Nrf2 and apoptotic signals of caspase 3 and 9 were downregulated [190]. Trials carried out on *Drosophila melanogaster* with 9-cis-β-carotene obtained from *Dunaliella salina* showed that this carotenoid improved the mitochondrial function in terms of organelle mobility and ATP production, leading to the extension of the mean lifespan [192]. On the other side, adverse effects concerning cardiovascular disease were observed in smoker subjects treated with β-carotene [193]. Furthermore, according to the meta-analysis proposed by Pecollo et al. [194], an increased risk of lung and gastric cancer was observed in smokers and asbestos workers treated with β-carotene at a dosage equal to or above 20 mg/day, whereas no protective effect on other kinds of cancer was observed at lower dosages. However, this topic remains the object of discussion, and some evidence of protective effects at physiological dosages was proposed for breast cancer [195,196], colon cancer [197], esophageal cancer [198] and others.

Astaxanthin and fucoxanthin are xanthophylls, i.e., oxygen-containing carotenoids, which derive from carotenes through the carotenoid synthesis pathway [199]. They act by upregulating peroxisome proliferator-activated receptors (PPARs) [188]. Importantly, PPARγ increases the PGC1α, NRF1/2, and TFAM transcription factors, with consequent positive effects on mitochondrial biogenesis, oxygen consumption, mitochondrial membrane potential, antioxidant defenses, etc. [200].

Table 5. Carotenoids detected in microalgae species. Some reported data are significantly higher than values expected from standard cultures because of referred biomasses cultivated under stressing conditions or adopting modified methods (including heterotrophic cultures), in order to maximize the synthesis and accumulation of the desired metabolite. Some species names used in the cited references have been updated according to the current taxonomic status reported in AlgaeBase [126].

Major Component	Species	Compound Concentration	Ref.	Total Carotenoid Concentration	Ref.
β-carotene	Dunaliella salina	Up to 10–13% DW	[201]	up to 29%	[188]
	Tetraselmis suecica	0.1% DW		0.35–1.1% DW	[202]
	Vischeria stellata	5.9% DW	[203]	7.7% DW	[203]
	Chromochloris zofingiensis	0.9% DW	[201]	0.7–0.88% DW	[204,205]
Astaxanthin	Haematococcus pluvialis	2.3–7.7% DW	[206]	astaxanthin accounts for 85–90% of total carotenoids [207]	
		Up to 5% DW	[188]		
	Chromochloris zofingiensis	0.3–0.6% DW	[208]	0.7% DW	[204]
		0.53–0.6% DW	[188]	0.7% DW	[204]
Canthaxanthin	Coelastrella striolata var. multistriata	4.75% DW	[205]	5.6% DW	[205]
Fucoxanthin	Isochrysis aff. galbana	1.7–2.1% DW	[209]	2% DW	[209]
	Mallomonas sp. SBV13	2.6%	[210]		
	Isochrysis galbana	0.22–1.35% DW	[130,211]	1.76% DW	[211]
	Odontella aurita	up to 2.2% DW	[201]	~1.5% DW	[212]
	Phaeodactylum tricornutum	0.78–1.65% DW	[201,211]	0.61–1% DW	[151,211]
Lutein	Auxenochlorella protothecoides	0.54 DW	[201]	0.8% DW	[213]
	Chlorella sorokiniana	0.21–0.32% DW	[158]	0.4% DW	[214]
	Coelastrella sp.	0.69% DW	[201]		
	Desmodesmus sp.	0.51% DW	[158]	0.67% DW	[158]
	Chromochloris zofingiensis (mutant strain)	1.38% DW	[215]	2.74% DW	[215]
	Scenedesmus almeriensis	0.54% DW	[201]		
Violaxanthin	Nannochloropsis sp.	0.12–0.58% DW	[117]	0.30–0.86% DW	[117]
Zeaxanthin	Chloroidium saccharophila	1.1% DW	[216]	1.6% DW	[217]
	Chloroidium ellipsoideum	0.42% DW	[216]		
	Chromochloris zofingiensis (mutant strain)	0.7% DW	[215]	2.74% DW	[215]
	Dunaliella salina (mutant strain)	0.42–0.59% DW	[218]	1.1–1.28% DW	[218]

Astaxanthin is one of the most studied carotenoids for its high antioxidant power, effective anti-inflammatory activity, and many other effects due to the modulation of several enzymes and genetic factors. Moreover, it was reported to inhibit the generation of mitochondrial-derived ROS by protecting its membranes from lipid peroxidation [219]. The cystic form of *Haematococcus pluvialis* is the richest source in nature of this compound with about 3% DW [19], which can reach 5–7% DW under special culture conditions (cf. Table 5). Astaxanthin has been shown to significantly extend the lifespan by affecting the biogenesis of the mitochondrial respiratory complex III (CIII), in plants, *Caenorhabditis elegans* (a nematode often used as a model organism), rodents and humans [220]. Mutant-lines of the animal model *Drosophila melanogaster* with reduced levels of SOD1, SOD2 and catalase were fed with experimental diets comprising *Haematococcus pluvialis* extracts, which, at specific concentrations (1 mg/mL), have shown a significant lifespan extension and amelioration of age-related decline of motility [221].

Astaxanthin appears to act on various biochemical pathways, and, in many cases, its action is not attributable to the mere antioxidant activity, of which the review by Sztretye et al. [222] proposed a perusal analysis. Under some experimental conditions, astaxanthin has been shown to protect mitochondrial functionality, possibly by protecting membranes from oxidative damage rather than by preventing excessive ROS production [223]. At the same time, it increased the expression of the PINK-parkin pathway, thus promoting the mitophagic degradation of damaged mitochondria or their dysfunctional parts [42]. In addition to the scavenging of free radicals and membrane integrity preservation, an important activity of astaxanthin as a neuroprotector was observed. This was explained as due to the modulation of Nrf2, FOXO3 (a transcriptional activator which has been shown to promote mtDNA transcription under reduction of nutrient intake [224]) and SIRT1, i.e., key regulators which control the metabolic mechanisms of longevity, directly or indirectly involving mitochondria [225]. It was also reported that, under hypoxic stress, i.e., conditions of special interest for cardiovascular diseases, astaxanthin promoted the phosphorylation of ERK1/2 in response to the concomitant administration of acetyl-L-carnitine and was able to stimulate mitochondrial biogenesis by upregulating PGC-1α, or NRF-1 via upregulation of Nrf2 [156]. Furthermore, several studies show that this carotenoid was able to effectively protect mitochondria from the damage resulting from oxidative stress in experimental models of pathologies, such as myocardial ischemia, homocysteine-induced cardiotoxicity, pulmonary fibrosis, hyperglycemia, hepatic inflammation and fibrosis, and nonalcoholic steatosis [226]. In another study on cells subjected to stress, astaxanthin was shown to stimulate both the mitophagy of dysfunctional mitochondria via the PINK-Parkin pathway and organelle biogenesis for maintaining the overall mitochondrial efficiency via upregulation of TFAM and PGC-1α [42]. Moreover, astaxanthin increased the oxidative metabolism of lipids by promoting the activation of carnitine palmitoyl-transferase I (CPT I) in the muscle cells of endurance athletes, protecting this enzyme from alterations induced by hexanoyl-lysine (an oxidative stress marker) produced during prolonged physical exercise [227]. This mitochondrial enzyme catalyzes the transfer of the acyl group of a long-chain fatty acyl-CoA from coenzyme A to L-carnitine, producing acyl carnitine that is suitable to be moved from the cytosol into the mitochondria and to undergo the oxidative degradation. For this reason, astaxanthin is adopted by athletes to improve their performances, even if the effectiveness can depend on the muscle effort required. In addition to this, several genes suitable for protecting mitochondrial functionality from oxidative stress are upregulated by lycopene and astaxanthin, thanks to the activation of Nrf2 via different pathways, only partially elucidated and possibly including the dissociation of Nrf2 from the Keap1 repressor [219]. KEAP1 forms part of an E3 ubiquitin ligase, which binds NRF2 by targeting it for ubiquitination and proteasome-dependent degradation. The action of lycopene and astaxanthin, if confirmed, would be interesting since it would support the assumption that, under oxidative stress conditions, their reaction with ROS attributes an electrophilic property to these carotenoids. These reaction products could be sufficiently electrophilic to react with cysteine thiol groups of Keap1, which in turn will act as an oxidative stress sensor, weakening its binding to Nrf2. Upon dissociation from Keap1, Nrf2 evades proteasome degradation, accumulates in the cytosol, and finally translocates to the nucleus, where it exerts its regulatory activities.

Among the most important activities of astaxanthin and fucoxanthin, the regulation of apoptosis should be mentioned, with relevant implications for the prevention or reduction of tumors. Although it is generally accepted that carotenoids help cancer prevention, their interaction with several biochemical pathways producing both proapoptotic and antiapoptotic effects, depending on the cell environment, was reported. Sathasivam and Ki [201] reviewed the bioactivities of carotenoids and, within a complex network of reactions, pointed out three key metabolic pathways involving MAP kinases and mitochondrion as organelle effectors:

- Activation of the PI3K/Akt (phosphatidylinositol 3-kinase; AKT-serine/threonine kinase also known as PKB, protein kinase B) survival pathway, which inactivates Bax by phosphorylation and reduces the release of Cyt-c (antiapoptotic effect). Indeed, according to Kale et al. [105], the phosphorylation at residue S184 by Akt inhibits Bax, thus preventing its translocation into the mitochondrion.
- Activation of the p38 MAPK signaling pathway, which promotes the release of Cyt-c and activates the apoptosome (apoptotic effect). Specifically, p38 MAPK can act on the mitochondrial permeability by activating Bim by phosphorylation, which in turn activates Bax or, alternatively, it can phosphorylate p53, which induces the expression of death receptors and can activate members of the BCL-2 family to promote

apoptosis [228]. Other proapoptotic mechanisms of action have been hypothesized for p38MAPK, beyond the scope of the present review.
- Stimulation of MEK1/2–ERK1/2 signaling pathway, which in turn activates the pro-survival BCL-2 proteins (antiapoptotic effect), as shortly explained in the first part of this contribution.

Interestingly, the activation of ERK1/2 can also stimulate DRP1 expression and, thus, promote mitochondrial fission [106], which is functional to the segregation of mitochondria between the two daughter cells during mitosis, but also to the separation and subsequent mitophagy of dysfunctional parts of the mitochondrial reticulum. On the other side, a massive activation of mitochondrial fission is consistent with a proapoptotic effect described for ERK1/2 by activation of the pro-death BCL-2 protein, NOXA, which can occur as an alternative route to the classic pro-survival Ras/Raf/MEK/ERK signaling [106]. Therefore, as already remarked concerning the activities of phenolic compounds, it should be noted that carotenoids can produce a complex and variable range of effects, depending on both the considered molecule and the metabolic situation of the cell. For example, it has been shown that fucoxanthin and siphonaxanthin were able to inhibit the activation of ERK1/2 by phosphorylation mediated by FGF-2, in vascular endothelial cells [229]. However, astaxanthin stimulated the activation of ERK1/2 in HCT-116 colon cancer cells as part of an overall pro-apoptotic effect [230]. Again, astaxanthin prevented apoptosis induced by cytotoxic treatments aimed at increasing ROS in the *substantia nigra* neurons in a mouse model of Parkinson's disease and in human neuroblastoma SH-SY5Y cells [72]. This effect was due to the increased expression of BCL-2 protein, the downregulation of α-synuclein and Bax, and the inhibition of the cleavage of caspase-3. However, the administration of a diet supplemented with astaxanthin showed pro-apoptotic activity in Syrian hamsters treated with carcinogenic stimuli, producing protective effects against the onset of squamous cell carcinomas [231]. The study showed an antiproliferative effect of astaxanthin by inhibiting the MEK/ERK and PI3K/Akt pathways and the related downstream IKKβ/NF-κB and GSK-3β/Wnt-catenin signaling, promoting intrinsic apoptosis as a final outcome. Notably, in this study, astaxanthin showed opposite effects with respect to the above-reported stimulations of MEK/ERK and PI3/Akt, suggesting that the same receptors can produce alternative modulations on the underling pathways depending on the cellular environmental context. According to Kavitha et al. [231], astaxanthin prevented the inactivation of GSK-3β by phosphorylation, which, therefore, can constitute, with other proteins, the "destruction complex" responsible for the phosphorylation and subsequent degradation of β-catenin. This last protein, therefore, interrupts its translocation into the nucleus and its activation of genes involved in cell proliferation and apoptosis evasion. Besides, in the same context, astaxanthin also inhibited the Akt kinase, responsible, among other activities, for the inactivating phosphorylation of Bad (in addition to the inhibiting phosphorylation of Bax, above mentioned). Bad, in the dephosphorylated form, can translocate to the mitochondrial membrane, selectively displacing Bax from the inhibiting binding to antiapoptotic BCL-2 proteins. In this free form, Bax is then able to initiate the mitochondrial membrane permeability process by inducing the release of Cyt-c and Smac/DIABLO proteins, which in turn trigger the caspase cascade and, finally, apoptosis. Similarly, astaxanthin has shown pro-apototic activities by inhibiting NF-κB and Wnt/β-catenin in human hepatoma cell lines [232]. These cases are of special interest in order to point out the complexity of the response characterizing the intra-cell secondary messages and the related biochemical pathways.

Considering the above-reported studies, it should be noted that NF-kB, a typical pro-inflammatory factor, can act as a pro- or anti-apoptotic intermediate depending on the upstream stimulus [233], with relevant implications on the efficacy of some anticancer chemotherapies [234]. More generally, the pleiotropic action of astaxanthin and its ability to act in different cellular contexts as a promoter of biogenesis and mitochondrial functionality or as a pro-apoptotic and anticarcinogenic agent, depends on its ability to interact with a high number of enzymes involved in cell cycle regulation. The different outcomes depend on the cell metabolic condition and on the concomitant presence of other stimuli. Recent studies suggested that astaxanthin can interact with a number of proteins involved in cell growth pathways, including EGFR (epidermal growth factor receptor), IGF1R (insulin-like growth factor 1 receptor), AKT1, AKT2, ERK1, and ERK2 [235].

Fucoxanthin, another carotenoid synthesized by several microalgae, has been shown to protect mitochondrial function in a cell model treated with pro-inflammatory stimuli, specifically by preserving the membrane potential and by modulating mitochondrial dynamics, i.e., by promoting the mitophagy of dysfunctional mitochondria and, at the same time, stimulating their renewal via biogenesis [49]. This carotenoid is known for its peculiar ability to modulate the metabolism of adipocytes and to reduce the accumulation of fat by promoting the mitochondrial expression of UCP1 and the uptake of glucose in the muscles via increased expression of GLUT4 glucose transporter [236,237]. In addition to this, the improved metabolism of fat also appeared due to the upregulation of PGC-1α and improved mitochondrial dynamics [47]. Importantly, the combination of the antioxidant activity with the regulation of glucose uptake makes fucoxanthin an ideal candidate for the treatment of metabolic syndrome, since there is strong evidence of the important role played by ROS in various types of insulin resistances [238]. Moreover, fucoxanthin has shown neuroprotective activity, in vivo and in vitro, upregulating the expression of the DJ-1 stress-sensing protein in rats and protecting mitochondria from oxidative stress following the treatment with hydrogen peroxide [239].

3.6. Other Bioactive Compounds

Some microalgal compounds have shown important bioactivities, possibly influencing the biology of the mitochondria, although their mechanisms of action are still not sufficiently known. Many of these have been characterized as anticarcinogens [17,240–242], even if often by tests conducted only on cell lines, as already pointed out in many above-reported examples. In this regard, it should be kept in mind that if the microalgal preparation has to be taken orally, as happens with functional foods, the data obtained by treating cell cultures should be confirmed in vivo since active molecules may not be absorbed or can be modified during digestion or after absorption. These compounds include, by way of example, polysaccharides (often sulfated), glycosides, terpenoids and galactolipids.

Among polysaccharides, β-glucans or chrysolaminarins are produced by several microalgae and especially by Bacillariophyta [189]. In particular, 1,3-1,6 β-glucans have been shown to improve mitochondrial respiration and functionality in a model of Duchenne muscular dystrophy [243]. A fatty alcohol ester isolated from *Phaeodactylum tricornutum*, nonyl 8-acetoxy-6-methyloctanoate, was described to promote intrinsic apoptosis in promyeloblast HL-60 cells by activating the pro-apoptotic Bax protein and by suppressing the anti-apoptotic BCL-2-like protein 1 (alias BCL-xL) [244].

Cyclic peptides synthesized by some marine cyanobacteria, such as cyclic depsipeptides aurilide B and C produced by *Lyngbya majusculus*, or the cyclic depsipeptide Coibamade A produced by *Leptolyngbya* sp., showed cytotoxicity in several human tumor cell lines. A perusal revision was proposed by Mondal et al. [240]. Some of these compounds, e.g., aurilides isolated from the cyanobacterium *Moorena bouillonii*, have been shown to act on mitochondria by binding prohibitin 1 (PHB1) and by stimulating OPA1 synthesis, thus promoting mitochondrial fission and apoptosis [240]. PHB1 regulates the organization and maintenance of the mitochondrial genome by the accurate organization of mitochondrial nucleoids and controls the copy number of mtDNA by stabilizing TFAM [245].

4. Discussion and Conclusions

The interest in the use of microalgae as a source of active compounds is grounded on their ability to produce and concentrate bioactive substances suitable to protect the cell from harmful processes and to preserve some needful functionalities, many of which are related to the functional integrity of mitochondria. As shown in many cases discussed above, the preservation of mitochondrial functionality is essential to prevent damages due to oxidative stress, the main cause of aging. Oxidative stress also promotes many chronic and degenerative diseases, such as cardiovascular diseases, diseases of the nervous system, diabetes, and many types of cancer. In addition to this, these single-cell organisms assume high economic interest because they can be industrially cultivated in purity by means of bioreactors or in semi-purity in suitable open-pond plants [246]. Their culture does not require the use of pesticides or drugs and can also occur in infertile soils, ensuring the logistical and insolation conditions to successfully manage bioreactor plants. Furthermore, microalgae can be produced in wastewater treatment plants, even with some applicative limitations on the use of the biomasses obtained [247]. From a technical point of view, therefore, microalgae are perfect candidates to play a relevant role in the development of an innovative, sustainable and green economy. Moreover, microalgae can be processed in order to obtain dehydrated flours, which can be commercialized as raw materials and easily mixed to obtain a balanced combination of desirable actives. In this sense, they represent an ideal source of ingredients for functional foods and nutritional supplements. In 2020, the global microalgae market was estimated at USD 3.4 billion, and the annual growth rate is estimated at 4.3%, so in 2027, this value is expected to reach USD 4.6 billion [248]. The attention paid to the antioxidant properties of many microalgal active compounds, such as carotenoids, PUFAs, polyphenols, etc., is consistent with the fact that aging is largely derived from molecular damage due to oxidative reactions triggered by free radicals. Importantly, even if many of these active compounds are industrially synthesized at lower costs, there is evidence that the biological activity of synthetic analogs is different, and in some cases considerably lower, than that of natural compounds [249–251].

On the other hand, mitochondria, due to their function as cell "powerhouses" and sites of high-intensity redox reactions, represent a fundamental target to protect the functional integrity of the cell. However, from the above-reported data, it is evident that the protective activity exerted by the mentioned bio-actives is only partly related to their antioxidant properties. Indeed, it seems that the relevance of their biological action is broader and correlated with their ability to interact with some biochemical pathways involving inflammation, gene expression of antioxidant enzymes, intrinsic apoptosis and mitochondrial dynamics. Simplified synthesis of some key pathways involving mitochondria as final organelle executors and affected by microalgal compounds are shown in Figure 2. Interestingly, the regulatory action exerted by microalgal bioactive compounds on cell signaling explains how they can be effective, even if taken in limited quantities, compatible with dietary intake. Works currently available in the literature are often focused on the beneficial properties of individual compounds present in microalgae, but studies aimed at verifying the benefits deriving from the natural combination of different active compounds are very scarce.

Nevertheless, multifunctionality is one of the most interesting characteristics of microalgae and suggests that they can represent excellent functional foods, potentially suitable for simultaneously providing protection against different types of metabolic disorders and for delaying cellular aging through complementary and synergistic mechanisms of action. However, multifunctional actions can hardly be evaluated using in vitro experimental models, while they would require the execution of long-term clinical trials. Another aspect in which the study of microalgae is still unsatisfactory concerns the chemical characterization of their composition, containing different compounds potentially active in human metabolism. For example, the quantitative comparison between the identified phenolic compounds and the total phenolic content observed in many case studies shows that most of the compounds have not been characterized yet. This is probably due to the fact that analyses were carried out looking for phenolic compounds already known in terrestrial plants, whereas it is known that these microorganisms produce molecules (e.g., carotenoids and long-chain fatty acids) that are rare or even absent in the terrestrial biomes.

Importantly, the use of microalgae for foods would require further development of the downstream processing of cell-mass and products in order to improve the bioavailability of active compounds of interest and, in addition, to ensure preservation until consumption [252]. Indeed, the cell wall of some strains can represent an important impairment to intestinal absorption of part of the actives [119,253–255], which, due to their reducing properties, are also susceptible to being modified during their processing or storage. In any case, the potential of microalgae as sources of active compounds deserves intense research efforts.

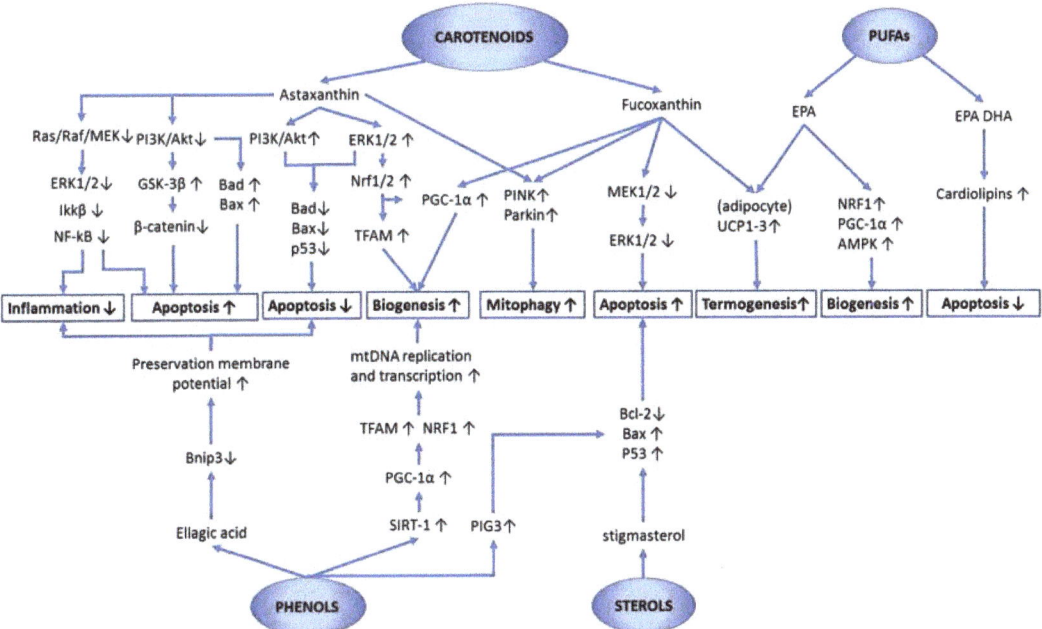

Figure 2. Simplified scheme of relevant interactions of microalgal bioactive compounds acting on mitochondrial functionality and apoptosis. The direction of the arrows indicates the modulation of enzyme/compound activity, not of gene expression. Abbreviations: AMPK, 5′-AMP-activated protein kinase; Bad, Bcl-2-associated death promoter; Bax, BCL-2-associated X protein; BCL-2, B-cell lymphoma 2; Bnip3, BCL2 interacting protein 3; DHA, docosahexaenoic acid; EPA, eicosapentaenoic acid; ERKs, extracellular signal-regulated kinases; MEK, MAPK/ERK kinase; NF-kB, nuclear factor kappa-light-chain-enhancer of activated B cells; Nrf1, nuclear respiratory factor-1; Nrf2, nuclear factor erythroid 2-related factor 2; p53, cellular tumor antigen p53; PGC-1α, peroxisome proliferator-activated receptor-γ coactivator-1α; PINK, PTEN-induced kinase; Raf, RAF proto-oncogene serine/threonine-protein kinase (alias rapidly accelerated fibrosarcoma kinase); Ras, KRAS Proto-Oncogene, GTPase; SIRT1, silent information regulator-1; TFAM, transcription factor A mitochondrial; UCPs, uncoupling proteins.

Even if the chemical characterization of algal biomass is still insufficient, the most important deficiency relies on the current lack of an overall evaluation of the nutraceutical functions attributable to the different microalgal species already authorized for food use and the relative recommended rations. To date, trials on humans are available for a few microalgae and are often based on dietary treatments for a few weeks. In this regard, some relevant findings are available for *Phaeodactylum tricornutum* (Bacillariophyta) [256], species of the genus *Chlorella* (Trebouxiophyceae) [257–262], *Haematococcus pluvialis* (Chlorophyceae) [263–266], species of the genus *Tetraselmis* (Chlorodendrophyceae) [267], *Euglena gracilis* (Euglenophyceae) [268], species of the genus *Nannochloropsis* (Eustigmatophyceae) [269] and cyanobacteria of the genus *Arthrospira* (Cyanophyceae) [270,271].

In conclusion, authors considered of particular interest the promotion of further trials involving significant numbers of subjects and carried out over a long period of time. Indeed, the effects of functional foods based on the response of biochemical markers can be very useful, but unlike the behavior of drugs for the treatment of specific pathologies, the assessment of a preventive approach requires long-term studies and data based on large sample sizes in order to support robust statistical analyses.

Author Contributions: All authors contributed equally to this work. All authors have read and agreed to the published version of the manuscript.

Funding: This work did not receive external funding.

Institutional Review Board Statement: Not applicable.

Informed Consent Statement: Not applicable.

Data Availability Statement: Not applicable.

Conflicts of Interest: The authors declare no conflict of interest.

References

1. Bloom, D.E.; Luca, D.L. Chapter 1—The Global Demography of Aging: Facts, Explanations, Future. In *Handbook of the Economics of Population Aging*; Piggott, J., Woodland, A., Eds.; North-Holland: Amsterdam, The Netherlands, 2016; Volume 1, pp. 3–56.
2. de Meijer, C.; Wouterse, B.; Polder, J.; Koopmanschap, M. The Effect of Population Aging on Health Expenditure Growth: A Critical Review. *Eur. J. Ageing* **2013**, *10*, 353–361. [CrossRef] [PubMed]
3. Han, Y.; He, Y.; Lyu, J.; Yu, C.; Bian, M.; Lee, L. Aging in China: Perspectives on Public Health. *Glob. Health J.* **2020**, *4*, 11–17. [CrossRef]
4. Kaplan, M.; Inguanzo, M. The Social, Economic, and Public Health Consequences of Global Population Aging: Implications for Social Work Practice and Public Policy. *J. Soc. Work Glob. Community* **2017**, *2*, 1–12. [CrossRef]
5. Vancea, M.; Solé-Casals, J. Population Aging in the European Information Societies: Towards a Comprehensive Research Agenda in EHealth Innovations for Elderly. *Aging Dis.* **2015**, *7*, 526–539. [CrossRef]
6. Meydani, M. Nutrition Interventions in Aging and Age-Associated Disease. *Ann. N. Y. Acad. Sci.* **2001**, *928*, 226–235. [CrossRef] [PubMed]
7. Miyazawa, T.; Abe, C.; Burdeos, G.C.; Matsumoto, A.; Toda, M. Food Antioxidants and Aging: Theory, Current Evidence and Perspectives. *Nutraceuticals* **2022**, *2*, 181–204. [CrossRef]
8. García-Montero, C.; Fraile-Martínez, O.; Gómez-Lahoz, A.M.; Pekarek, L.; Castellanos, A.J.; Noguerales-Fraguas, F.; Coca, S.; Guijarro, L.G.; García-Honduvilla, N.; Asúnsolo, A.; et al. Nutritional Components in Western Diet Versus Mediterranean Diet at the Gut Microbiota–Immune System Interplay. Implications for Health and Disease. *Nutrients* **2021**, *13*, 699. [CrossRef]
9. Cordain, L.; Eaton, S.B.; Sebastian, A.; Mann, N.; Lindeberg, S.; Watkins, B.A.; O'Keefe, J.H.; Brand-Miller, J. Origins and Evolution of the Western Diet: Health Implications for the 21st Century. *Am. J. Clin. Nutr.* **2005**, *81*, 341–354. [CrossRef]
10. Castillo, M.; Iriondo-DeHond, A.; Martirosyan, D. Are Functional Foods Essential for Sustainable Health? *Ann. Nutr. Food Sci.* **2018**, *2*, 1015.
11. Milner, J.A. Functional Foods and Health Promotion. *J. Nutr.* **1999**, *129*, 1395S–1397S. [CrossRef]
12. Meléndez-Martínez, A.J.; Böhm, V.; Borge, G.I.A.; Cano, M.P.; Fikselová, M.; Gruskiene, R.; Lavelli, V.; Loizzo, M.R.; Mandić, A.I.; Brahm, P.M.; et al. Carotenoids: Considerations for Their Use in Functional Foods, Nutraceuticals, Nutricosmetics, Supplements, Botanicals, and Novel Foods in the Context of Sustainability, Circular Economy, and Climate Change. *Annu. Rev. Food Sci. Technol.* **2021**, *12*, 433–460. [CrossRef]
13. Barkia, I.; Saari, N.; Manning, S.R. Microalgae for High-Value Products Towards Human Health and Nutrition. *Mar. Drugs* **2019**, *17*, 304. [CrossRef]
14. Basheer, S.; Huo, S.; Zhu, F.; Qian, J.; Xu, L.; Cui, F.; Zou, B. Microalgae in Human Health and Medicine. In *Microalgae Biotechnology for Food, Health and High Value Products*; Alam, M.A., Xu, J.-L., Wang, Z., Eds.; Springer: Singapore, 2020; pp. 149–174. ISBN 9789811501692.
15. Del Mondo, A.; Smerilli, A.; Sané, E.; Sansone, C.; Brunet, C. Challenging Microalgal Vitamins for Human Health. *Microb. Cell Factories* **2020**, *19*, 201. [CrossRef]
16. Matos, J.; Cardoso, C.; Bandarra, N.M.; Afonso, C. Microalgae as Healthy Ingredients for Functional Food: A Review. *Food Funct.* **2017**, *8*, 2672–2685. [CrossRef]
17. Abd El-Hack, M.E.; Abdelnour, S.; Alagawany, M.; Abdo, M.; Sakr, M.A.; Khafaga, A.F.; Mahgoub, S.A.; Elnesr, S.S.; Gebriel, M.G. Microalgae in Modern Cancer Therapy: Current Knowledge. *Biomed. Pharmacother.* **2019**, *111*, 42–50. [CrossRef] [PubMed]
18. Andrade, L.M.; Andrade, C.J.; Dias, M.; Nascimento, C.A.O.; Mendes, M.A. *Chlorella* and *Spirulina* Microalgae as Sources of Functional Foods, Nutraceuticals, and Food Supplements; an Overview. *MOJ Food Process. Technol.* **2018**, *6*, 45–58. [CrossRef]
19. Guerin, M.; Huntley, M.E.; Olaizola, M. *Haematococcus* Astaxanthin: Applications for Human Health and Nutrition. *Trends Biotechnol.* **2003**, *21*, 210–216. [CrossRef]
20. Napolitano, G.; Fasciolo, G.; Salbitani, G.; Venditti, P. *Chlorella sorokiniana* Dietary Supplementation Increases Antioxidant Capacities and Reduces ROS Release in Mitochondria of Hyperthyroid Rat Liver. *Antioxidants* **2020**, *9*, 883. [CrossRef] [PubMed]

21. Wells, M.L.; Potin, P.; Craigie, J.S.; Raven, J.A.; Merchant, S.S.; Helliwell, K.E.; Smith, A.G.; Camire, M.E.; Brawley, S.H. Algae as Nutritional and Functional Food Sources: Revisiting Our Understanding. *J. Appl. Phycol.* **2017**, *29*, 949–982. [CrossRef] [PubMed]
22. Chatterjee, S. Chapter Two—Oxidative Stress, Inflammation, and Disease. In *Oxidative Stress and Biomaterials*; Dziubla, T., Butterfield, D.A., Eds.; Academic Press: Cambridge, MA, USA, 2016; pp. 35–58. ISBN 978-0-12-803269-5.
23. Rani, V.; Deep, G.; Singh, R.K.; Palle, K.; Yadav, U.C.S. Oxidative Stress and Metabolic Disorders: Pathogenesis and Therapeutic Strategies. *Life Sci.* **2016**, *148*, 183–193. [CrossRef]
24. Hajam, Y.A.; Rani, R.; Ganie, S.Y.; Sheikh, T.A.; Javaid, D.; Qadri, S.S.; Pramodh, S.; Alsulimani, A.; Alkhanani, M.F.; Harakeh, S.; et al. Oxidative Stress in Human Pathology and Aging: Molecular Mechanisms and Perspectives. *Cells* **2022**, *11*, 552. [CrossRef] [PubMed]
25. Murphy, E.; Ardehali, H.; Balaban, R.S.; DiLisa, F.; Dorn, G.W.; Kitsis, R.N.; Otsu, K.; Ping, P.; Rizzuto, R.; Sack, M.N.; et al. Mitochondrial Function, Biology, and Role in Disease. *Circ. Res.* **2016**, *118*, 1960–1991. [CrossRef]
26. Murphy, M.P.; Hartley, R.C. Mitochondria as a Therapeutic Target for Common Pathologies. *Nat. Rev. Drug Discov.* **2018**, *17*, 865–886. [CrossRef]
27. Sukhorukov, V.M.; Dikov, D.; Reichert, A.S.; Meyer-Hermann, M. Emergence of the Mitochondrial Reticulum from Fission and Fusion Dynamics. *PLoS Comput. Biol.* **2012**, *8*, e1002745. [CrossRef]
28. Hock, M.B.; Kralli, A. Transcriptional Control of Mitochondrial Biogenesis and Function. *Annu. Rev. Physiol.* **2009**, *71*, 177–203. [CrossRef]
29. Gureev, A.P.; Shaforostova, E.A.; Popov, V.N. Regulation of Mitochondrial Biogenesis as a Way for Active Longevity: Interaction Between the Nrf2 and PGC-1α Signaling Pathways. *Front. Genet.* **2019**, *10*, 435. [CrossRef]
30. Yun, J.; Finkel, T. Mitohormesis. *Cell Metab.* **2014**, *19*, 757–766. [CrossRef] [PubMed]
31. Westermann, B. Bioenergetic Role of Mitochondrial Fusion and Fission. *Biochim. Biophys. Acta BBA Bioenerg.* **2012**, *1817*, 1833–1838. [CrossRef]
32. Robb, E.L.; Moradi, F.; Maddalena, L.A.; Valente, A.J.F.; Fonseca, J.; Stuart, J.A. Resveratrol Stimulates Mitochondrial Fusion by a Mechanism Requiring Mitofusin-2. *Biochem. Biophys. Res. Commun.* **2017**, *485*, 249–254. [CrossRef]
33. Nicholls, T.J.; Gustafsson, C.M. Separating and Segregating the Human Mitochondrial Genome. *Trends Biochem. Sci.* **2018**, *43*, 869–881. [CrossRef] [PubMed]
34. Mallat, A.; Uchiyama, L.F.; Lewis, S.C.; Fredenburg, R.A.; Terada, Y.; Ji, N.; Nunnari, J.; Tseng, C.C. Discovery and Characterization of Selective Small Molecule Inhibitors of the Mammalian Mitochondrial Division Dynamin, DRP1. *Biochem. Biophys. Res. Commun.* **2018**, *499*, 556–562. [CrossRef]
35. Otera, H.; Ishihara, N.; Mihara, K. New Insights into the Function and Regulation of Mitochondrial Fission. *Biochim. Biophys. Acta BBA Mol. Cell Res.* **2013**, *1833*, 1256–1268. [CrossRef]
36. Kageyama, Y.; Zhang, Z.; Sesaki, H. Mitochondrial Division: Molecular Machinery and Physiological Functions. *Curr. Opin. Cell Biol.* **2011**, *23*, 427–434. [CrossRef] [PubMed]
37. Frank, M.; Duvezin-Caubet, S.; Koob, S.; Occhipinti, A.; Jagasia, R.; Petcherski, A.; Ruonala, M.O.; Priault, M.; Salin, B.; Reichert, A.S. Mitophagy Is Triggered by Mild Oxidative Stress in a Mitochondrial Fission Dependent Manner. *Biochim. Biophys. Acta BBA Mol. Cell Res.* **2012**, *1823*, 2297–2310. [CrossRef]
38. Youle, R.J.; Narendra, D.P. Mechanisms of Mitophagy. *Nat. Rev. Mol. Cell Biol.* **2011**, *12*, 9–14. [CrossRef]
39. Tanaka, K. The PINK1–Parkin Axis: An Overview. *Neurosci. Res.* **2020**, *159*, 9–15. [CrossRef] [PubMed]
40. Ding, W.-X.; Yin, X.-M. Mitophagy: Mechanisms, Pathophysiological Roles, and Analysis. *Biol. Chem.* **2012**, *393*, 547–564. [CrossRef]
41. Liu, P.H.; Aoi, W.; Takami, M.; Terajima, H.; Tanimura, Y.; Naito, Y.; Itoh, Y.; Yoshikawa, T. The Astaxanthin-Induced Improvement in Lipid Metabolism during Exercise Is Mediated by a PGC-1α Increase in Skeletal Muscle. *J. Clin. Biochem. Nutr.* **2014**, *54*, 86–89. [CrossRef] [PubMed]
42. Chen, Y.; Li, S.; Guo, Y.; Yu, H.; Bao, Y.; Xin, X.; Yang, H.; Ni, X.; Wu, N.; Jia, D. Astaxanthin Attenuates Hypertensive Vascular Remodeling by Protecting Vascular Smooth Muscle Cells from Oxidative Stress-Induced Mitochondrial Dysfunction. *Oxidative Med. Cell. Longev.* **2020**, *2020*, 4629189. [CrossRef]
43. Laiglesia, L.M.; Lorente-Cebrián, S.; Prieto-Hontoria, P.L.; Fernández-Galilea, M.; Ribeiro, S.M.R.; Sáinz, N.; Martínez, J.A.; Moreno-Aliaga, M.J. Eicosapentaenoic Acid Promotes Mitochondrial Biogenesis and Beige-like Features in Subcutaneous Adipocytes from Overweight Subjects. *J. Nutr. Biochem.* **2016**, *37*, 76–82. [CrossRef]
44. Flachs, P.; Horakova, O.; Brauner, P.; Rossmeisl, M.; Pecina, P.; Franssen-van Hal, N.; Ruzickova, J.; Sponarova, J.; Drahota, Z.; Vlcek, C.; et al. Polyunsaturated Fatty Acids of Marine Origin Upregulate Mitochondrial Biogenesis and Induce β-Oxidation in White Fat. *Diabetologia* **2005**, *48*, 2365–2375. [CrossRef]
45. Gibellini, L.; Bianchini, E.; De Biasi, S.; Nasi, M.; Cossarizza, A.; Pinti, M. Natural Compounds Modulating Mitochondrial Functions. *Evid.-Based Complement. Altern. Med. ECAM* **2015**, *2015*, 527209. [CrossRef]
46. Lepretti, M.; Martucciello, S.; Burgos Aceves, M.A.; Putti, R.; Lionetti, L. Omega-3 Fatty Acids and Insulin Resistance: Focus on the Regulation of Mitochondria and Endoplasmic Reticulum Stress. *Nutrients* **2018**, *10*, 350. [CrossRef] [PubMed]
47. Wu, M.-T.; Chou, H.-N.; Huang, C. Dietary Fucoxanthin Increases Metabolic Rate and Upregulated MRNA Expressions of the PGC-1alpha Network, Mitochondrial Biogenesis and Fusion Genes in White Adipose Tissues of Mice. *Mar. Drugs* **2014**, *12*, 964–982. [CrossRef] [PubMed]

48. Mao, G.-X.; Xu, X.-G.; Wang, S.-Y.; Li, H.-F.; Zhang, J.; Zhang, Z.-S.; Su, H.-L.; Chen, S.-S.; Xing, W.-M.; Wang, Y.-Z.; et al. Salidroside Delays Cellular Senescence by Stimulating Mitochondrial Biogenesis Partly through a MiR-22/SIRT-1 Pathway. *Oxid. Med. Cell. Longev.* **2019**, *2019*, e5276096. [CrossRef]
49. Li, S.; Ren, X.; Wang, Y.; Hu, J.; Wu, H.; Song, S.; Yan, C. Fucoxanthin Alleviates Palmitate-Induced Inflammation in RAW 264.7 Cells through Improving Lipid Metabolism and Attenuating Mitochondrial Dysfunction. *Food Funct.* **2020**, *11*, 3361–3370. [CrossRef]
50. Zhang, J.; Xu, P.; Wang, Y.; Wang, M.; Li, H.; Lin, S.; Mao, C.; Wang, B.; Song, X.; Lv, C. Astaxanthin Prevents Pulmonary Fibrosis by Promoting Myofibroblast Apoptosis Dependent on Drp1-Mediated Mitochondrial Fission. *J. Cell. Mol. Med.* **2015**, *19*, 2215–2231. [CrossRef]
51. Varghese, N.; Werner, S.; Grimm, A.; Eckert, A. Dietary Mitophagy Enhancer: A Strategy for Healthy Brain Aging? *Antioxidants* **2020**, *9*, 932. [CrossRef] [PubMed]
52. Gleyzer, N.; Vercauteren, K.; Scarpulla, R.C. Control of Mitochondrial Transcription Specificity Factors (TFB1M and TFB2M) by Nuclear Respiratory Factors (NRF-1 and NRF-2) and PGC-1 Family Coactivators. *Mol. Cell. Biol.* **2005**, *25*, 1354–1366. [CrossRef]
53. Nicholls, D.G. Mitochondrial Function and Dysfunction in the Cell: Its Relevance to Aging and Aging-Related Disease. *Int. J. Biochem. Cell Biol.* **2002**, *34*, 1372–1381. [CrossRef]
54. Ortiz, G.G.; Mireles-Ramírez, M.A.; González-Usigli, H.; Macías-Islas, M.A.; Bitzer-Quintero, O.K.; DheniTorres-Sánchez, E.; Sánchez-López, A.L.; Ramírez-Jirano, J.; Ríos-Silva, M.; Torres-Mendoza, B. *Mitochondrial Aging and Metabolism: The Importance of a Good Relationship in the Central Nervous System*; IntechOpen: London, UK, 2018; ISBN 978-1-78984-266-1.
55. Srivastava, S. The Mitochondrial Basis of Aging and Age-Related Disorders. *Genes* **2017**, *8*, 398. [CrossRef]
56. Brand, M.D.; Orr, A.L.; Perevoshchikova, I.V.; Quinlan, C.L. The Role of Mitochondrial Function and Cellular Bioenergetics in Ageing and Disease. *Br. J. Dermatol.* **2013**, *169*, 1–8. [CrossRef] [PubMed]
57. Hamon, M.-P.; Bulteau, A.-L.; Friguet, B. Mitochondrial Proteases and Protein Quality Control in Ageing and Longevity. *Ageing Res. Rev.* **2015**, *23*, 56–66. [CrossRef] [PubMed]
58. Sastre, J.; Serviddio, G.; Pereda, J.; Minana, J.B.; Arduini, A.; Vendemiale, G.; Poli, G.; Pallardo, F.V.; Vina, J. Mitochondrial Function in Liver Disease. *Front. Biosci.-Landmark* **2007**, *12*, 1200–1209. [CrossRef]
59. Serviddio, G.; Bellanti, F.; Vendemiale, G.; Altomare, E. Mitochondrial Dysfunction in Nonalcoholic Steatohepatitis. *Expert Rev. Gastroenterol. Hepatol.* **2011**, *5*, 233–244. [CrossRef] [PubMed]
60. Song, B.-J.; Moon, K.-H.; Olsson, N.U.; Salem, N. Prevention of Alcoholic Fatty Liver and Mitochondrial Dysfunction in the Rat by Long-Chain Polyunsaturated Fatty Acids. *J. Hepatol.* **2008**, *49*, 262–273. [CrossRef]
61. Videla, L.A.; Rodrigo, R.; Araya, J.; Poniachik, J. Oxidative Stress and Depletion of Hepatic Long-Chain Polyunsaturated Fatty Acids May Contribute to Nonalcoholic Fatty Liver Disease. *Free Radic. Biol. Med.* **2004**, *37*, 1499–1507. [CrossRef]
62. Hirabara, S.M.; Curi, R.; Maechler, P. Saturated Fatty Acid-Induced Insulin Resistance Is Associated with Mitochondrial Dysfunction in Skeletal Muscle Cells. *J. Cell. Physiol.* **2010**, *222*, 187–194. [CrossRef]
63. Jheng, H.-F.; Tsai, P.-J.; Guo, S.-M.; Kuo, L.-H.; Chang, C.-S.; Su, I.-J.; Chang, C.-R.; Tsai, Y.-S. Mitochondrial Fission Contributes to Mitochondrial Dysfunction and Insulin Resistance in Skeletal Muscle. *Mol. Cell. Biol.* **2012**, *32*, 309–319. [CrossRef]
64. Che, R.; Yuan, Y.; Huang, S.; Zhang, A. Mitochondrial Dysfunction in the Pathophysiology of Renal Diseases. *Am. J. Physiol.-Ren. Physiol.* **2014**, *306*, F367–F378. [CrossRef]
65. Paradies, G.; Paradies, V.; Ruggiero, F.M.; Petrosillo, G. Role of Cardiolipin in Mitochondrial Function and Dynamics in Health and Disease: Molecular and Pharmacological Aspects. *Cells* **2019**, *8*, 728. [CrossRef] [PubMed]
66. Zharikov, S.; Shiva, S. Platelet Mitochondrial Function: From Regulation of Thrombosis to Biomarker of Disease. *Biochem. Soc. Trans.* **2013**, *41*, 118–123. [CrossRef] [PubMed]
67. Jenner, P. Altered Mitochondrial Function, Iron Metabolism and Glutathione Levels in Parkinson's Disease. *Acta Neurol. Scand.* **1993**, *87*, 6–13. [CrossRef]
68. Turner, C.; Cooper, J.M.; Schapira, A.H.V. Clinical Correlates of Mitochondrial Function in Huntington's Disease Muscle. *Mov. Disord.* **2007**, *22*, 1715–1721. [CrossRef]
69. Eckert, G.P.; Renner, K.; Eckert, S.H.; Eckmann, J.; Hagl, S.; Abdel-Kader, R.M.; Kurz, C.; Leuner, K.; Muller, W.E. Mitochondrial Dysfunction—A Pharmacological Target in Alzheimer's Disease. *Mol. Neurobiol.* **2012**, *46*, 136–150. [CrossRef] [PubMed]
70. Catalgol, B.; Batirel, S.; Taga, Y.; Ozer, N. Resveratrol: French Paradox Revisited. *Front. Pharmacol.* **2012**, *3*, 141. [CrossRef]
71. Kodydková, J.; Vávrová, L.; Kocík, M.; Žák, A. Human Catalase, Its Polymorphisms, Regulation and Changes of Its Activity in Different Diseases. *Folia Biol.* **2014**, *60*, 153–167.
72. Lee, D.-H.; Kim, C.-S.; Lee, Y.J. Astaxanthin Protects against MPTP/MPP+-Induced Mitochondrial Dysfunction and ROS Production in Vivo and in Vitro. *Food Chem. Toxicol. Int. J. Publ. Br. Ind. Biol. Res. Assoc.* **2011**, *49*, 271–280. [CrossRef]
73. Zhang, Y.; Liu, L.; Sun, D.; He, Y.; Jiang, Y.; Cheng, K.-W.; Chen, F. DHA Protects against Monosodium Urate-Induced Inflammation through Modulation of Oxidative Stress. *Food Funct.* **2019**, *10*, 4010–4021. [CrossRef]
74. Kang, M.Y.; Kim, H.-B.; Piao, C.; Lee, K.H.; Hyun, J.W.; Chang, I.-Y.; You, H.J. The Critical Role of Catalase in Prooxidant and Antioxidant Function of P53. *Cell Death Differ.* **2013**, *20*, 117–129. [CrossRef]
75. Haque, R.; Chun, E.; Howell, J.C.; Sengupta, T.; Chen, D.; Kim, H. MicroRNA-30b-Mediated Regulation of Catalase Expression in Human ARPE-19 Cells. *PLoS ONE* **2012**, *7*, e42542. [CrossRef]

76. Xu, Y.; Porntadavity, S.; St Clair, D.K. Transcriptional Regulation of the Human Manganese Superoxide Dismutase Gene: The Role of Specificity Protein 1 (Sp1) and Activating Protein-2 (AP-2). *Biochem. J.* 2002, *362*, 401–412. [CrossRef]
77. Kim, Y.S.; Gupta Vallur, P.; Phaëton, R.; Mythreye, K.; Hempel, N. Insights into the Dichotomous Regulation of SOD2 in Cancer. *Antioxidants* 2017, *6*, 86. [CrossRef]
78. Miao, L.; St. Clair, D.K. Regulation of Superoxide Dismutase Genes: Implications in Diseases. *Free Radic. Biol. Med.* 2009, *47*, 344–356. [CrossRef]
79. Rui, T.; Kvietys, P.R. NFkappaB and AP-1 Differentially Contribute to the Induction of Mn-SOD and ENOS during the Development of Oxidant Tolerance. *FASEB J. Off. Publ. Fed. Am. Soc. Exp. Biol.* 2005, *19*, 1908–1910. [CrossRef]
80. Drane, P.; Bravard, A.; Bouvard, V.; May, E. Reciprocal Down-Regulation of P53 and SOD2 Gene Expression–Implication in P53 Mediated Apoptosis. *Oncogene* 2001, *20*, 430–439. [CrossRef] [PubMed]
81. Ji, G.; Lv, K.; Chen, H.; Wang, T.; Wang, Y.; Zhao, D.; Qu, L.; Li, Y. MiR-146a Regulates SOD2 Expression in H2O2 Stimulated PC12 Cells. *PLoS ONE* 2013, *8*, e69351. [CrossRef] [PubMed]
82. Röhrdanz, E.; Bittner, A.; Tran-Thi, Q.-H.; Kahl, R. The Effect of Quercetin on the MRNA Expression of Different Antioxidant Enzymes in Hepatoma Cells. *Arch. Toxicol.* 2003, *77*, 506–510. [CrossRef]
83. Zhang, J.; Bai, K.W.; He, J.; Niu, Y.; Lu, Y.; Zhang, L.; Wang, T. Curcumin Attenuates Hepatic Mitochondrial Dysfunction through the Maintenance of Thiol Pool, Inhibition of MtDNA Damage, and Stimulation of the Mitochondrial Thioredoxin System in Heat-Stressed Broilers. *J. Anim. Sci.* 2018, *96*, 867–879. [CrossRef] [PubMed]
84. Milani, P.; Amadio, M.; Laforenza, U.; Dell'Orco, M.; Diamanti, L.; Sardone, V.; Gagliardi, S.; Govoni, S.; Ceroni, M.; Pascale, A.; et al. Posttranscriptional Regulation of SOD1 Gene Expression under Oxidative Stress: Potential Role of ELAV Proteins in Sporadic ALS. *Neurobiol. Dis.* 2013, *60*, 51–60. [CrossRef] [PubMed]
85. Spanier, G.; Xu, H.; Xia, N.; Tobias, S.; Deng, S.; Wojnowski, L.; Forstermann, U.; Li, H. Resveratrol Reduces Endothelial Oxidative Stress by Modulating the Gene Expression of Superoxide Dismutase 1 (SOD1), Glutathione Peroxidase 1 (GPx1) and NADPH Oxidase Subunit (Nox4). *J. Physiol. Pharmacol. Off. J. Pol. Physiol. Soc.* 2009, *60* (Suppl. 4), 111–116.
86. Seo, S.J.; Kim, H.T.; Cho, G.; Rho, H.M.; Jung, G. Sp1 and C/EBP-Related Factor Regulate the Transcription of Human Cu/Zn SOD Gene. *Gene* 1996, *178*, 177–185. [CrossRef]
87. Minc, E.; de Coppet, P.; Masson, P.; Thiery, L.; Dutertre, S.; Amor-Guéret, M.; Jaulin, C. The Human Copper-Zinc Superoxide Dismutase Gene (SOD1) Proximal Promoter Is Regulated by Sp1, Egr-1, and WT1 via Non-Canonical Binding Sites*. *J. Biol. Chem.* 1999, *274*, 503–509. [CrossRef]
88. Okado-Matsumoto, A.; Fridovich, I. Subcellular Distribution of Superoxide Dismutases (SOD) in Rat Liver: Cu,Zn-SOD in Mitochondria. *J. Biol. Chem.* 2001, *276*, 38388–38393. [CrossRef]
89. Riera, H.; Afonso, V.; Collin, P.; Lomri, A. A Central Role for JNK/AP-1 Pathway in the Pro-Oxidant Effect of Pyrrolidine Dithiocarbamate through Superoxide Dismutase 1 Gene Repression and Reactive Oxygen Species Generation in Hematopoietic Human Cancer Cell Line U937. *PLoS ONE* 2015, *10*, e0127571. [CrossRef] [PubMed]
90. Ishii, T.; Yanagawa, T. Stress-Induced Peroxiredoxins. In *Peroxiredoxin Systems: Structures and Functions*; Flohé, L., Harris, J.R., Eds.; Subcellular Biochemistry; Springer: Dordrecht, The Netherlands, 2007; pp. 375–384. ISBN 978-1-4020-6051-9.
91. Lijnen, P.J.; Piccart, Y.; Coenen, T.; Prihadi, J.S. Angiotensin II-Induced Mitochondrial Reactive Oxygen Species and Peroxiredoxin-3 Expression in Cardiac Fibroblasts. *J. Hypertens.* 2012, *30*, 1986–1991. [CrossRef] [PubMed]
92. Kim, A.; Joseph, S.; Khan, A.; Epstein, C.J.; Sobel, R.; Huang, T.-T. Enhanced Expression of Mitochondrial Superoxide Dismutase Leads to Prolonged in Vivo Cell Cycle Progression and Up-Regulation of Mitochondrial Thioredoxin. *Free Radic. Biol. Med.* 2010, *48*, 1501–1512. [CrossRef] [PubMed]
93. Li, K.-Y.; Xiang, X.-J.; Song, L.; Chen, J.; Luo, B.; Wen, Q.-X.; Zhong, B.-R.; Zhou, G.-F.; Deng, X.-J.; Ma, Y.-L.; et al. Mitochondrial TXN2 Attenuates Amyloidogenesis via Selective Inhibition of BACE1 Expression. *J. Neurochem.* 2021, *157*, 1351–1365. [CrossRef]
94. Suzuki, K.; Koike, H.; Matsui, H.; Ono, Y.; Hasumi, M.; Nakazato, H.; Okugi, H.; Sekine, Y.; Oki, K.; Ito, K.; et al. Genistein, a Soy Isoflavone, Induces Glutathione Peroxidase in the Human Prostate Cancer Cell Lines LNCaP and PC-3. *Int. J. Cancer* 2002, *99*, 846–852. [CrossRef] [PubMed]
95. Lu, S.C. Regulation of Glutathione Synthesis. *Mol. Aspects Med.* 2009, *30*, 42–59. [CrossRef] [PubMed]
96. Rodríguez-Ramiro, I.; Ramos, S.; Bravo, L.; Goya, L.; Martín, M.Á. Procyanidin B2 Induces Nrf2 Translocation and Glutathione S-Transferase P1 Expression via ERKs and P38-MAPK Pathways and Protect Human Colonic Cells against Oxidative Stress. *Eur. J. Nutr.* 2012, *51*, 881–892. [CrossRef] [PubMed]
97. Ribas, V.; García-Ruiz, C.; Fernández-Checa, J.C. Glutathione and Mitochondria. *Front. Pharmacol.* 2014, *5*, 151. [CrossRef]
98. Wang, H.-M.; Cheng, K.-C.; Lin, C.-J.; Hsu, S.-W.; Fang, W.-C.; Hsu, T.-F.; Chiu, C.-C.; Chang, H.-W.; Hsu, C.-H.; Lee, A.Y.-L. Obtusilactone A and (−)-Sesamin Induce Apoptosis in Human Lung Cancer Cells by Inhibiting Mitochondrial Lon Protease and Activating DNA Damage Checkpoints. *Cancer Sci.* 2010, *101*, 2612–2620. [CrossRef]
99. Luciakova, K.; Sokolikova, B.; Chloupkova, M.; Nelson, B.D. Enhanced Mitochondrial Biogenesis Is Associated with Increased Expression of the Mitochondrial ATP-Dependent Lon Protease. *FEBS Lett.* 1999, *444*, 186–188. [CrossRef] [PubMed]
100. Bota, D.A.; Davies, K.J.A. Mitochondrial Lon Protease in Human Disease and Aging: Including an Etiologic Classification of Lon-Related Diseases and Disorders. *Free Radic. Biol. Med.* 2016, *100*, 188–198. [CrossRef]
101. Nouri, K.; Feng, Y.; Schimmer, A.D. Mitochondrial ClpP Serine Protease-Biological Function and Emerging Target for Cancer Therapy. *Cell Death Dis.* 2020, *11*, 841. [CrossRef]

102. Peña-Blanco, A.; García-Sáez, A.J. Bax, Bak and beyond—Mitochondrial Performance in Apoptosis. *FEBS J.* **2018**, *285*, 416–431. [CrossRef] [PubMed]
103. Roufayel, R.; Younes, K.; Al-Sabi, A.; Murshid, N. BH3-Only Proteins Noxa and Puma Are Key Regulators of Induced Apoptosis. *Life* **2022**, *12*, 256. [CrossRef]
104. Happo, L.; Strasser, A.; Cory, S. BH3-Only Proteins in Apoptosis at a Glance. *J. Cell Sci.* **2012**, *125*, 1081–1087. [CrossRef]
105. Kale, J.; Osterlund, E.J.; Andrews, D.W. BCL-2 Family Proteins: Changing Partners in the Dance towards Death. *Cell Death Differ.* **2018**, *25*, 65–80. [CrossRef]
106. Cook, S.J.; Stuart, K.; Gilley, R.; Sale, M.J. Control of Cell Death and Mitochondrial Fission by ERK1/2 MAP Kinase Signalling. *FEBS J.* **2017**, *284*, 4177–4195. [CrossRef] [PubMed]
107. Henry, C.J. Functional Foods. *Eur. J. Clin. Nutr.* **2010**, *64*, 657–659. [CrossRef]
108. Domínguez Díaz, L.; Fernández-Ruiz, V.; Cámara, M. The Frontier between Nutrition and Pharma: The International Regulatory Framework of Functional Foods, Food Supplements and Nutraceuticals. *Crit. Rev. Food Sci. Nutr.* **2020**, *60*, 1738–1746. [CrossRef]
109. Kalra, E.K. Nutraceutical-Definition and Introduction. *AAPS PharmSci* **2003**, *5*, 27–28. [CrossRef] [PubMed]
110. Hardy, G. Nutraceuticals and Functional Foods: Introduction and Meaning. *Nutrition* **2000**, *16*, 688–689. [CrossRef]
111. Basu, S.; Thomas, J.; Acharya, S. Prospects for Growth in Global Nutraceutical and Functional Food Markets: A Canadian Perspective. *Aust. J. Basic Appl. Sci.* **2007**, *1*, 637–649.
112. Kwak, N.-S.; Jukes, D.J. Functional Foods. Part 1: The Development of a Regulatory Concept. *Food Control* **2001**, *12*, 99–107. [CrossRef]
113. Guleri, S.; Tiwari, A. Algae and Ageing. In *Microalgae Biotechnology for Food, Health and High Value Products*; Alam, M.A., Xu, J.-L., Wang, Z., Eds.; Springer: Singapore, 2020; pp. 267–293. ISBN 9789811501692.
114. Hachicha, R.; Elleuch, F.; Ben Hlima, H.; Dubessay, P.; de Baynast, H.; Delattre, C.; Pierre, G.; Hachicha, R.; Abdelkafi, S.; Michaud, P.; et al. Biomolecules from Microalgae and Cyanobacteria: Applications and Market Survey. *Appl. Sci.* **2022**, *12*, 1924. [CrossRef]
115. Remize, M.; Brunel, Y.; Silva, J.L.; Berthon, J.-Y.; Filaire, E. Microalgae N-3 PUFAs Production and Use in Food and Feed Industries. *Mar. Drugs* **2021**, *19*, 113. [CrossRef]
116. Ampofo, J.; Abbey, L. Microalgae: Bioactive Composition, Health Benefits, Safety and Prospects as Potential High-Value Ingredients for the Functional Food Industry. *Foods* **2022**, *11*, 1744. [CrossRef] [PubMed]
117. Zanella, L.; Vianello, F. Microalgae of the Genus *Nannochloropsis*: Chemical Composition and Functional Implications for Human Nutrition. *J. Funct. Foods* **2020**, *68*, 103919. [CrossRef]
118. Chen, C.; Tang, T.; Shi, Q.; Zhou, Z.; Fan, J. The Potential and Challenge of Microalgae as Promising Future Food Sources. *Trends Food Sci. Technol.* **2022**, *126*, 99–112. [CrossRef]
119. Bernaerts, T.M.M.; Gheysen, L.; Kyomugasho, C.; Jamsazzadeh Kermani, Z.; Vandionant, S.; Foubert, I.; Hendrickx, M.E.; Van Loey, A.M. Comparison of Microalgal Biomasses as Functional Food Ingredients: Focus on the Composition of Cell Wall Related Polysaccharides. *Algal Res.* **2018**, *32*, 150–161. [CrossRef]
120. Raposo, M.F.D.J.; De Morais, A.M.M.B.; De Morais, R.M.S.C. Carotenoids from Marine Microalgae: A Valuable Natural Source for the Prevention of Chronic Diseases. *Mar. Drugs* **2015**, *13*, 5128–5155. [CrossRef] [PubMed]
121. Dehghani, J.; Movafeghi, A.; Mathieu-Rivet, E.; Mati-Baouche, N.; Calbo, S.; Lerouge, P.; Bardor, M. Microalgae as an Efficient Vehicle for the Production and Targeted Delivery of Therapeutic Glycoproteins against SARS-CoV-2 Variants. *Mar. Drugs* **2022**, *20*, 657. [CrossRef] [PubMed]
122. Torres-Tiji, Y.; Fields, F.J.; Mayfield, S.P. Microalgae as a Future Food Source. *Biotechnol. Adv.* **2020**, *41*, 107536. [CrossRef]
123. Prüser, T.F.; Braun, P.G.; Wiacek, C. Microalgae as a novel food. Potential and legal framework. *Ernahrungs Umsch.* **2021**, *68*, 78–85.
124. Cecchin, M.; Cazzaniga, S.; Martini, F.; Paltrinieri, S.; Bossi, S.; Maffei, M.E.; Ballottari, M. Astaxanthin and Eicosapentaenoic Acid Production by S4, a New Mutant Strain of *Nannochloropsis gaditana*. *Microb. Cell Factories* **2022**, *21*, 117. [CrossRef]
125. Novoveská, L.; Ross, M.E.; Stanley, M.S.; Pradelles, R.; Wasiolek, V.; Sassi, J.-F. Microalgal Carotenoids: A Review of Production, Current Markets, Regulations, and Future Direction. *Mar. Drugs* **2019**, *17*, 640. [CrossRef]
126. Guiry, M.D.; Guiry, G.M. AlgaeBase World-Wide Electronic Publication, National University of Ireland, Galway. Available online: https://www.algaebase.org (accessed on 23 December 2022).
127. Sansone, C.; Galasso, C.; Orefice, I.; Nuzzo, G.; Luongo, E.; Cutignano, A.; Romano, G.; Brunet, C.; Fontana, A.; Esposito, F.; et al. The Green Microalga *Tetraselmis suecica* Reduces Oxidative Stress and Induces Repairing Mechanisms in Human Cells. *Sci. Rep.* **2017**, *7*, 41215. [CrossRef]
128. Cha, Y.; Kim, T.; Jeon, J.; Jang, Y.; Kim, P.B.; Lopes, C.; Leblanc, P.; Cohen, B.M.; Kim, K.-S. SIRT2 Regulates Mitochondrial Dynamics and Reprogramming via MEK1-ERK-DRP1 and AKT1-DRP1 Axes. *Cell Rep.* **2021**, *37*, 110155. [CrossRef]
129. Nacer, W.; Baba Ahmed, F.Z.; Merzouk, H.; Benyagoub, O.; Bouanane, S. Evaluation of the Anti-Inflammatory and Antioxidant Effects of the Microalgae *Nannochloropsis gaditana* in Streptozotocin-Induced Diabetic Rats. *J. Diabetes Metab. Disord.* **2020**, *19*, 1483–1490. [CrossRef]
130. Gupta, S.P.; Siddiqi, N.J.; Khan, H.A.; Alrokayan, S.H.; Alhomida, A.S.; Singh, R.K.; Verma, P.K.; Kumar, S.; Acharya, A.; Sharma, B. Phytochemical Profiling of Microalgae *Euglena tuba* and Its Anticancer Activity in Dalton's Lymphoma Cells. *Front. Biosci.-Landmark* **2022**, *27*, 120. [CrossRef] [PubMed]

131. Lin, P.-Y.; Tsai, C.-T.; Chuang, W.-L.; Chao, Y.-H.; Pan, I.-H.; Chen, Y.-K.; Lin, C.-C.; Wang, B.-Y. *Chlorella sorokiniana* Induces Mitochondrial-Mediated Apoptosis in Human Non-Small Cell Lung Cancer Cells and Inhibits Xenograft Tumor Growth In Vivo. *BMC Complement. Altern. Med.* **2017**, *17*, 88. [CrossRef] [PubMed]
132. Abolhasani, M.H.; Safavi, M.; Goodarzi, M.T.; Kassaee, S.M.; Azin, M. Identification and Anti-Cancer Activity in 2D and 3D Cell Culture Evaluation of an Iranian Isolated Marine Microalgae *Picochlorum* sp. RCC486. *DARU J. Pharm. Sci.* **2018**, *26*, 105–116. [CrossRef] [PubMed]
133. Suh, S.-S.; Kim, S.-M.; Kim, J.E.; Hong, J.-M.; Lee, S.G.; Youn, U.J.; Han, S.J.; Kim, I.-C.; Kim, S. Anticancer Activities of Ethanol Extract from the Antarctic Freshwater Microalga, *Botryidiopsidaceae* sp. *BMC Complement. Altern. Med.* **2017**, *17*, 509. [CrossRef]
134. Ebrahimi Nigjeh, S.; Yusoff, F.M.; Mohamed Alitheen, N.B.; Rasoli, M.; Keong, Y.S.; bin Omar, A.R. Cytotoxic Effect of Ethanol Extract of Microalga, *Chaetoceros calcitrans*, and Its Mechanisms in Inducing Apoptosis in Human Breast Cancer Cell Line. *BioMed Res. Int.* **2012**, *2013*, e783690. [CrossRef]
135. Guo, B.; Zhou, Y.; Liu, B.; He, Y.; Chen, F.; Cheng, K.-W. Lipid-Lowering Bioactivity of Microalga *Nitzschia laevis* Extract Containing Fucoxanthin in Murine Model and Carcinomic Hepatocytes. *Pharmaceuticals* **2021**, *14*, 1004. [CrossRef]
136. Campiche, R.; Sandau, P.; Kurth, E.; Massironi, M.; Imfeld, D.; Schuetz, R. Protective Effects of an Extract of the Freshwater Microalga *Scenedesmus rubescens* on UV-Irradiated Skin Cells. *Int. J. Cosmet. Sci.* **2018**, *40*, 187–192. [CrossRef]
137. Nawrocka, D.; Kornicka, K.; Śmieszek, A.; Marycz, K. *Spirulina platensis* Improves Mitochondrial Function Impaired by Elevated Oxidative Stress in Adipose-Derived Mesenchymal Stromal Cells (ASCs) and Intestinal Epithelial Cells (IECs), and Enhances Insulin Sensitivity in Equine Metabolic Syndrome (EMS) Horses. *Mar. Drugs* **2017**, *15*, 237. [CrossRef] [PubMed]
138. Stanley, W.C.; Khairallah, R.J.; Dabkowski, E.R. Update on Lipids and Mitochondrial Function: Impact of Dietary n-3 Polyunsaturated Fatty Acids. *Curr. Opin. Clin. Nutr. Metab. Care* **2012**, *15*, 122–126. [CrossRef]
139. Khairallah, R.J.; Sparagna, G.C.; Khanna, N.; O'Shea, K.M.; Hecker, P.A.; Kristian, T.; Fiskum, G.; Des Rosiers, C.; Polster, B.M.; Stanley, W.C. Dietary Supplementation with Docosahexaenoic Acid, but Not Eicosapentaenoic Acid, Dramatically Alters Cardiac Mitochondrial Phospholipid Fatty Acid Composition and Prevents Permeability Transition. *Biochim. Biophys. Acta BBA Bioenerg.* **2010**, *1797*, 1555–1562. [CrossRef] [PubMed]
140. Singer, P.; Honigmann, G.; Schliack, V. Decrease of Eicosapentaenoic Acid in Fatty Liver of Diabetic Subjects. *Prostaglandins Med.* **1980**, *5*, 183–200. [CrossRef] [PubMed]
141. Wensaas, A.J.; Rustan, A.C.; Just, M.; Berge, R.K.; Drevon, C.A.; Gaster, M. Fatty Acid Incubation of Myotubes From Humans With Type 2 Diabetes Leads to Enhanced Release of β-Oxidation Products Because of Impaired Fatty Acid Oxidation: Effects of Tetradecylthioacetic Acid and Eicosapentaenoic Acid. *Diabetes* **2009**, *58*, 527–535. [CrossRef] [PubMed]
142. Zhao, M.; Chen, X. Eicosapentaenoic Acid Promotes Thermogenic and Fatty Acid Storage Capacity in Mouse Subcutaneous Adipocytes. *Biochem. Biophys. Res. Commun.* **2014**, *450*, 1446–1451. [CrossRef]
143. Zhou, L.; Li, K.; Duan, X.; Hill, D.; Barrow, C.; Dunshea, F.; Martin, G.; Suleria, H. Bioactive Compounds in Microalgae and Their Potential Health Benefits. *Food Biosci.* **2022**, *49*, 101932. [CrossRef]
144. Randhir, A.; Laird, D.W.; Maker, G.; Trengove, R.; Moheimani, N.R. Microalgae: A Potential Sustainable Commercial Source of Sterols. *Algal Res.* **2020**, *46*, 101772. [CrossRef]
145. Fithriani, D.; Ambarwaty, D.; Nurhayati, N. Identification of Bioactive Compounds from *Nannochloropsis* sp. *IOP Conf. Series: Earth Environ. Sci.* **2020**, *404*, 012064. [CrossRef]
146. Kim, Y.-S.; Li, X.-F.; Kang, K.-H.; Ryu, B.; Kim, S.K. Stigmasterol Isolated from Marine Microalgae *Navicula incerta* Induces Apoptosis in Human Hepatoma HepG2 Cells. *BMB Rep.* **2014**, *47*, 433–438. [CrossRef]
147. Cilla, A.; Attanzio, A.; Barberá, R.; Tesoriere, L.; Livrea, M.A. Anti-Proliferative Effect of Main Dietary Phytosterols and β-Cryptoxanthin Alone or Combined in Human Colon Cancer Caco-2 Cells through Cytosolic Ca+2–and Oxidative Stress-Induced Apoptosis. *J. Funct. Foods* **2015**, *12*, 282–293. [CrossRef]
148. Mamari, H.H.A. *Phenolic Compounds: Classification, Chemistry, and Updated Techniques of Analysis and Synthesis*; IntechOpen: London, UK, 2021; ISBN 978-1-83969-347-2.
149. Alara, O.R.; Abdurahman, N.H.; Ukaegbu, C.I. Extraction of Phenolic Compounds: A Review. *Curr. Res. Food Sci.* **2021**, *4*, 200–214. [CrossRef] [PubMed]
150. Kapoor, S.; Singh, M.; Srivastava, A.; Chavali, M.; Chandrasekhar, K.; Verma, P. Extraction and Characterization of Microalgae-Derived Phenolics for Pharmaceutical Applications: A Systematic Review. *J. Basic Microbiol.* **2021**, *62*, 1044–1063. [CrossRef]
151. Goiris, K.; Muylaert, K.; Fraeye, I.; Foubert, I.; De Brabanter, J.; De Cooman, L. Antioxidant Potential of Microalgae in Relation to Their Phenolic and Carotenoid Content. *J. Appl. Phycol.* **2012**, *24*, 1477–1486. [CrossRef]
152. Rodis, P.S.; Karathanos, V.T.; Mantzavinou, A. Partitioning of Olive Oil Antioxidants between Oil and Water Phases. *J. Agric. Food Chem.* **2002**, *50*, 596–601. [CrossRef] [PubMed]
153. Scaglioni, P.T.; Quadros, L.; de Paula, M.; Furlong, V.B.; Abreu, P.C.; Badiale-Furlong, E. Inhibition of Enzymatic and Oxidative Processes by Phenolic Extracts from *Spirulina* sp. and *Nannochloropsis* sp. *Food Technol. Biotechnol.* **2018**, *56*, 344–353. [CrossRef]
154. Goh, S.-H.; Yusoff, F.M.; Loh, S.P. A Comparison of the Antioxidant Properties and Total Phenolic Content in a Diatom, *Chaetoceros* sp. and a Green Microalga, *Nannochloropsis* sp. *J. Agric. Sci.* **2010**, *2*, p123. [CrossRef]
155. Parcheta, M.; Świsłocka, R.; Orzechowska, S.; Akimowicz, M.; Choińska, R.; Lewandowski, W. Recent Developments in Effective Antioxidants: The Structure and Antioxidant Properties. *Materials* **2021**, *14*, 1984. [CrossRef] [PubMed]

156. Andriopoulos, V.; Gkioni, M.D.; Koutra, E.; Mastropetros, S.G.; Lamari, F.N.; Hatziantoniou, S.; Kornaros, M. Total Phenolic Content, Biomass Composition, and Antioxidant Activity of Selected Marine Microalgal Species with Potential as Aquaculture Feed. *Antioxidants* **2022**, *11*, 1320. [CrossRef] [PubMed]
157. Muñoz-Almagro, N.; Gilbert-López, B.M.; Carmen, P.-R.; García-Fernandez, Y.; Almeida, C.; Villamiel, M.; Mendiola, J.A.; Ibáñez, E. Exploring the Microalga *Euglena cantabrica* by Pressurized Liquid Extraction to Obtain Bioactive Compounds. *Mar. Drugs* **2020**, *18*, 308. [CrossRef]
158. Safafar, H.; Van Wagenen, J.; Møller, P.; Jacobsen, C. Carotenoids, Phenolic Compounds and Tocopherols Contribute to the Antioxidative Properties of Some Microalgae Species Grown on Industrial Wastewater. *Mar. Drugs* **2015**, *13*, 7339–7356. [CrossRef] [PubMed]
159. Massa, M.; Buono, S.; Langellotti, A.L.; Martello, A.; Russo, G.L.; Troise, D.A.; Sacchi, R.; Vitaglione, P.; Fogliano, V. Biochemical Composition and in Vitro Digestibility of *Galdieria sulphuraria* Grown on Spent Cherry-Brine Liquid. *New Biotechnol.* **2019**, *53*, 9–15. [CrossRef]
160. Machu, L.; Misurcova, L.; Vavra Ambrozova, J.; Orsavova, J.; Mlcek, J.; Sochor, J.; Jurikova, T. Phenolic Content and Antioxidant Capacity in Algal Food Products. *Molecules* **2015**, *20*, 1118–1133. [CrossRef]
161. Michael, A.; Kyewalyanga, M.S.; Mtolera, M.S.; Lugomela, C.V. Antioxidants Activity of the Cyanobacterium, *Arthrospira* (*Spirulina*) *fusiformis* Cultivated in a Low-Cost Medium. *Afr. J. Food Sci.* **2018**, *12*, 188–195. [CrossRef]
162. Martinez-Goss, M.R.; Arguelles, E.D.L.R.; Sapin, A.B.; Almeda, R.A. Chemical Composition and In Vitro Antioxidant and Antibacterial Properties of the Edible Cyanobacterium, *Nostoc commune* Vaucher. *Philipp. Sci. Lett.* **2021**, *14*, 25–35.
163. Lima, G.P.P.; Vianello, F.; Corrêa, C.R.; Campos, R.A.D.S.; Borguini, M.G. Polyphenols in Fruits and Vegetables and Its Effect on Human Health. *Food Nutr. Sci.* **2014**, *5*, 1065–1082. [CrossRef]
164. Chodari, L.; Dilsiz Aytemir, M.; Vahedi, P.; Alipour, M.; Vahed, S.Z.; Khatibi, S.M.H.; Ahmadian, E.; Ardalan, M.; Eftekhari, A. Targeting Mitochondrial Biogenesis with Polyphenol Compounds. *Oxid. Med. Cell. Longev.* **2021**, *2021*, e4946711. [CrossRef]
165. Sandoval-Acuña, C.; Ferreira, J.; Speisky, H. Polyphenols and Mitochondria: An Update on Their Increasingly Emerging ROS-Scavenging Independent Actions. *Arch. Biochem. Biophys.* **2014**, *559*, 75–90. [CrossRef] [PubMed]
166. Naoi, M.; Wu, Y.; Shamoto-Nagai, M.; Maruyama, W. Mitochondria in Neuroprotection by Phytochemicals: Bioactive Polyphenols Modulate Mitochondrial Apoptosis System, Function and Structure. *Int. J. Mol. Sci.* **2019**, *20*, 2451. [CrossRef]
167. Howitz, K.T.; Bitterman, K.J.; Cohen, H.Y.; Lamming, D.W.; Lavu, S.; Wood, J.G.; Zipkin, R.E.; Chung, P.; Kisielewski, A.; Zhang, L.-L.; et al. Small Molecule Activators of Sirtuins Extend *Saccharomyces cerevisiae* Lifespan. *Nature* **2003**, *425*, 191–196. [CrossRef]
168. Davis, J.M.; Murphy, E.A.; Carmichael, M.D.; Davis, B. Quercetin Increases Brain and Muscle Mitochondrial Biogenesis and Exercise Tolerance. *Am. J. Physiol. Regul. Integr. Comp. Physiol.* **2009**, *296*, R1071–R1077. [CrossRef] [PubMed]
169. Hao, J.; Shen, W.; Yu, G.; Jia, H.; Li, X.; Feng, Z.; Wang, Y.; Weber, P.; Wertz, K.; Sharman, E.; et al. Hydroxytyrosol Promotes Mitochondrial Biogenesis and Mitochondrial Function in 3T3-L1 Adipocytes. *J. Nutr. Biochem.* **2010**, *21*, 634–644. [CrossRef] [PubMed]
170. Signorile, A.; Micelli, L.; De Rasmo, D.; Santeramo, A.; Papa, F.; Ficarella, R.; Gattoni, G.; Scacco, S.; Papa, S. Regulation of the Biogenesis of OXPHOS Complexes in Cell Transition from Replicating to Quiescent State: Involvement of PKA and Effect of Hydroxytyrosol. *Biochim. Biophys. Acta* **2014**, *1843*, 675–684. [CrossRef]
171. Feillet-Coudray, C.; Sutra, T.; Fouret, G.; Ramos, J.; Wrutniak-Cabello, C.; Cabello, G.; Cristol, J.P.; Coudray, C. Oxidative Stress in Rats Fed a High-Fat High-Sucrose Diet and Preventive Effect of Polyphenols: Involvement of Mitochondrial and NAD(P)H Oxidase Systems. *Free Radic. Biol. Med.* **2009**, *46*, 624–632. [CrossRef] [PubMed]
172. Zimermann, J.D.F.; Sydney, E.B.; Cerri, M.L.; de Carvalho, I.K.; Schafranski, K.; Sydney, A.C.N.; Vitali, L.; Gonçalves, S.; Micke, G.A.; Soccol, C.R.; et al. Growth Kinetics, Phenolic Compounds Profile and Pigments Analysis of *Galdieria sulphuraria* Cultivated in Whey Permeate in Shake-Flasks and Stirred-Tank Bioreactor. *J. Water Process Eng.* **2020**, *38*, 101598. [CrossRef]
173. Hwang, J.M.; Cho, J.S.; Kim, T.H.; Lee, Y.I. Ellagic Acid Protects Hepatocytes from Damage by Inhibiting Mitochondrial Production of Reactive Oxygen Species. *Biomed. Pharmacother.* **2010**, *64*, 264–270. [CrossRef] [PubMed]
174. Firdaus, F.; Zafeer, M.F.; Waseem, M.; Anis, E.; Hossain, M.M.; Afzal, M. Ellagic Acid Mitigates Arsenic-Trioxide-Induced Mitochondrial Dysfunction and Cytotoxicity in SH-SY5Y Cells. *J. Biochem. Mol. Toxicol.* **2018**, *32*, e22024. [CrossRef]
175. Dhingra, A.; Jayas, R.; Afshar, P.; Guberman, M.; Maddaford, G.; Gerstein, J.; Lieberman, B.; Nepon, H.; Margulets, V.; Dhingra, R.; et al. Ellagic Acid Antagonizes Bnip3-Mediated Mitochondrial Injury and Necrotic Cell Death of Cardiac Myocytes. *Free Radic. Biol. Med.* **2017**, *112*, 411–422. [CrossRef]
176. Larrosa, M.; Tomás-Barberán, F.A.; Espín, J.C. The Dietary Hydrolysable Tannin Punicalagin Releases Ellagic Acid That Induces Apoptosis in Human Colon Adenocarcinoma Caco-2 Cells by Using the Mitochondrial Pathway. *J. Nutr. Biochem.* **2006**, *17*, 611–625. [CrossRef]
177. Salimi, A.; Roudkenar, M.H.; Sadeghi, L.; Mohseni, A.; Seydi, E.; Pirahmadi, N.; Pourahmad, J. Ellagic Acid, a Polyphenolic Compound, Selectively Induces ROS-Mediated Apoptosis in Cancerous B-Lymphocytes of CLL Patients by Directly Targeting Mitochondria. *Redox Biol.* **2015**, *6*, 461–471. [CrossRef]
178. Ho, C.-C.; Huang, A.-C.; Yu, C.-S.; Lien, J.-C.; Wu, S.-H.; Huang, Y.-P.; Huang, H.-Y.; Kuo, J.-H.; Liao, W.-Y.; Yang, J.-S.; et al. Ellagic Acid Induces Apoptosis in TSGH8301 Human Bladder Cancer Cells through the Endoplasmic Reticulum Stress- and Mitochondria-Dependent Signaling Pathways. *Environ. Toxicol.* **2014**, *29*, 1262–1274. [CrossRef]

179. Edderkaoui, M.; Odinokova, I.; Ohno, I.; Gukovsky, I.; Go, V.L.W.; Pandol, S.J.; Gukovskaya, A.S. Ellagic Acid Induces Apoptosis through Inhibition of Nuclear Factor Kappa B in Pancreatic Cancer Cells. *World J. Gastroenterol.* **2008**, *14*, 3672–3680. [CrossRef] [PubMed]
180. Duan, J.; Li, Y.; Gao, H.; Yang, D.; He, X.; Fang, Y.; Zhou, G. Phenolic Compound Ellagic Acid Inhibits Mitochondrial Respiration and Tumor Growth in Lung Cancer. *Food Funct.* **2020**, *11*, 6332–6339. [CrossRef] [PubMed]
181. Gorlach, S.; Fichna, J.; Lewandowska, U. Polyphenols as Mitochondria-Targeted Anticancer Drugs. *Cancer Lett.* **2015**, *366*, 141–149. [CrossRef] [PubMed]
182. Zhang, Q.; Cheng, G.; Qiu, H.; Zhu, L.; Ren, Z.; Zhao, W.; Zhang, T.; Liu, L. The P53-Inducible Gene 3 Involved in Flavonoid-Induced Cytotoxicity through the Reactive Oxygen Species-Mediated Mitochondrial Apoptotic Pathway in Human Hepatoma Cells. *Food Funct.* **2015**, *6*, 1518–1525. [CrossRef]
183. de Oliveira, M.R.; Nabavi, S.F.; Manayi, A.; Daglia, M.; Hajheydari, Z.; Nabavi, S.M. Resveratrol and the Mitochondria: From Triggering the Intrinsic Apoptotic Pathway to Inducing Mitochondrial Biogenesis, a Mechanistic View. *Biochim. Biophys. Acta BBA Gen. Subj.* **2016**, *1860*, 727–745. [CrossRef]
184. Goiris, K.; Muylaert, K.; Voorspoels, S.; Noten, B.; De Paepe, D.; E Baart, G.J.; De Cooman, L. Detection of Flavonoids in Microalgae from Different Evolutionary Lineages. *J. Phycol.* **2014**, *50*, 483–492. [CrossRef] [PubMed]
185. Mapoung, S.; Arjsri, P.; Thippraphan, P.; Semmarath, W.; Yodkeeree, S.; Chiewchanvit, S.; Piyamongkol, W.; Limtrakul, P. Photochemoprotective Effects of *Spirulina platensis* Extract against UVB Irradiated Human Skin Fibroblasts. *S. Afr. J. Bot.* **2020**, *130*, 198–207. [CrossRef]
186. Seghiri, R.; Kharbach, M.; Essamri, A. Functional Composition, Nutritional Properties, and Biological Activities of Moroccan *Spirulina* Microalga. *J. Food Qual.* **2019**, *2019*, e3707219. [CrossRef]
187. Niranjana, R.; Gayathri, R.; Nimish Mol, S.; Sugawara, T.; Hirata, T.; Miyashita, K.; Ganesan, P. Carotenoids Modulate the Hallmarks of Cancer Cells. *J. Funct. Foods* **2015**, *18*, 968–985. [CrossRef]
188. Le Goff, M.; Le Ferrec, E.; Mayer, C.; Mimouni, V.; Lagadic-Gossmann, D.; Schoefs, B.; Ulmann, L. Microalgal Carotenoids and Phytosterols Regulate Biochemical Mechanisms Involved in Human Health and Disease Prevention. *Biochimie* **2019**, *167*, 106–118. [CrossRef]
189. Zanella, L.; Alam, M.A. Extracts and Bioactives from Microalgae (Sensu Stricto): Opportunities and Challenges for a New Generation of Cosmetics. In *Microalgae Biotechnology for Food, Health and High Value Products*; Alam, M.A., Xu, J.-L., Wang, Z., Eds.; Springer: Singapore, 2020; pp. 295–349. ISBN 9789811501692.
190. Lesmana, R.; Yusuf, I.F.; Goenawan, H.; Achadiyani, A.; Khairani, A.F.; Fatimah, S.N.; Supratman, U. Low Dose of β-Carotene Regulates Inflammation, Reduces Caspase Signaling, and Correlates with Autophagy Activation in Cardiomyoblast Cell Lines. *Med. Sci. Monit. Basic Res.* **2020**, *26*, e928648-1. [CrossRef]
191. Yamamoto, H.; Itoh, N.; Kawano, S.; Yatsukawa, Y.; Momose, T.; Makio, T.; Matsunaga, M.; Yokota, M.; Esaki, M.; Shodai, T.; et al. Dual Role of the Receptor Tom20 in Specificity and Efficiency of Protein Import into Mitochondria. *Proc. Natl. Acad. Sci. USA* **2011**, *108*, 91–96. [CrossRef]
192. Weinrich, T.; Xu, Y.; Wosu, C.; Harvey, P.J.; Jeffery, G. Mitochondrial Function, Mobility and Lifespan Are Improved in *Drosophila melanogaster* by Extracts of 9-Cis-β-Carotene from *Dunaliella salina*. *Mar. Drugs* **2019**, *17*, 279. [CrossRef] [PubMed]
193. Voutilainen, S.; Nurmi, T.; Mursu, J.; Rissanen, T.H. Carotenoids and Cardiovascular Health. *Am. J. Clin. Nutr.* **2006**, *83*, 1265–1271. [CrossRef]
194. Druesne-Pecollo, N.; Latino-Martel, P.; Norat, T.; Barrandon, E.; Bertrais, S.; Galan, P.; Hercberg, S. Beta-Carotene Supplementation and Cancer Risk: A Systematic Review and Metaanalysis of Randomized Controlled Trials. *Int. J. Cancer* **2010**, *127*, 172–184. [CrossRef] [PubMed]
195. Sowmya Shree, G.; Yogendra Prasad, K.; Arpitha, H.S.; Deepika, U.R.; Nawneet Kumar, K.; Mondal, P.; Ganesan, P. β-Carotene at Physiologically Attainable Concentration Induces Apoptosis and down-Regulates Cell Survival and Antioxidant Markers in Human Breast Cancer (MCF-7) Cells. *Mol. Cell. Biochem.* **2017**, *436*, 1–12. [CrossRef]
196. He, J.; Gu, Y.; Zhang, S. Vitamin A and Breast Cancer Survival: A Systematic Review and Meta-Analysis. *Clin. Breast Cancer* **2018**, *18*, e1389–e1400. [CrossRef]
197. Lee, K.E.; Kwon, M.; Kim, Y.S.; Kim, Y.; Chung, M.G.; Heo, S.C.; Kim, Y. KoreaMed Synapse. *Nutr. Res. Pract.* **2021**, *16*, 161–172. [CrossRef]
198. Li, K.; Zhang, B. The Association of Dietary β-Carotene and Vitamin A Intake on the Risk of Esophageal Cancer: A Meta-Analysis. *Rev. Espanola Enfermedades Dig. Organo Of. Soc. Espanola Patol. Dig.* **2020**, *112*, 620–626. [CrossRef] [PubMed]
199. Tamaki, S.; Mochida, K.; Suzuki, K. Diverse Biosynthetic Pathways and Protective Functions against Environmental Stress of Antioxidants in Microalgae. *Plants* **2021**, *10*, 1250. [CrossRef]
200. Corona, J.C.; Duchen, M.R. PPARγ as a Therapeutic Target to Rescue Mitochondrial Function in Neurological Disease. *Free Radic. Biol. Med.* **2016**, *100*, 153–163. [CrossRef]
201. Sathasivam, R.; Ki, J.-S. A Review of the Biological Activities of Microalgal Carotenoids and Their Potential Use in Healthcare and Cosmetic Industries. *Mar. Drugs* **2018**, *16*, 26. [CrossRef]
202. Patel, A.K.; Albarico, F.P.J.B.; Perumal, P.K.; Vadrale, A.P.; Nian, C.T.; Chau, H.T.B.; Anwar, C.; Wani, H.M.U.D.; Pal, A.; Saini, R.; et al. Algae as an Emerging Source of Bioactive Pigments. *Bioresour. Technol.* **2022**, *351*, 126910. [CrossRef]

203. Li, Z.; Sun, M.; Li, Q.; Li, A.; Zhang, C. Profiling of Carotenoids in Six Microalgae (Eustigmatophyceae) and Assessment of Their β-Carotene Productions in Bubble Column Photobioreactor. *Biotechnol. Lett.* **2012**, *34*, 2049–2053. [CrossRef] [PubMed]
204. Del Campo, J.A.; Rodríguez, H.; Moreno, J.; Vargas, M.Á.; Rivas, J.; Guerrero, M.G. Accumulation of Astaxanthin and Lutein in *Chlorella zofingiensis* (Chlorophyta). *Appl. Microbiol. Biotechnol.* **2004**, *64*, 848–854. [CrossRef]
205. Abe, K.; Hattori, H.; Hirano, M. Accumulation and Antioxidant Activity of Secondary Carotenoids in the Aerial Microalga *Coelastrella striolata* var. *multistriata*. *Food Chem.* **2007**, *100*, 656–661. [CrossRef]
206. Kang, C.D.; Lee, J.S.; Park, T.H.; Sim, S.J. Comparison of Heterotrophic and Photoautotrophic Induction on Astaxanthin Production by *Haematococcus pluvialis*. *Appl. Microbiol. Biotechnol.* **2005**, *68*, 237–241. [CrossRef] [PubMed]
207. Butler, T.; Golan, Y. Astaxanthin Production from Microalgae. In *Microalgae Biotechnology for Food, Health and High Value Products*; Springer: Singapore, 2020; pp. 175–242. [CrossRef]
208. Liu, J.; Sun, Z.; Gerken, H.; Liu, Z.; Jiang, Y.; Chen, F. *Chlorella zofingiensis* as an Alternative Microalgal Producer of Astaxanthin: Biology and Industrial Potential. *Mar. Drugs* **2014**, *12*, 3487–3515. [CrossRef] [PubMed]
209. Kim, S.M.; Kang, S.-W.; Kwon, O.-N.; Chung, D.; Pan, C.-H. Fucoxanthin as a Major Carotenoid in *Isochrysis aff. galbana*: Characterization of Extraction for Commercial Application. *J. Korean Soc. Appl. Biol. Chem.* **2012**, *55*, 477–483. [CrossRef]
210. Petrushkina, M.; Gusev, E.; Sorokin, B.; Zotko, N.; Mamaeva, A.; Filimonova, A.; Kulikovskiy, M.; Maltsev, Y.; Yampolsky, I.; Guglya, E.; et al. Fucoxanthin Production by Heterokont Microalgae. *Algal Res.* **2017**, *24*, 387–393. [CrossRef]
211. Di Lena, G.; Casini, I.; Lucarini, M.; Lombardi-Boccia, G. Carotenoid Profiling of Five Microalgae Species from Large-Scale Production. *Food Res. Int.* **2019**, *120*, 810–818. [CrossRef]
212. Li, Z.; Li, A.-F.; Zhang, C.-W. High Performance Liquid Chromatography Analysis and Supercritical Carbon Dioxide Extraction of Pigments from the Diatom *Odontella aurita*. *Nat. Prod. Res. Dev.* **2012**, *24*, 814–818.
213. Campenni', L.; Nobre, B.P.; Santos, C.A.; Oliveira, A.C.; Aires-Barros, M.R.; Palavra, A.M.F.; Gouveia, L. Carotenoid and Lipid Production by the Autotrophic Microalga *Chlorella protothecoides* under Nutritional, Salinity, and Luminosity Stress Conditions. *Appl. Microbiol. Biotechnol.* **2013**, *97*, 1383–1393. [CrossRef] [PubMed]
214. Diprat, A.B.; Silveira Thys, R.C.; Rodrigues, E.; Rech, R. *Chlorella sorokiniana*: A New Alternative Source of Carotenoids and Proteins for Gluten-Free Bread. *LWT* **2020**, *134*, 109974. [CrossRef]
215. Huang, W.; Lin, Y.; He, M.; Gong, Y.; Huang, J. Induced High-Yield Production of Zeaxanthin, Lutein, and β-Carotene by a Mutant of *Chlorella zofingiensis*. *J. Agric. Food Chem.* **2018**, *66*, 891–897. [CrossRef] [PubMed]
216. Bourdon, L.; Jensen, A.A.; Kavanagh, J.M.; McClure, D.D. Microalgal Production of Zeaxanthin. *Algal Res.* **2021**, *55*, 102266. [CrossRef]
217. Singh, D.; Puri, M.; Wilkens, S.; Mathur, A.S.; Tuli, D.K.; Barrow, C.J. Characterization of a New Zeaxanthin Producing Strain of *Chlorella saccharophila* Isolated from New Zealand Marine Waters. *Bioresour. Technol.* **2013**, *143*, 308–314. [CrossRef]
218. Jin, E.; Feth, B.; Melis, A. A Mutant of the Green Alga *Dunaliella salina* Constitutively Accumulates Zeaxanthin under All Growth Conditions. *Biotechnol. Bioeng.* **2003**, *81*, 115–124. [CrossRef] [PubMed]
219. Nishida, Y.; Nawaz, A.; Hecht, K.; Tobe, K. Astaxanthin as a Novel Mitochondrial Regulator: A New Aspect of Carotenoids, beyond Antioxidants. *Nutrients* **2022**, *14*, 107. [CrossRef]
220. Hoffman, R.; Sultan, L.D.; Saada, A.; Hirschberg, J.; Osterzetser-Biran, O.; Gruenbaum, Y. Astaxanthin Extends Lifespan via Altered Biogenesis of the Mitochondrial Respiratory Chain Complex III. *bioRxiv* 2019. [CrossRef]
221. Huangfu, J.; Liu, J.; Sun, Z.; Wang, M.; Jiang, Y.; Chen, Z.-Y.; Chen, F. Antiaging Effects of Astaxanthin-Rich Alga *Haematococcus pluvialis* on Fruit Flies under Oxidative Stress. *J. Agric. Food Chem.* **2013**, *61*, 7800–7804. [CrossRef]
222. Sztretye, M.; Dienes, B.; Gönczi, M.; Czirják, T.; Csernoch, L.; Dux, L.; Szentesi, P.; Keller-Pintér, A. Astaxanthin: A Potential Mitochondrial-Targeted Antioxidant Treatment in Diseases and with Aging. *Oxid. Med. Cell. Longev.* **2019**, *2019*, e3849692. [CrossRef] [PubMed]
223. Wolf, A.M.; Asoh, S.; Hiranuma, H.; Ohsawa, I.; Iio, K.; Satou, A.; Ishikura, M.; Ohta, S. Astaxanthin Protects Mitochondrial Redox State and Functional Integrity against Oxidative Stress. *J. Nutr. Biochem.* **2010**, *21*, 381–389. [CrossRef] [PubMed]
224. Peserico, A.; Chiacchiera, F.; Grossi, V.; Matrone, A.; Latorre, D.; Simonatto, M.; Fusella, A.; Ryall, J.G.; Finley, L.W.S.; Haigis, M.C.; et al. A Novel AMPK-Dependent FoxO3A-SIRT3 Intramitochondrial Complex Sensing Glucose Levels. *Cell. Mol. Life Sci. CMLS* **2013**, *70*, 2015–2029. [CrossRef] [PubMed]
225. Sorrenti, V.; Davinelli, S.; Scapagnini, G.; Willcox, B.J.; Allsopp, R.C.; Willcox, D.C. Astaxanthin as a Putative Geroprotector: Molecular Basis and Focus on Brain Aging. *Mar. Drugs* **2020**, *18*, 351. [CrossRef]
226. Kim, S.H.; Kim, H. Inhibitory Effect of Astaxanthin on Oxidative Stress-Induced Mitochondrial Dysfunction-A Mini-Review. *Nutrients* **2018**, *10*, 1137. [CrossRef]
227. Aoi, W.; Naito, Y.; Takanami, Y.; Ishii, T.; Kawai, Y.; Akagiri, S.; Kato, Y.; Osawa, T.; Yoshikawa, T. Astaxanthin Improves Muscle Lipid Metabolism in Exercise via Inhibitory Effect of Oxidative CPT I Modification. *Biochem. Biophys. Res. Commun.* **2008**, *366*, 892–897. [CrossRef] [PubMed]
228. Gräb, J.; Rybniker, J. The Expanding Role of P38 Mitogen-Activated Protein Kinase in Programmed Host Cell Death. *Microbiol. Insights* **2019**, *12*, 1178636119864594. [CrossRef]
229. Ganesan, P.; Matsubara, K.; Sugawara, T.; Hirata, T. Marine Algal Carotenoids Inhibit Angiogenesis by Down-Regulating FGF-2-Mediated Intracellular Signals in Vascular Endothelial Cells. *Mol. Cell. Biochem.* **2013**, *380*, 1–9. [CrossRef]

230. Palozza, P.; Torelli, C.; Boninsegna, A.; Simone, R.; Catalano, A.; Mele, M.C.; Picci, N. Growth-Inhibitory Effects of the Astaxanthin-Rich Alga *Haematococcus pluvialis* in Human Colon Cancer Cells. *Cancer Lett.* **2009**, *283*, 108–117. [CrossRef]
231. Kavitha, K.; Kowshik, J.; Kishore, T.K.K.; Baba, A.B.; Nagini, S. Astaxanthin Inhibits NF-KB and Wnt/β-Catenin Signaling Pathways via Inactivation of Erk/MAPK and PI3K/Akt to Induce Intrinsic Apoptosis in a Hamster Model of Oral Cancer. *Biochim. Biophys. Acta* **2013**, *1830*, 4433–4444. [CrossRef]
232. Li, J.; Dai, W.; Xia, Y.; Chen, K.; Li, S.; Liu, T.; Zhang, R.; Wang, J.; Lu, W.; Zhou, Y.; et al. Astaxanthin Inhibits Proliferation and Induces Apoptosis of Human Hepatocellular Carcinoma Cells via Inhibition of Nf-Kb P65 and Wnt/B-Catenin in Vitro. *Mar. Drugs* **2015**, *13*, 6064–6081. [CrossRef] [PubMed]
233. Kaltschmidt, B.; Kaltschmidt, C.; Hofmann, T.G.; Hehner, S.P.; Dröge, W.; Schmitz, M.L. The Pro- or Anti-Apoptotic Function of NF-KB Is Determined by the Nature of the Apoptotic Stimulus. *Eur. J. Biochem.* **2000**, *267*, 3828–3835. [CrossRef] [PubMed]
234. Luo, J.-L.; Kamata, H.; Karin, M. IKK/NF-KB Signaling: Balancing Life and Death—A New Approach to Cancer Therapy. *J. Clin. Investig.* **2005**, *115*, 2625–2632. [CrossRef]
235. Gardaneh, M.; Nayeri, Z.; Akbari, P.; Gardaneh, M.; Tahermansouri, H. Molecular Simulations Identify Target Receptor Kinases Bound by Astaxanthin to Induce Breast Cancer Cell Apoptosis. *Arch. Breast Cancer* **2020**, *7*, 72–82. [CrossRef]
236. Gammone, M.A.; D'Orazio, N. Anti-Obesity Activity of the Marine Carotenoid Fucoxanthin. *Mar. Drugs* **2015**, *13*, 2196–2214. [CrossRef] [PubMed]
237. Maeda, H. Nutraceutical Effects of Fucoxanthin for Obesity and Diabetes Therapy: A Review. *J. Oleo Sci.* **2015**, *64*, 125–132. [CrossRef]
238. Houstis, N.; Rosen, E.D.; Lander, E.S. Reactive Oxygen Species Have a Causal Role in Multiple Forms of Insulin Resistance. *Nature* **2006**, *440*, 944–948. [CrossRef] [PubMed]
239. Ferdous, K.A.; Burnett, G.; Scott, M.; Amjad, E.; Bannerman, S.; Park, H.-A. Neuroprotective Function of Fucoxanthin in Oxidative Stress-Mediated Mitochondrial Dysfunction. *Curr. Dev. Nutr.* **2022**, *6*, 787. [CrossRef]
240. Mondal, A.; Bose, S.; Banerjee, S.; Patra, J.K.; Malik, J.; Mandal, S.K.; Kilpatrick, K.L.; Das, G.; Kerry, R.G.; Fimognari, C.; et al. Marine Cyanobacteria and Microalgae Metabolites—A Rich Source of Potential Anticancer Drugs. *Mar. Drugs* **2020**, *18*, 476. [CrossRef]
241. Gugulothu, P.; Bajhaiya, A.K. Bioactive Compound from Micro Algae and Their Anti-Cancer Properties. *Biomed. J. Sci. Tech. Res.* **2022**, *42*, 33928–33931. [CrossRef]
242. Saxena, A.; Raj, A.; Tiwari, A.; Saxena, A.; Raj, A.; Tiwari, A. *Exploring the Anti-Cancer Potential of Microalgae*; IntechOpen: London, UK, 2022; ISBN 978-1-80356-024-3.
243. Brogi, L.; Marchese, M.; Cellerino, A.; Licitra, R.; Naef, V.; Mero, S.; Bibbiani, C.; Fronte, B. β-Glucans as Dietary Supplement to Improve Locomotion and Mitochondrial Respiration in a Model of Duchenne Muscular Dystrophy. *Nutrients* **2021**, *13*, 1619. [CrossRef]
244. Samarakoon, K.W.; Ko, J.-Y.; Lee, J.-H.; Kwon, O.-N.; Kim, S.-W.; Jeon, Y.-J. Apoptotic Anticancer Activity of a Novel Fatty Alcohol Ester Isolated from Cultured Marine Diatom, *Phaeodactylum tricornutum*. *J. Funct. Foods* **2014**, *6*, 231–240. [CrossRef]
245. Kasashima, K.; Sumitani, M.; Satoh, M.; Endo, H. Human Prohibitin 1 Maintains the Organization and Stability of the Mitochondrial Nucleoids. *Exp. Cell Res.* **2008**, *314*, 988–996. [CrossRef]
246. Tredici, M.R. Mass Production of Microalgae: Photobioreactors. In *Handbook of Microalgal Culture: Biotechnology and Applied Phycology*; Blackwell Publishing Ltd.: Oxford, UK, 2004; pp. 178–214.
247. Vishwakarma, R.; Dhaka, V.; Ariyadasa, T.U.; Malik, A. Exploring Algal Technologies for a Circular Bio-Based Economy in Rural Sector. *J. Clean. Prod.* **2022**, *354*, 131653. [CrossRef]
248. Loke Show, P. Global Market and Economic Analysis of Microalgae Technology: Status and Perspectives. *Bioresour. Technol.* **2022**, *357*, 127329. [CrossRef]
249. Brendler, T.; Williamson, E.M. Astaxanthin: How Much Is Too Much? A Safety Review. *Phytother. Res.* **2019**, *33*, 3090–3111. [CrossRef] [PubMed]
250. Sun, W.; Xing, L.; Lin, H.; Leng, K.; Zhai, Y.; Liu, X. Assessment and Comparison of in Vitro Immunoregulatory Activity of Three Astaxanthin Stereoisomers. *J. Ocean Univ. China* **2016**, *15*, 283–287. [CrossRef]
251. Becker, W. Microalgae in Human and Animal Nutrition. In *Handbook of Microalgal Culture*; Blackwell: Oxford, UK, 2004; pp. 312–351.
252. Muhammad, G.; Alam, M.A.; Xiong, W.; Lv, Y.; Xu, J.-L. Microalgae Biomass Production: An Overview of Dynamic Operational Methods. In *Microalgae Biotechnology for Food, Health and High Value Products*; Alam, M.A., Xu, J.-L., Wang, Z., Eds.; Springer: Singapore, 2020; pp. 415–432. ISBN 9789811501692.
253. Teuling, E.; Wierenga, P.A.; Agboola, J.O.; Gruppen, H.; Schrama, J.W. Cell Wall Disruption Increases Bioavailability of *Nannochloropsis gaditana* Nutrients for Juvenile Nile Tilapia (*Oreochromis niloticus*). *Aquaculture* **2019**, *499*, 269–282. [CrossRef]
254. Machado, L.; Carvalho, G.; Pereira, R.N. Effects of Innovative Processing Methods on Microalgae Cell Wall: Prospects towards Digestibility of Protein-Rich Biomass. *Biomass* **2022**, *2*, 80–102. [CrossRef]
255. Mendes-Pinto, M.M.; Raposo, M.F.J.; Bowen, J.; Young, A.J.; Morais, R. Evaluation of Different Cell Disruption Processes on Encysted Cells of *Haematococcus pluvialis*: Effects on Astaxanthin Recovery and Implications for Bio-Availability. *J. Appl. Phycol.* **2001**, *13*, 19–24. [CrossRef]

256. Stiefvatter, L.; Lehnert, K.; Frick, K.; Montoya-Arroyo, A.; Frank, J.; Vetter, W.; Schmid-Staiger, U.; Bischoff, S.C. Oral Bioavailability of Omega-3 Fatty Acids and Carotenoids from the Microalgae *Phaeodactylum tricornutum* in Healthy Young Adults. *Mar. Drugs* **2021**, *19*, 700. [CrossRef]
257. Merchant, R.E.; Andre, C.A. A Review of Recent Clinical Trials of the Nutritional Supplement *Chlorella pyrenoidosa* in the Treatment of Fibromyalgia, Hypertension, and Ulcerative Colitis. *Altern. Ther. Health Med.* **2001**, *7*, 79–91.
258. Panahi, Y.; Darvishi, B.; Jowzi, N.; Beiraghdar, F.; Sahebkar, A. *Chlorella vulgaris*: A Multifunctional Dietary Supplement with Diverse Medicinal Properties. *Curr. Pharm. Des.* **2016**, *22*, 164–173.
259. Ebrahimi-Mameghani, M.; Sadeghi, Z.; Abbasalizad Farhangi, M.; Vaghef-Mehrabany, E.; Aliashrafi, S. Glucose Homeostasis, Insulin Resistance and Inflammatory Biomarkers in Patients with Non-Alcoholic Fatty Liver Disease: Beneficial Effects of Supplementation with Microalgae *Chlorella vulgaris*: A Double-Blind Placebo-Controlled Randomized Clinical Trial. *Clin. Nutr.* **2017**, *36*, 1001–1006. [CrossRef]
260. Panahi, Y.; Ghamarchehreh, M.E.; Beiraghdar, F.; Zare, R.; Jalalian, H.R.; Sahebkar, A. Investigation of the Effects of *Chlorella vulgaris* Supplementation in Patients with Non-Alcoholic Fatty Liver Disease: A Randomized Clinical Trial. *Hepatogastroenterology* **2012**, *59*, 2099–2103. [CrossRef] [PubMed]
261. Talebi Pour, B.; Jameshorani, M.; Salmani, R.; Chiti, H. The Effect of *Chlorella vulgaris* vs. Artichoke on Patients with Non-Alcoholic Fatty Liver Disease (NAFLD): A Randomized Clinical Trial. *J. Adv. Med. Biomed. Res.* **2015**, *23*, 36–44.
262. Chiu, H.-F.; Lee, H.-J.; Han, Y.-C.; Venkatakrishnan, K.; Golovinskaia, O.; Wang, C.-K. Beneficial Effect of *Chlorella pyrenoidosa* Drink on Healthy Subjects: A Randomized, Placebo-Controlled, Double-Blind, Cross-over Clinical Trial. *J. Food Biochem.* **2021**, *45*, e13665. [CrossRef] [PubMed]
263. Spiller, G.A.; Dewell, A. Safety of an Astaxanthin-Rich *Haematococcus pluvialis* Algal Extract: A Randomized Clinical Trial. *J. Med. Food* **2003**, *6*, 51–56. [CrossRef] [PubMed]
264. Katagiri, M.; Satoh, A.; Tsuji, S.; Shirasawa, T. Effects of Astaxanthin-Rich *Haematococcus pluvialis* Extract on Cognitive Function: A Randomised, Double-Blind, Placebo-Controlled Study. *J. Clin. Biochem. Nutr.* **2012**, *51*, 102–107. [CrossRef]
265. Kim, J.H.; Chang, M.J.; Choi, H.D.; Youn, Y.-K.; Kim, J.T.; Oh, J.M.; Shin, W.G. Protective Effects of *Haematococcus* Astaxanthin on Oxidative Stress in Healthy Smokers. *J. Med. Food* **2011**, *14*, 1469–1475. [CrossRef]
266. Kidd, P. Astaxanthin, Cell Membrane Nutrient with Diverse Clinical Benefits and Anti-Aging Potential. *Altern. Med. Rev. J. Clin. Ther.* **2011**, *16*, 355–364.
267. García, Á.; Toro-Román, V.; Siquier-Coll, J.; Bartolomé, I.; Muñoz, D.; Maynar-Mariño, M. Effects of *Tetraselmis chuii* Microalgae Supplementation on Anthropometric, Hormonal and Hematological Parameters in Healthy Young Men: A Double-Blind Study. *Int. J. Environ. Res. Public. Health* **2022**, *19*, 6060. [CrossRef] [PubMed]
268. Nakashima, A.; Yasuda, K.; Murata, A.; Suzuki, K.; Miura, N. Effects of *Euglena gracilis* Intake on Mood and Autonomic Activity under Mental Workload, and Subjective Sleep Quality: A Randomized, Double-Blind, Placebo-Controlled Trial. *Nutrients* **2020**, *12*, 3243. [CrossRef] [PubMed]
269. Rao, A.; Briskey, D.; Nalley, J.O.; Ganuza, E. Omega-3 Eicosapentaenoic Acid (EPA) Rich Extract from the Microalga *Nannochloropsis* Decreases Cholesterol in Healthy Individuals: A Double-Blind, Randomized, Placebo-Controlled, Three-Month Supplementation Study. *Nutrients* **2020**, *12*, 1869. [CrossRef]
270. Karkos, P.D.; Leong, S.C.; Karkos, C.D.; Sivaji, N.; Assimakopoulos, D.A. *Spirulina* in Clinical Practice: Evidence-Based Human Applications. *Evid. Based Complement. Alternat. Med.* **2010**, *2011*, 531053. [CrossRef] [PubMed]
271. de la Jara, A.; Ruano-Rodriguez, C.; Polifrone, M.; Assunçao, P.; Brito-Casillas, Y.; Wägner, A.M.; Serra-Majem, L. Impact of Dietary *Arthrospira* (*Spirulina*) Biomass Consumption on Human Health: Main Health Targets and Systematic Review. *J. Appl. Phycol.* **2018**, *30*, 2403–2423. [CrossRef]

Disclaimer/Publisher's Note: The statements, opinions and data contained in all publications are solely those of the individual author(s) and contributor(s) and not of MDPI and/or the editor(s). MDPI and/or the editor(s) disclaim responsibility for any injury to people or property resulting from any ideas, methods, instructions or products referred to in the content.

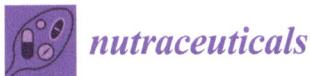

Review

Food Antioxidants and Aging: Theory, Current Evidence and Perspectives

Taiki Miyazawa [1,*], Chizumi Abe [1], Gregor Carpentero Burdeos [2], Akira Matsumoto [3,4] and Masako Toda [1,5]

[1] New Industry Creation Hatchery Center (NICHe), Tohoku University, Sendai 980-8579, Japan; chizumi.abe.e5@tohoku.ac.jp (C.A.); masako.toda.a7@tohoku.ac.jp (M.T.)
[2] Institute for Animal Nutrition and Physiology, Christian Albrechts University Kiel, Hermann-Rodewald Street, 9, 24118 Kiel, Germany; burdeos@aninut.uni-kiel.de
[3] Institute of Biomaterials and Bioengineering, Tokyo Medical and Dental University (TMDU), Chiyoda-ku, Tokyo 101-0062, Japan; matsumoto.bsr@tmd.ac.jp
[4] Kanagawa Institute of Industrial Science and Technology (KISTEC), Ebina 243-0435, Japan
[5] Graduate School of Agricultural Science, Tohoku University, Sendai 980-8555, Japan
* Correspondence: taiki.miyazawa.b3@tohoku.ac.jp; Tel.: +81-22-795-3205

Abstract: The concept of food and aging is of great concern to humans. So far, more than 300 theories of aging have been suggested, and approaches based on these principles have been investigated. It has been reported that antioxidants in foods might play a role in human aging. To clarify the current recognition and positioning of the relationship between these food antioxidants and aging, this review is presented in the following order: (1) aging theories, (2) food and aging, and (3) individual food antioxidants and aging. Clarifying the significance of food antioxidants in the field of aging will lead to the development of strategies to achieve healthy human aging.

Keywords: antioxidants; aging theories; cohort study; healthy diet; longevity; nutraceuticals; oxidative stress; reactive oxygen species; senescence; vitamins

Introduction

Aging is regarded as a biological phenomenon that results in decreasing biological function and increasing mortality over time, in terms of personal, organ, and tissue levels. The concept of aging in terms of individual aging has been recognized since ancient times, but the new view of aging as a "population scenario" that focuses on the overall population has only appeared in the last century [1]. There is also still a debate over the definition of the relationship between aging and disease [2,3]. Although research related to aging continues the trends of the past and present for many researchers, it seems to be difficult to define the concept of aging because it is an ambiguous and changing term that changes its view at different times. Numerous mechanisms related to the induction of aging have been reported, and there are currently more than 300 existing theories [4]. Among them, the recognition and positioning of the relationship between foods, food antioxidants, and the aging process remain vague, even though there has been interest in this topic in the past. Therefore, this review aims to organize the recognition of the relationship between food antioxidants and the aging process by considering: (1) aging theories, (2) food and aging, and (3) individual food antioxidants and aging, in that order, and to clarify the current status of knowledge and the problems in the field.

1. Aging Theories

Since it is difficult to cover all these aging theories in this review, the most fundamental of those that have been proposed to date are outlined in Figure 1. Although it is difficult to clarify the classification of aging theories as they are complementary to other theories, this chapter will categorize them into two major groups: (1) genetic factors associated with aging, and (2) non-genetic factors associated with aging, along with the presentation of the relevant molecular reactions and examples of the aging characteristics associated with each theory.

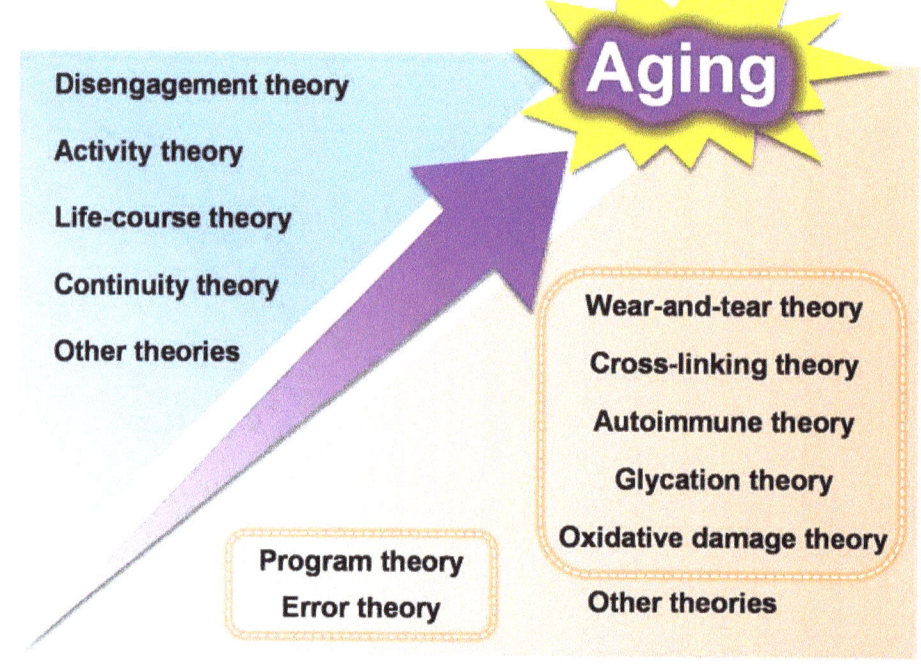

Figure 1. The biological and psychosocial aging theories that are mentioned in this review.

1.1. Genetic Factors Associated with Aging

1.1.1. Program Theory

The program theory proposes that aging is not a random occurrence but is instead inherent in our genetic information. This theory is based on a discovery by Hayflick et al. in 1961 that there is a limitation on the number of divisions of and the proliferation of human and animal cells (the so-called Hayflick limit) [5]. Telomeres and telomerase are closely related to the program theory. DNA loses its replicative ability when its terminal bases are lost during replication. Mammals have a TTAGGG repeat structure called a telomere at the end of their DNA, which protects the genetic information and allows replication. Telomeres are elongated by telomerase. Therefore, telomere length is believed to be a determinant of the number of cell divisions and is thus a factor in aging and lifespan [6]. However, telomeres are shortened with age and affect the process of aging because they are regenerated with each replication, but not completely. More recently, telomerase-deficient mice have been shown to demonstrate impaired neuronal differentiation and neurogenesis [7]. The recovery of telomere function and length has also been reported to extend the lifespan of mammals and can delay physical aging in mouse experiments [8,9].

1.1.2. Error Theory

The error theory states that random errors in DNA transcription and translation lead to the accumulation of mutant proteins, which causes cellular dysfunction and aging [10].

To date, no direct evidence of the age-dependent dysfunction of protein synthesis has been reported [11]. Furthermore, another study using *Escherichia coli* showed that the induction of errors in the gene increased the frequency of error generation but did not induce bacterial death [12]. Therefore, the number of recent reports supporting this theory has relatively decreased.

1.2. Non-Genetic Factors Associated with Aging

1.2.1. Wear-and-Tear Theory

The wear-and-tear theory, which was proposed by Weismann in 1882, states that aging progresses when cells and tissues are worn down by risk factors over the years [13]. However, this theory was invalidated by several phenomena. For instance, hyperactive mice wore down their tissues but can live longer than normal mice [14]. Caterpillars that have lost the ability to express antioxidant enzymes can live longer [15]. Recently, there seems to be increasing evidence that the wearing down is not simply explainable as a physical inevitability in aging and needs to be considered in terms of natural selection from an evolutionary aspect.

1.2.2. Cross-Linking Theory

The cross-linking theory states that the accumulation of molecules with multiple reactive units due to the cross-linking of poorly degradable macromolecules impairs cellular function and promotes aging. Increased viscosity of the extracellular environment is induced by decreased solubility, elasticity, and permeability, due to the cross-linking of collagens and other molecules. As a result, the circulation of nutrients and wastes in the cells is delayed and, thus, aging progresses [16]. The cross-linking products of glucose and collagen (products of the Maillard reaction) are widely recognized as products that increase along with aging in the body [17]. Bjorksten et al. pointed out that the free radical theory is also a form of cross-linking theory because free radicals that are generated in the body induce cross-linking reactions in collagen and other molecules [18]. Despite qualitative and quantitative evidence of cross-linked molecules that has been provided to support this theory, it is still not clear whether the molecules are crucial in biological aging.

1.2.3. Autoimmune Theory

The autoimmune system has been regarded as being at least indirectly associated with aging. Higher vertebrates have two major immune mechanisms, innate and acquired immunity. The dysfunction of acquired immunity is particularly significant in terms of aging. Innate immunity captures antigens via pattern recognition receptors and presents them to T cells, while acquired immunity is characterized by the antigen-specific effector and memory responses of T cells and B cells (T cells: directives, antigen memory, antigen destruction; B cells: antibody production). Involution of the thymus, the primary lymphoid tissues for T-cell education and development, starts at a relatively early age in different species [19]. In an aged thymus, biological processes for the elimination of self-reactive T cells and the induction of regulatory T cells, namely, central tolerance, are seen to decline [20]. In addition, aging is associated with a decline in B cell production in the bone marrow, along with increased self-reactive B cell populations. Taken together, aged adaptive immunity promotes development that results in damage to the body's own tissues and is one of the major causes of death in women under 65 years of age in the US [21,22].

1.2.4. Glycation Theory

In 1912, the aminocarbonyl reaction (Maillard reaction) was reported by Maillard; it is considered part of the phenomenon of biological body aging [23]. The glucose and lysine residues of proteins react at body temperature, to form advanced glycation end products (AGEs) through a condensation reaction. The formed AGEs are accumulated in various tissues, such as the blood vessel walls, and induce tissue inflexibility, leading to vasodilator dysfunction and hypertension, which is regarded as a trigger of aging [24].

1.2.5. Oxidative Damage Theory

Aerobic organisms consume oxygen for the purposes of energy metabolism, which produces reactive oxygen species (ROS) in the metabolic process. In 1956, Harman proposed that ROS leads to aging by causing damage to cells and tissues [25]. Older individuals have higher concentrations of oxidized products, such as proteins, DNA, and lipids, than younger individuals, whereas antioxidants have often been highlighted as molecules that reduce ROS generation and contribute toward extending the lifespan [26–28]. Among cellular organelles, especially in mitochondria, which are involved in aerobic energy metabolism, there is a higher level of ROS in aging individuals. Furthermore, in mammals, there is an inverse correlation between the concentration of ROS in mitochondria and the lifespan, suggesting that damage to mitochondrial DNA and membrane lipids is also a factor closely related to aging [29]. However, ROS also plays a role in the mammalian immune system for biological defense that eliminates intracellular pathogens [30]. Therefore, it is widely recognized that dysfunction of the redox balance induces inflammatory reactions. Related to this, the term "inflammaging" has developed to describe the concept of aging as it is related to innate immunity, which corresponds to (1) chronically, (2) no contact with bacteria, etc., and (3) weak inflammation [31]. Recently, based on the concept of "inflammaging," it has been shown that chronic tissue inflammation caused by ROS has a significant impact on the regulatory systems of the nervous system and immune system, as well as the aging process; it can be induced by suppressing the regulation of the inflammatory factors of the immune system [32,33].

1.2.6. Other Biological Aging-Related Theories

The existence of "senescent cells," which accelerate aging in the body, has been the topic of growing attention among gerontologists. In general, aged cells that have stopped dividing are removed from the body through cell death or the phagocytosis of immune cells. However, there are senescent cells that accumulate in the tissues despite the cell division having stopped. Recent studies have shown that these accumulated senescent cells release inflammatory substances that accelerate the senescence of neighboring cells, trigger excessive inflammation, and lead to tissue dysfunction [34]. Since the immune system in the body cannot eliminate all the senescent cells, some anti-aging approaches have begun to be developed that target these senescent cells [35]. Since there is still a lack of direct information on the relationship of these senescent cells with aging, further elucidation of the physiological phenomenon may be necessary.

In contrast to the theory that certain factor(s) accelerate the rate of aging, there is a theory stating that the rate of aging is unchanged by any factor. Colchero et al. reported strong linearity between life expectancy and lifespan equality in various primates, mainly connected to infant mortality or age-independent mortality improvement, with no impact on the aging rate [36]. This result suggests that only the biological limit determines longevity.

1.3. Sociology of Aging

The concept of aging exists not only from a biological viewpoint but also from a sociological one. Social animals, such as humans, are thought to be influenced by their surroundings in their biological development. Theories of aging in social gerontology can be broadly classified into four categories: (1) disengagement theory, (2) activity theory, (3) life-course theory, and (4) continuity theory.

1.3.1. Disengagement Theory

The disengagement theory posits that aging is a process of disengagement from being a part of society. The ultimate stage of disengagement is incurable illness or death. This is the concept that elderly people who contribute less to society could leave and give up their roles to young people who will contribute more to society, leading to the sustainability of the social system to which they belong [37,38].

1.3.2. Activity Theory

Activity theory is the concept that maintaining activities and attitudes in middle age for as long as possible is the key to healthy aging. This concept has existed previously but was given this name as a contrast to the disengagement theory proposed earlier. The difference between this theory and the disengagement theory is that the elderly may or may not be considered to be at a developmental stage. Disengagement theory describes old age as a natural developmental process, while activity theory describes the period after middle age as a completed stage [39].

1.3.3. Life-Course Theory

Life-course theory is the theory that human aging is part of the growth (development) process, with earlier experiences being important for later life adaptability [40]. More recently, based on this concept, an epidemiologic assessment of the relationship between aging, physical activity, and cognitive function has been conducted [41,42].

1.3.4. Continuity Theory

Continuity theory arose from discussions of disengagement theory and activity theory. Humans tend to keep their personalities for the long term, but they become more introspective with age, focusing their attention and interest inward to their individual selves. This theory proposes that healthy aging is the state of keeping a mature and integrated personality during aging [43].

1.4. Aging and Senescence

Living biological organisms age with time. With regard to this concept of aging, some researchers use the term "senescence" as a subgroup to distinguish between harmless changes and changes associated with mortality risk [1]. Dodig et al. defined senescence as an "irreversible form of long-term cell-cycle arrest, caused by excessive intracellular or extracellular stress or damage," which is regarded as influencing various biological events related to aging, such as metabolism, immune function, autophagy changes, and chromatin development [44]. These investigations with the keyword "cellular senescence" and "biological senescence" are one of the most significant issues in the field of molecular biology and gerontology.

2. Food and Aging

2.1. Potential Foods for Anti-Aging

To make the relationship between food and lifespan clearer, there has been an ongoing discussion for some years, based on the theories of aging as described in the previous chapter [45,46]. Foods contain numerous bioactive compounds that are essential for maintaining human health. Therefore, dietary consumption is the most common and routine way for humans to supply nutrients to the body. Although there is still no proven relationship with the theory of aging, it has traditionally been suggested that certain foods themselves or certain compounds in foods have preventive and curative functions against diseases. Although no specific foods or nutrients in foods related to longevity have yet been identified, it is worth pointing out that a number of reports have suggested that the consumption of foods relatively rich in antioxidants has the ability to reduce mortality. Against this background, this section describes previous reports made in cohort studies on the relationship between diet and aging as it contributes to lifespan (Table 1).

Table 1. Cohort studies examining diet and lifespan.

Target	Diet	Country	Populations Analyzed/Total	Age	Follow-Up Time	Reducing Mortality/Increasing Life Span	Ref.
Mortality	Mediterranean diet	Greece	22,043/28,572 (M, F)	20–86	3.7 years	Yes	[47]
Mortality	Mediterranean diet	US	3215/(F) (with heart failure)	50–79	4.6 years	Yes	[48]
Mortality	Traditional Nordic foods	Denmark	2383/27,178 (M) 1743/29,875 (F)	50–64	12 years	Yes (especially in middle-aged men)	[49]
Mortality	Nordic foods	Sweden	44,961/49,259 (F)	29–49	21.3 years	Yes (especially by cancer, non-cancer, non-cardiovascular, non-injury/suicide)	[50]
Longevity	Japanese diet	Japan	14,764/32,126 (M, F)	40–79	20 years	Yes	[51]
Mortality	Japanese diet	Japan	23,162 (M) and 34,232 (F) /110,585 (M, F)	40–79	18.9 years (M) 19.4 years (F)	Yes (especially in females)	[52]
Mortality risk of CVD	fruits, vegetables	US	9608/14,407 (M, F)	25–74	19 years	Yes	[53]
Mortality	fresh fruits, vegetables	Europe (DNK, FRA, DEU, GRC, ITA, NLD, NOR, ESP, SWE, GBR)	129,882 (M) and 321,269 (F)/ 521,448	25–70	13 years	Yes (especially by CVD)	[54]
Mortality	21 fruits, 24 vegetables	POL, RUS, CZE	19,333/28,945 (M, F)	Middle age	7.1 years	Yes (especially by CVD in smokers/hypertension)	[55]
Mortality	8 fruits, 33 vegetables	China	73,360/74,942 (F) 61,436/61,500 (M)	40–70 (F) 40–74 (M)	10.2 years (F) 4.6 (M)	Yes (by CVD), no (by cancer)	[56]
Mortality	fruits, vegetables	Europe (FRA, DU, ITA, HUN, POL, PRT, ROU, ESP, SWE, TUR) and ARG	8078/9757 (M, F) (with hemodialysis)	mean 63	2.7 years	Yes (except by CVD)	[57]
Mortality	Meat, fish, dairy products, eggs, and vegetables	UK	11,140 (M, F) (Vegetarians and meat-eaters)	mean 38.7 (V), mean 39.3 (NV)	12 years	No	[58]
			65,411 (M, F) (Meat/fish eaters, vegetarians and vegans)	20–97	15 years		
Mortality	Nuts (peanuts and tree nuts)	U.S.	39,167/39,876 (F)	≥45	19 years	Yes (except by CVD)	[59]
Mortality	Nuts (peanuts and others)	U.S.	47,299/51,529 (M) (PCa patients)	40–75	26 years	No (except in men diagnosed with non-metastatic PCa)	[60]
Mortality	Nuts (walnuts, hazelnuts, almonds and peanuts)	Italy	19,386/24,325 (M, F)	≥35	4.3 years	Yes	[61]
Mortality	Nuts (peanut butter, nut bread and rice cooked with chestnuts)	Japan	13,355 (M) 15,724 (F) /36,990	≥35	17 years	Yes	[62]
Mortality	Nuts (peanuts, tree nuts and overall nuts consumption)	Iran	20,855 (M) 28,257 (F) /50,045	40–87	7 years	Yes	[63]
Mortality risk of type-2 diabetes risk of CVD (meta-analysis)	Nuts	US	134,486 (F)	55–69	11 years	Yes	[64]
		China	64,227 (F)	40–70	4.6 years		
		US	20,224 (M)	41–87	21.1 years		
		US	1,164,248 (F)	30–55	22 years		
		US	1,599,667 (F)	20–45	18 years		
		US	31,208 (M, F)	>25	6 years		
		US	21,454 (M)	40–84	17 years		
		US	31,778 (F)	55–69	15 years		

Table 1. *Cont.*

Target	Diet	Country	Populations Analyzed/Total	Age	Follow-Up Time	Reducing Mortality/Increasing Life Span	Ref.
		US	6309 (F)	52.8 ± 8.5	22 years		
		US	34,492 (F)	30–55	26 years		
		US	21,078 (M)	41–87	21.1 years		
		US	43,150 (M) 84,010 (F)	40–75 (M) 30–55 (F)	26 years (M) 22 years (F)		
		US	87,025 (F)	50–79	4 years		
		US	NS (M, F)	>25	–		
		US	NS (M, F)	>85	12 years		
		UK	10,802 (M, F)	16–79	13.3 years		
		Netherlands	NS (M, F)	55–69	24 years		
		US	3,038,853 (M, F)	30–55 (NHS) 40–75 (HPFS)	30 years (NHS) 24 years (HPFS)		
		Spain	31,077 (M, F)	55–80	4.8 years		
Mortality	Mediterranean diet, (especially nuts)	Spain	7216/7447 (M, F)	55–80 (M) 60–80 (F)	4.8 years	Yes	[65]
Mortality	Nuts (peanuts, walnuts and other nuts)	China	3449/5042 (F)	20–75	8.27 years	Yes	[66]
		Japan	22,597 (M) 25,382 (F)	40–59	20.25 years		
		Japan	27,941 (M) 31,415 (F)	40–69	17.3 years		
		Japan	28,258 (M) 39,446 (F)	40–79	16.1 years		
Mortality	Green tea	Japan	16,874 (M) 18,077 (F)	40–64	20.52 years	Yes (especially by HD and CVD)	[67]
		Japan	12,152 (M) 13,194 (F)	40–79	11.66 years		
		Japan	16,749 (M) 18,185 (F)	≥40	10.98 years		
		Japan	8663 (M) 9951 (F)	40–103	11.67 years		
		Japan	11,516 (M) 12,981 (F)	40–97	12.56 years		
Mortality	Green tea	Japan	42,836/68,722 (M) 48,078/71,698 (F)	40–69	18.7 years	Yes	[68]
	Tea	China	51,668/65,212 (M, F)	≥65	3.5–3.8 years		
Longevity	Elements in food and water	China	NA	≥65, ≥90	-	Yes	[69]
		China	3139 (M, F)	≥65	9.1 years		
		China	61,414 (M) 73,232 (F)	40–74 (M) 40–70 (F)	5.5 years (M) 11 years (F)		
		Canada	9033 (M, F)	≥25	10 years		
		Sweden	61,433 (F)	39–74	19 years		
Mortality CVD mortality	Calcium	US	388,229 (M, F)	50–71	12 years	Yes (except high dose > 900 mg calcium/day)	[70]
		US	18,714 (M, F)	≥17	18 years		
		Germany	23,980 (M, F)	35–64	11 years		
		US	38,772 (F)	55–69	11 years		
		Sweden	23,366 (M)	45–79	10 years		
		Japan	21,068 (M) 32,319 (F)	40–59	9.6 years		
		Netherlands	1340 (M) 1265 (F)	40–65	28 years		

Table 1. Cont.

Target	Diet	Country	Populations Analyzed/Total	Age	Follow-Up Time	Reducing Mortality/Increasing Life Span	Ref.
Mortality	Coffee	Spain	19,888/22,320 (M, F)	Middle age	10 years	Yes ($\geq$54 years)	[71]
Longevity	Coffee	US	27,480/93,676 (F) (postmenopausal)	65–81	25 years	No	[72]
Morality	Meat intake	China	61,128/61,483 (M) 73,162/74,941 (F)	40–74 (M) 40–70 (F)	5.5 years (M) 11.2 years (F)	No (increased mortality in men)	[73]
Mortality	Dietary diversity (meat, fish and seafood, eggs, beans, fruits, salty vegetables, tea, garlic, and fresh vegetables)	China	28,790/43,487	$\geq$80	3.4 years	Yes (especially by consumption of protein-rich food)	[74]
Mortality	Eastern European diet	Eastern Europe (RUS, POL and CZE)	18,852/29,845 (M, F)	45–70	8–15 years	No (rather than increased)	[75]
Mortality	Ultra-processed food	France	44,551/158,361 (M, F)	$\geq$45	7.1 years	No (rather than increased)	[76]
Mortality	Ultra-processed food	Italy	22,475/24,325 (M, F)	$\geq$35	8.2 years	No (rather than increased)	[77]
Mortality	Ultra-processed food	Spain	11,898/12,948	$\geq$18	7.7 years	No (rather than increased)	[78]
Mortality	Fried food	US	106,966/373,092 (F) (postmenopausal)	50–79	17.9 years	No (rather than increased by CVD)	[79]
Mortality	Potato	North America	4400/4796 (M, F)	45–79	8 years	No (rather than increased)	[80]

2.2. Mediterranean Diet

Among the diets associated with health and longevity, the traditional Mediterranean diet is widely recognized as one of the most popular. Mediterranean diets are rich in vegetables, legumes, fruits, nuts, grains, seafood, and olive oil; they are also low in saturated fats, dairy products, and meat. Drinking wine and other alcoholic beverages is also popular. Attention regarding the dietary functions of the Mediterranean diet was greatly increased in the early 1990s, with (1) growing concerns that large doses of simple carbohydrates might not be beneficial to health, and (2) growing interest in the use of the Mediterranean diet score to quantify the health benefits of the food [81]. In a cohort study of Greek adults, mortality related to cardiovascular (coronary heart) disease and cancer was examined using the Mediterranean diet score as a criterion and reported that Mediterranean diet ingestion was correlated with lower overall mortality [47]. This may support the report by Crous-Bou et al. that higher dietary Mediterranean diet scores tend to result in longer telomeres in healthy women [82]. Other research institutes also suggested that the Mediterranean diet is beneficial in reducing mortality among heart failure patients as well as healthy subjects [48].

2.3. Other Traditional Foods

The Nordic diet is characterized by low levels of processed foods and includes yogurt, berries, whole grain bread, oatmeal, apples/pears, root vegetables, cabbage, fish/shellfish, etc., It has also been reported that consumption of the Nordic diet lowers mortality in humans. A cohort study of Danes showed that consumption of the Nordic diet was associated with lower mortality, especially among middle-aged men [49]. Another cohort study of Swedish women indicated that all-cause mortality was significantly lower when on a diet with higher Nordic diet scores [50].

Japan is one of the leading countries of longevity in the world. With the "Japanese diet" being registered as a World Intangible Heritage in 2013, attention has been attracted by the relationship between the Japanese diet and aging. In a cohort study of Japanese subjects, the consumption of Japanese food (including rice, miso soup, seaweed, cucumber, green and yellow vegetables, fish, green tea, beef, pork, and coffee) was associated with prolonged survival [51]. Other cohort studies of Japanese people have also reported that consumption of the Japanese diet reduces mortality from all causes, especially among women [52]. On the other hand, the definition of Japanese food in cohort studies is still unclear and varies. Furthermore, the diet of Japanese people has been changing in recent years. Therefore, there is a consideration that the longevity of Japanese people in recent years might be related to other factors besides the Japanese diet [83].

2.4. Individual Foodstuffs

2.4.1. Fruits and Vegetables

Individual fruits and vegetables that are abundant in the Mediterranean diet have also been found to be related to aging. A cohort study of US adults showed that consumption of fruits and vegetables may reduce the risk of cardiovascular disease and all-cause mortality [53]. Cohort studies of adults in ten European countries have also indicated that an increased intake of fruits and vegetables tends to reduce mortality [54]. In a cohort study of participants from the Czech Republic, Poland, and Russia, an increased intake of fruits and vegetables was associated with lower mortality, especially among smokers and hypertensive patients [55]. Among vegetables, cruciferous vegetables are widely consumed in the general diet. A cohort study of Chinese adults indicated that fruit and vegetable intake was inversely associated with the risk of total mortality in both women and men, with a dose-response pattern that was particularly evident in the intake of cruciferous vegetables [56]. A multinational cohort study of adults in eleven countries who were being treated with hemodialysis has also indicated that a higher vegetable intake is associated with lower all-cause and non-cardiovascular mortality [57]. As mentioned in this section, vegetable consumption seems to be associated with longevity; however, the consumption of only vegetables may not result in longevity. For instance, a large-scale cohort study of adults in the United Kingdom observed that all-cause mortality rates for vegetarians and non-vegetarians were almost the same [58].

2.4.2. Nuts

Nuts, which are abundant in the Mediterranean diet, are consumed worldwide. A cohort study of U.S. women indicates that the consumption of nuts led to changes in plasma lipids, inflammation, and glucose metabolism, resulting in an association with a reduced risk of death from cardiovascular disease [59]. In another cohort study of US men, it was observed that subjects who consumed nuts five or more times per week had a 34% lower all-cause mortality rate than those who consumed nuts less than once per month [60]. Several types of nuts (walnuts, hazelnuts, almonds, and peanuts) were also reported to show a significant reduction in cancer death [61]. One Japanese cohort study showed that total nut intake (peanuts and chestnuts) was inversely associated with all-cause mortality in men [62]. Interestingly, the Golestan Cohort Study conducted in Iran evidenced that reduced mortality by nut consumption (peanuts, tree nuts, and overall nuts) is independent of a healthy lifestyle [63]. Among nuts, there are relatively numerous studies on walnuts, examining their relationship with longevity. Several cohort studies have found that walnut consumption may reduce mortality [64,65]. On the other hand, a cohort study in China reported that nut consumption dose-dependently induced better survival in long-term breast cancer survivors, regardless of the types of nuts [66]. Thus, further investigation and scientific evidence on the components of each nut type is warranted to clarify the essential factor in reduced mortality that is induced by various types of nuts.

2.4.3. Beverages

It is considered that daily beverage intake may also have an impact on aging. Among Japanese diets, green tea is one of the most widely studied beverages for aging. Several cohort studies of Japanese have reported that the consumption of green tea has the potential to reduce the risk of mortality from heart disease and cardiovascular disease [67,68]. Hao et al. compared the effects of minerals in food and drinking water on life expectancy, using the database of demographics from eighteen counties in the Chinese census [69]. As a result, the amount of Cu, Se, and Zn ingested from the diet and drinking water was positively correlated with longevity, while Pb was negatively correlated in Hainan Province, which is known for its longevity. In a meta-analysis of 757,304 individuals from 12 independent cohorts, Wang et al. reported that low to moderate doses of Ca were associated with reduced mortality, but not at higher doses, and concluded that each individual should consume the appropriate amount [70]. Navarro et al. reported an inverse linear association between total coffee consumption and the risk of death from all causes in Spaniards, which was particularly pronounced in those over 54 years old [71].

2.5. Age and Food Intake

The nutritional function that can be expected from the intake of food seems to differ significantly, depending on age at the time of intake. A cohort study of elderly women (65 to 81 years old) in the US tried to determine the association between coffee and tea consumption and survival to age 90 [72]. The results showed that coffee and tea consumption may not prolong survival until later life in women. Concerning protein intake, a cohort study of Chinese people aged 40 to 74 reported that in healthy people, red meat (a rich source of protein) intake increases the risk of death [73]. In contrast, a cohort study of Chinese people over 80 indicated that the consumption of protein-rich foods reduced the risk of death [74]. Such changes in dietary effects are considered to occur due to the various dysfunctions associated with aging, such as alteration of the gut microbiota, the decreased absorption of nutrients in the gastrointestinal tract, decreased chewing strength, decreased exercise, etc. The relationship between caloric restriction and lifespan has become a major topic in the field of gerontology, with reports indicating that caloric restriction may prevent aging in various species [84,85]. Caloric restriction is thought to have a significant impact on human aging. However, the effect of caloric restriction might be challenging to verify, as it would require very long-term, large-scale human lifestyle intervention studies.

2.6. Potential Foods That May Accelerate Aging

While food intake has been associated with longer life expectancy, others have also reported that it may contribute to accelerated aging and increased mortality. For example, there are cases in which traditional diets increase mortality. A cohort study of people in Russia, Poland, and the Czech Republic showed that the high mortality from cardiovascular disease in Eastern Europe is related to the traditional dietary habits in target regions, with lard consumption most likely to be responsible for increased mortality [75]. With the development of food processing technology in modern society, the concept of "ultra-processed food (UPF)" has increased in importance. It gradually became clear that the consumption of UPF might increase the risk of death [86]. UPF is defined as "formulations of ingredients, mostly of exclusive industrial use, typically created by a series of industrial techniques and processes" in the NOVA classification and is considered a different group from unprocessed and minimally processed foods, processed culinary ingredients, and processed foods [87]. UPF refers to ready-to-eat industrially formulated products that contain high levels of additives such as sugar, salt, hardened oil, flavorings, emulsifiers, and preservatives [88]. A large prospective cohort study in France (French NutriNet-Santé cohort), of subjects with a median age of 42.8 years, from 2009 to 2017 reported that the consumption of a diet classified as UPF according to the NOVA classification was associated with increased overall cancer risk [89]. A cohort study of French people indicated that the increased consumption of UPF was associated with an increased risk of total mortality in this adult population [76]. A cohort study of Italians also showed that UPFs, particularly those rich in sugar, were associated with an increased risk of death [77]. In addition, a cohort study of Spaniards, conducted by other research institutions, showed that replacing UPF with non- or low-processed foods with the same calories may reduce mortality [78]. Fried foods are highly palatable and popular but have been known to increase the risk of diseases that lead to death, such as type 2 diabetes and cardiovascular disease. A cohort study of postmenopausal women in the US indicated that the consumption of fried foods, especially fried chicken and fried seafood, was associated with mortality risk among US women, including from cardiovascular disease [79]. Furthermore, a cohort study of elderly people in the US also observed changes in mortality due to the consumption of fried and non-fried potatoes and indicated that the consumption of fried potatoes more than twice a week increased the risk of death [80]. As this section has shown, an evaluation of food and aging suggests that it is necessary to consider not only information on foodstuffs but also changes in certain foods' properties due to processing in factories.

3. Individual Food Antioxidants and Aging

Based on the results of the numerous cohort studies described in the previous chapter that have examined the impact of diet on the risk of aging and death, it seems almost certain that the content of the human diet has a significant effect on aging. However, there is still no clear evidence on which molecular, cellular, and physiological changes are the most important factors of aging in individual organisms and on how they affect each other [90]. With current scientific technology, it seems hard to quantify the effect of "whole foods," which are composed of many molecules, on aging. However, numerous studies have suggested that a variety of individual antioxidants in foods are related to aging: for example, the autoimmune theory [91]; cross-linking theory [92]; glycation theory [93]; and KEAP1-NRF2 theory [94].

Most of these previous studies are based on the concept of "oxidative damage theory," as described in the first half of this review. Among the various theories of aging, the oxidative damage theory has been one of the most popular theories in aging research, with much quantitative experimental evidence being reported from the past to the present [4]. There is growing evidence that ROS may act as signaling molecules that not only induce oxidative stress but also ultimately extend the lifespan [95]. Such trends led to the concept of "mitohormesis", which states that ROS promotes aging but, in the appropriate concentrations, can enhance the biological defense system [96,97]. The regulation of redox balance in the body is a crucial factor in aging, as ATP production in mitochondria with ROS generation is an essential factor for energy acquisition in aerobic organisms. It is also expected that individual antioxidants in foods also contribute to the regulation of the redox balance (Figure 2). Cell signaling pathways involved with this balance, such as MAPKs, NF-κB, and Nrf2 seem important in the anti-aging effects of antioxidants [98–102]. However, a description of the detailed mechanism for this process will not be discussed here because that goes beyond the remit of this review. Please refer to Maleki et al. [103] and Luo et al. [104] for a review of this topic.

However, with the current state of scientific technology, it is difficult to identify the effects of individual antioxidants on "aging" and "mortality," which involve complex factors, and there are few direct reports. On the other hand, there have been several reports on the effects of these individual antioxidants on "various diseases related to aging and mortality" [28,105,106]. This chapter focuses on the relationship between individual antioxidants in foods, which have been reported and relatively well investigated, and diseases related to aging and mortality.

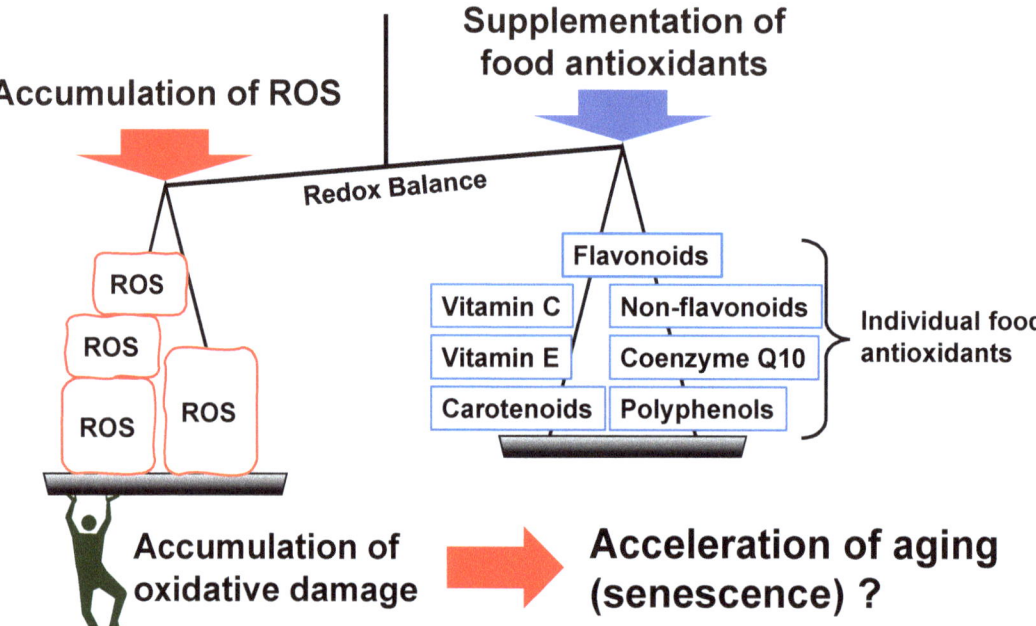

Figure 2. A typical illustration showing food antioxidants in the redox balance of the body, as mentioned in this review. Reactive oxygen species (ROS) are produced by mitochondria, drugs, oxidized foods, etc., and are considered to induce the redox balance toward an oxidized state, resulting in accelerated aging that is caused by the accumulation of oxidative damage. It is considered that food antioxidants regulate the redox balance and aging.

3.1. Vitamins

Vitamins are substances that are essential to animals and humans; they act as the cofactors and precursors of enzymes in the regulation of metabolic processes, do not provide energy, and are essential to the human body [107,108]. The body needs a supply of vitamins through the diet, among which vitamins A, C, and E are called the "antioxidant vitamins", and their relationship with aging is of great interest [109].

3.1.1. Vitamin C

Vitamin C, also known as L-ascorbic acid, is a lipophobic compound that is involved in collagen synthesis in the body. Vitamin C exists in the human body at the highest concentration among all vitamins and is considered to regulate redox status in the body [110–112]. In a cohort study of 17,304 middle-aged and elderly Europeans aged 42 to 82 years old, Lewis et al. reported that an adequate intake of Vitamin C is necessary to reduce the progression of frailty and sarcopenia caused by increased oxidative stress due to aging [113]. Qu et al. reported that Vitamin C inhibited prelamin A expression and the secretion of inflammatory mediators that induce cellular aging in subchondral bone mesenchymal stem cells [114]. Laboratory mice lifespans were increased with an amount of Vitamin C in drinking water, in a study using gluconolactone oxidase-deficient mice [115]. This report suggested that Vitamin C modulates the stress response in the endoplasmic reticulum and the lifespan of mice. Oxidative damage to the brain due to aging is regarded as one of the factors that cause brain dysfunction. Experiments in mouse models of Alzheimer's disease indicate that Vitamin C deficiency in the brain may affect the redox balance and accelerate the generation of amyloid-beta, an initiator of oxidative stress in Alzheimer's disease [116]. On the other hand, a review by Kaźmierczak-Barańska et al. summarized that vitamin C is important as a pro-oxidant related to the upregulation of DNA repair and other biological functions [117]. They noted that the function of vitamin C varies in different cell lines and conditions, which makes research difficult. The "two faces" of vitamin C, consisting of its functions as both an anti- and pro-oxidant, may make it difficult to elucidate the detailed functions of such antioxidants [117]. With the continued advancement of science and technology in general, it is necessary to fully understand the effects of these antioxidants and pro-oxidants, and more progress should be achieved in the near future.

3.1.2. Vitamin E

Vitamin E, also known as α-tocopherol, is a lipophilic compound. There are other analogs, such as other tocopherols (β-, γ-, δ-) and tocotrienols (α-, β-, γ-, δ-), but only α-tocopherol can be called "vitamin E" [118]. Vitamin E is localized in cell membranes and is thought to play a role in protecting cells from oxidative damage [96]. The α-tocopherol, β-carotene cancer prevention (ATBC) study, a famous large-scale US trial that examined cancer prevention effects, found that an intake of α-tocopherol and β-carotene had no effect on mortality from liver cancer or chronic liver disease [119]. However, in 2019, Huang et al. reported on a 30-year cohort study of subjects in the ATBC study, which showed that plasma vitamin E levels were associated with a reduced risk of all-cause mortality and death from all major causes [120]. Vitamin E deficiency is thought to cause the increased fragility of red blood cells and the degeneration of neurons, especially peripheral axons, and dorsal horn neurons. Mangialasche et al. quantified vitamin E concentration in the serum of patients with Alzheimer's disease, mild cognitive impairment, and normal cognitive function, and reported that the concentration was significantly lower in patients with Alzheimer's disease and dementia than in subjects with normal cognitive function [121]. It has also been reported that the long-term intake of vitamin E suppressed the shortening of telomeres in the peripheral blood mononuclear cells of Alzheimer's patients [122]. It should also be noted that each vitamin E analog has different biological activities. Tucker compared serum leukocyte telomere length with vitamin E and gamma-tocopherol concentrations in 5768 US adults and explained that high levels of gamma-tocopherol in the blood accelerated telomere length loss (vitamin E was not significant) and may accelerate cellular senescence [123]. A cohort study of 580 American people by Hanson et al. showed that there was a positive correlation between dietary vitamin E intake and lung function, but an inverse correlation between serum γ-tocopherol levels and lung function [124]. The ratio of vitamin E and its analogs in foods, or the coexistence of various other compounds, may have an effect on aging.

3.1.3. Carotenoids

Carotenoids, also known as provitamin A, are lipophilic pigments that are classified into two groups, carotenes and xanthophylls, based on their polarity. The blood concentrations of carotenoids were found to be decreased in the elderly and in Alzheimer's disease patients [125]. Huang et al. confirmed the relationship between serum parameters and mortality in a cohort study of 29,103 men in the ATBC study and reported that higher serum β-carotene concentration was associated with lower mortality from cardiovascular disease, heart disease, stroke, cancer, and all causes of death [126]. Min et al. analyzed the plasma of 3660 people in the US and showed that elevated blood β-carotene levels were correlated positively with the length of leukocyte telomeres [127]. Experimental models using *Caenorhabditis elegans* show that the continuous intake of astaxanthin from a young age leads to the increased expression of genes encoding superoxide dismutase (SOD) and catalase and protects the mitochondria and nuclear organelle through the nuclear transfer of DAF-16 protein, resulting in lifespan extension [128]. Wu et al. reported that astaxanthin intake was associated with anti-aging in the D-galactose-induced rat brain aging model by the maintenance of antioxidant enzyme activity, the suppression of oxidative enzyme expression, and an increase in brain-derived neurotrophic factor (BDNF) [129].

3.2. Polyphenols

"Polyphenols" is a general term for compounds with multiple phenolic hydroxy groups in their molecules and are mainly present in plants. Polyphenols can be further classified, depending on their chemical structure, but most of the polyphenols in foods are flavonoids. Flavonoids are a group of phenyl compounds with a structure consisting of two benzene rings connected by three carbon atoms (diphenylpropane), and various reports have been made in recent years on their functional health properties. Although more than 5000 polyphenols have been reported, we will broadly classify them into flavonoids and non-flavonoids in this section and introduce the relationship between each typical compound and aging.

3.2.1. Flavonoids

Quercetin is one of the most recognized flavonoids and is reported to have antioxidant and anti-inflammatory effects. El-Far et al. investigated the effect of quercetin intake on an aged rat model induced by D-galactose [130]. As a result, they reported that quercetin intake suppressed apoptosis and the elevation of inflammatory markers by inducing the expression of anti-apoptotic markers related to aging in the pancreas and kidneys of rats. In a study using mouse oocytes, quercetin also contributed to oocyte maturation and embryo development by reducing age-related increases in mitochondrial oxidative stress and by regulating mitochondrial dysfunction [131]. Geng et al. used a Werner's syndrome model, based on human mesenchymal stem cells to screen for potential natural compounds with anti-aging effects, and identified quercetin. They also reported that quercetin may reduce cellular aging by improving cell proliferation and the repair of the heterochromatin structure [132].

Anthocyanins are polyphenols that are well known due to the presence of the French paradox. Using aged rat models, Li et al. found that anthocyanin intake improves total antioxidant capacity and may ameliorate aging caused by oxidative stress through the induction of autophagy [133]. As is the case with polyphenols in general, it is also important to consider the relationship between their absorption, metabolism, and aging. For example, when anthocyanins are administered orally, the majority of molecules are not transferred into the bloodstream via antioxidant activity, which is likely to be because of glucuronidation and/or sulfate conjugation in the liver and small intestine [134,135].

Isoflavones have been reported to exhibit estrogen-like effects due to their structural similarities, and to contribute to the regulation of hormones in women. Studies on age-related disorders have also reported that genistein prevents the acquisition of insulin resistance in aged rats, but the hormone replacement effect of genistein is only effective in early menopause, not in older age [136].

3.2.2. Non-Flavonoids

Chlorogenic acid is a type of monophenol recognized for its presence in beverages such as tea and coffee. Li et al. reported that the oral administration of a chlorogenic acid-phospholipid complex to senescence-accelerated mice (SAMP8) for two weeks suppressed the post-myocardial infarction response of the aged heart [137].

Resveratrol, a polyphenol that is prolific in fruit peels, is known for having a strong antioxidant capacity in in vitro studies. Gines et al. reported that the oral administration of resveratrol to senescence-accelerated mice (SAMP8) reduced inflammatory factor expression, inhibited apoptosis and oxidative stress in the mouse pancreas, and had a protective effect against age-related pancreatic damage [138]. Resveratrol switches the SIRT-1 gene, which is known as the longevity gene. Several cognitive function studies have reported that the long-term administration of resveratrol has a protective effect against hippocampal and neuronal damage [139,140]. Caldeira et al. reported that resveratrol has antioxidant and anti-inflammatory effects, but its mechanism of action varies with cell age [141]. The antioxidant effect of resveratrol was found to be mediated by the SIRT1/AMPK pathway in middle-aged mononuclear cells, but not in aged cells. Therefore, the biological activity of resveratrol may change with age. Semba et al. conducted a cohort study of 783 Italian seniors aged 65 years or older and noted that in the elderly, resveratrol metabolites were not associated with inflammatory markers, heart disease, cancer, or mortality and that the resveratrol levels reached in the Western diet had virtually no effect on health status or longevity [142]. Furthermore, recent findings have raised concerns that the intake of antioxidants such as resveratrol may rather inhibit the beneficial effect of exercise on improving vascular function in humans [143].

Curcumin is reported in terms of its functions of anti-aging via an anti-inflammatory effect [144,145]. The intake of curcumin for 6 months (200 mg/kg) suppressed the aging process by affecting anti-aging markers (decreased C-reactive protein levels, increased malondialdehyde levels, and nitric oxide levels) in aged albino rats. [146]. In vitro studies have shown that curcumin preserved endothelial cells (HUVEC) from H_2O_2-induced premature senescence via endothelial nitric oxide synthase phosphorylation and silent information regulator (SIRT)-1 expression [147]. Curcumin intake over several weeks (100 mg/kg/day) is reported to delay the aging process of oocytes in the mouse model through anti-aging-related genes (SIRT1 and SIRT3) [148]. Furthermore, 10–40 times higher absorbable and brain-accessible curcumin nanomicelles prevented the mitochondrial dysfunction involved in brain aging and neurodegeneration [149]. As a result of investigating curcumin intake on an obesity-related cognitive dysfunction mouse model, dietary curcumin and caloric restriction worked positively on the frontal cortical functions, regardless of effects on adiposity [150]. A combination of in vivo experiments and computer simulations revealed that curcumin upregulates antioxidant enzymes and improves memory by binding to β-secretase 1 and amine oxidase A [151]. In middle-aged monkeys, daily curcumin treatment for 14–18 months improved only the spatial memory, suggesting the anti-aging effect of curcumin might be dependent upon the stage of aging [152].

3.3. Coenzyme Q10

Endogenous antioxidants exist in the body to maintain the redox balance. One of the most widely recognized endogenous antioxidants is coenzyme Q10, which is also available as a supplement. Gutierrez-Mariscal et al. observed the effects on oxidative stress in 20 subjects who consumed three random, same-calorie diets (the Mediterranean diet, the Mediterranean diet plus coenzyme Q10, and a diet rich in saturated fatty acids) for four weeks and found that the DNA-protective effects of the Mediterranean diet were enhanced by coenzyme Q10 [153]. The supplementation of aged mice with coenzyme Q10 was found to delay the decay of ovarian reserves and restore mitochondrial gene expression in oocytes, with associated functional improvements in the body [154]. Zhang et al. reported that coenzyme Q10 inhibits aging through the Akt/mTOR signaling pathway in D-galactose-treated mesenchymal stem cells [155]. Aging models in which hydrogen peroxide was added to human vascular endothelial cells have also reported that coenzyme Q10 has an aging delay effect by suppressing the expression of genes related to the secretory phenotype associated with aging, inhibiting intracellular ROS production, increasing nitric oxide (NO) production by increasing endothelial nitric oxide synthase (eNOS) expression, and promoting mitochondrial function [156].

4. Limitations of the Current Investigations

In the first chapter of this review, the various theories of aging that have been reported were presented. From the past to the present, many theories have tried to explain the aging process, but no single theory can fully explain it because the process is essentially a complex scenario characterized by changes occurring at different levels of the biological system. However, it is noteworthy that today's research in the field of aging has developed based on these theories of aging. Existing theories of aging would help to inspire new approaches to further the current understanding of the relationship between food and the aging process. In the future, theories of aging based on new discoveries and perspectives may well be proposed to elucidate the reality of diet and food components in aging.

In the second chapter, research conducted to investigate the impact of foodstuffs on life expectancy and mortality was introduced. Diet plays an important role in aging because the human body is composed of compounds found in the foods that are consumed every day. Considering the research reports presented in the second chapter, it seems that dietary patterns may have a significant impact on mortality. On the other hand, the evaluation of the physiological effects of foods composed of multiple molecules, unlike single molecules, seems to be difficult to explain with the current technology. Therefore, it is difficult to connect and discuss the findings of the cohort studies presented in this chapter with the individual theories of aging presented in the first chapter. However, in very recent years, with the development of AI technology, new methods of dietary assessment and physiological effects have begun to be established [157–159]. In addition, with the development of nanotechnology, the concept of "smart food," in which food is processed at the nanoscale to enhance its bioavailability and shelf life, will also lead to significant progress in aging research [160]. Considering these concepts, it will be even more important to elucidate the detailed role of food-derived antioxidants in the regulation of aging. Aging is affected not only by the kinds of food human ingests but also by the surrounding environment; for example, the natural environment, air, climate, soil, artificial environment, social environment, urban green spaces, economic background, social cohesion, socioeconomic status, and physical activity [161]. These complex factors and their relationship to food and aging are extensive and are beyond the scope of this review, but they need to be considered and evaluated.

In the third chapter, individual antioxidants in the human dietary resources and their effects on aging and related diseases (including lifespan extension) were summarized. Most of the previous research on food-derived antioxidants and lifespan has been based on the theory of oxidative damage, as introduced in the first chapter, and many reports have suggested that antioxidative activity is a major factor in promoting longevity. The various foods presented in the second section that may extend the lifespan seem to be rich in the individual antioxidants discussed in this chapter. The concentrations of food-derived antioxidants in the body are found to decrease with aging (Figure 3). Therefore, it may be a possibility that individual antioxidants might contribute to lifespan extension, but a clear cause-and-effect relationship has not yet been elucidated. Current methods for elucidating the relationship between individual antioxidants and aging, such as those described in this chapter, may yet have some details to be elucidated. Although the mechanisms of the effects of individual antioxidants on individual diseases, including Alzheimer's disease and lifestyle-related diseases, are becoming clearer, it seems that experimental models and evaluation methods to explain "aging" are currently insufficient. For example, the quantification of DNA repair capacity in humans regarding age-related genomic instability has not yet been established [162]. Proteostasis defects have been identified as a novel mechanism of aging but, to date, there is no effective technology for this purpose [163]. Stem cell depletion may also be an important marker of aging, but methods for its evaluation have not yet been established [164]. Telomeres, which are an important indicator of aging, have not yet been put to practical use in clinical practice because the current evaluation methods have problems with the accuracy of analysis, such as heterogeneity among cells and individuals [1]. As the technology for such evaluation methods develops, the concept of food-derived antioxidants and aging will become more visible. It will also be necessary to try to bring the two separate interpretations of "food" as a whole and "individual nutrients" closer together.

What is the biological meaning of oxidative stress in aging? Although various reports have shown that techniques for measuring age-related ROS are available, their relationship with aging is still unclear [165]. As mentioned in the concept of mitohormesis introduced at the beginning of the third chapter, moderate oxidative stress in the body may have the potential to improve the lifespan. Based on the concept of the oxidative damage theory of aging, it seems that higher amounts of antioxidants in food would benefit longevity, but this may not necessarily be the case. Gladyshev et al. stated that excess antioxidant supplementation disrupts the redox balance of the organism and there is a risk of accelerated aging [166]. Pérez et al. reported that transgenic mice that produced more antioxidant enzymes in their bodies did not live as long as normal mice [167]. Furthermore, when using catalase-deficient mice, Pérez-Estrada et al. reported that catalase contributes to lifespan extension by regulating the lipid metabolism in the liver without contributing to oxidative stress [168]. Van Raamsdonk et al. found that *C. elegans* (sod-12345) without SOD activity had a normal lifespan, although it was more sensitive to all stresses [169]. Furthermore, whether superoxide extends or shortens the lifespan depends on the genotype of the strain and the initial concentration of superoxide, which raises questions about the oxidative damage theory. In addition to the oxidative damage theory, it will be important to consider food antioxidants and aging on the basis of other aging theories. Throughout this review, we can report that there is definitely a promising future for diets that control aging, although more research needs to be performed to clarify the relationship between food antioxidants and aging.

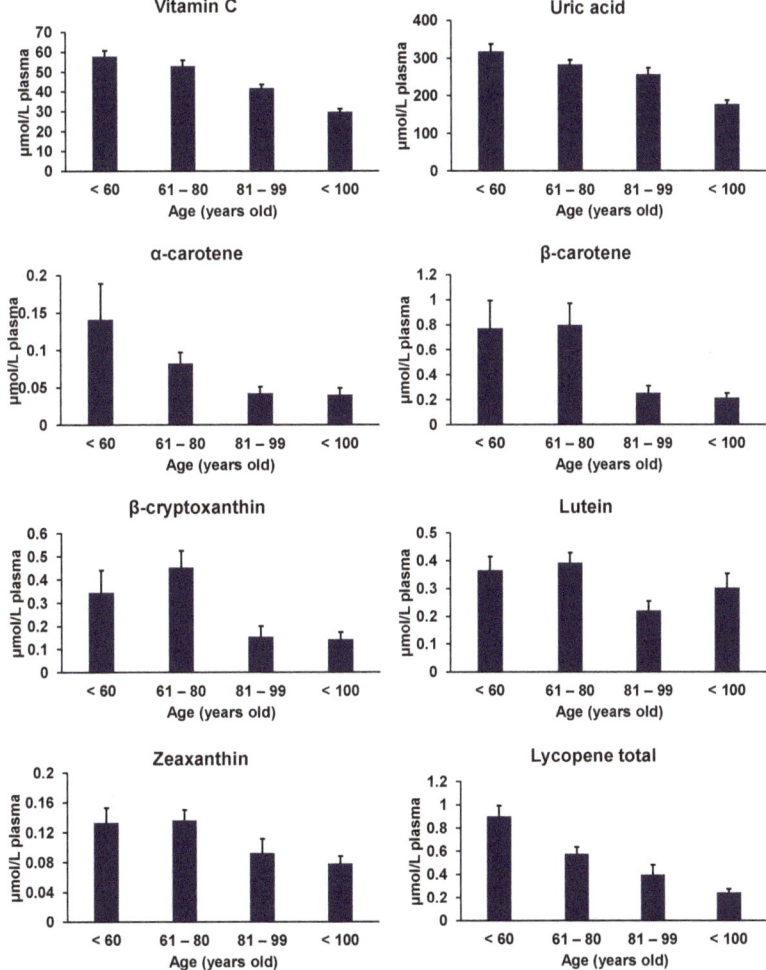

Figure 3. Age-related decline in the plasma concentrations of food antioxidants (vitamin C, uric acid, α-carotene, β-carotene, β-cryptoxanthin, lutein, zeaxanthin, and lycopene in total). (Figure modified from Miyazawa et al. [160]).

5. Conclusions and Outlook

Research on food antioxidants and aging has been widely based on the "oxidative damage theory" among the aging theories. Most of the previously reported cohort studies suggest that food antioxidant components may affect the lifespan; however, there is no direct evidence and the effect remains unclear. New technologies are expected to be developed in the future that can show that individual food antioxidants have the potential to extend the lifespan; moreover, the technology can evaluate the relationship between aging and the food as a whole, which is composed of various food antioxidants.

Author Contributions: Conceptualization, T.M. and C.A.; writing, review, and editing, T.M., C.A., G.C.B., A.M. and M.T.; supervision, T.M., A.M. and M.T. All authors have read and agreed to the published version of the manuscript.

Funding: This research received no external funding.

Institutional Review Board Statement: Not applicable.

Informed Consent Statement: Not applicable.

Data Availability Statement: Not applicable.

Conflicts of Interest: The authors declare no conflict of interest.

References

1. Colloca, G.; Di Capua, B.; Bellieni, A.; Fusco, D.; Ciciarello, F.; Tagliaferri, L.; Valentini, V.; Balducci, L. Biological and functional biomarkers of aging: Definition, characteristics, and how they can impact everyday cancer treatment. *Curr. Oncol. Rep.* **2020**, *22*, 115. [CrossRef]
2. Gladyshev, T.V.; Gladyshev, V.N. A disease or not a disease? Aging as a pathology. *Trends. Mol. Med.* **2016**, *22*, 995–996. [CrossRef] [PubMed]
3. López-Otín, C.; Blasco, M.A.; Partridge, L.; Serrano, M.; Kroemer, G. The hallmarks of aging. *Cell* **2013**, *153*, 1194–1217. [CrossRef]
4. Vina, J.; Borras, C.; Miquel, J. Theories of ageing. *IUBMB Life* **2007**, *59*, 249–254. [CrossRef] [PubMed]
5. Hayflick, L.; Moorhead, P.S. The serial cultivation of human diploid cell strains. *Exp. Cell Res.* **1961**, *25*, 585–621. [CrossRef]
6. Vidacek, N.S.; Nanic, L.; Ravlic, S.; Sopta, M.; Geric, M.; Gajski, G.; Garaj-Vrhovac, V.; Rubelj, I. Telomeres, Nutrition, and Longevity: Can We Really Navigate Our Aging? *J. Gerontol. A Biol. Sci. Med. Sci.* **2017**, *73*, 39–47. [CrossRef] [PubMed]
7. Ferron, S.R.; Marques-Torrejon, M.A.; Mira, H.; Flores, I.; Taylor, K.; Blasco, M.A.; Farinas, I. Telomere shortening in neural stem cells disrupts neuronal differentiation and neuritogenesis. *J. Neurosci.* **2009**, *29*, 14394–14407. [CrossRef]
8. Derevyanko, A.; Whittemore, K.; Schneider, R.P.; Jiménez, V.; Bosch, F.; Blasco, M.A. Gene therapy with the TRF1 telomere gene rescues decreased TRF1 levels with aging and prolongs mouse health span. *Aging Cell* **2017**, *16*, 1353–1368. [CrossRef] [PubMed]
9. de Jesus, B.B.; Vera, E.; Schneeberger, K.; Tejera, A.M.; Ayuso, E.; Bosch, F.; Blasco, M.A. Telomerase gene therapy in adult and old mice delays aging and increases longevity without increasing cancer. *EMBO Mol. Med.* **2012**, *4*, 691–704. [CrossRef] [PubMed]
10. Orgel, L.E. The maintenance of the accuracy of protein synthesis and its relevance to ageing. *Proc. Natl. Acad. Sci. USA* **1963**, *49*, 517–521. [CrossRef] [PubMed]
11. Troen, B.R. The biology of aging. *Mt. Sinai J. Med.* **2003**, *70*, 3–22. [PubMed]
12. Edelmann, P.; Gallant, J. On the translational error theory of aging. *Proc. Natl. Acad. Sci. USA* **1977**, *74*, 3396–3398. [CrossRef] [PubMed]
13. Weismann, A. *Essays Upon Heredity and Kindred Biological Problems*; Poulton, E.B., Selmar, S., Arthur, S.E., Eds.; Clarendon Press: Oxford, UK, 1889.
14. Hanson, R.W.; Hakimi, P. Born to run; the story of the PEPCK-Cmus mouse. *Biochimie* **2008**, *90*, 838–842. [CrossRef]
15. Van Raamsdonk, J.M.; Hekimi, S. Deletion of the mitochondrial superoxide dismutase sod-2 extends lifespan in Caenorhabditis elegans. *PLoS Genet.* **2009**, *5*, e1000361. [CrossRef] [PubMed]
16. Bjorksten, J. The Crosslinkage Theory of Aging. *Finska Kemists. Medd.* **1971**, *2*, 23–38. [CrossRef]
17. Monnier, V.M.; Mustata, G.T.; Biemel, K.L.; Reihl, O.; Lederer, M.O.; Dai, Y.; Sell, D.R. Cross-linking of the extracellular matrix by the maillard reaction in aging and diabetes: An update on "a puzzle nearing resolution". *Ann. N. Y. Acad. Sci.* **2005**, *1043*, 533–544. [CrossRef] [PubMed]
18. Bjorksten, J. *Theoretical Aspects of Aging*; Rockstein, M., Ed.; Academic Press: New York, NY, USA, 1974; p. 43.
19. Watad, A.; Bragazzi, N.L.; Adawi, M.; Amital, H.; Toubi, E.; Porat, B.-S.; Shoenfeld, Y. Autoimmunity in the elderly: Insights from basic science and clinics-a mini-review. *Gerontology* **2017**, *63*, 515–523. [CrossRef] [PubMed]
20. Ma, S.; Wang, C.; Mao, X.; Hao, Y. B cell dysfunction associated with aging and autoimmune diseases. *Front. Immunol.* **2019**, *10*, 318. [CrossRef]

21. Shanley, D.P.; Aw, D.; Manley, N.R.; Palmer, D.B. An evolutionary perspective on the mechanisms of immunosenescence. *Trends Immunol.* **2009**, *30*, 374–381. [CrossRef] [PubMed]
22. Cooper, G.S.; Stroehla, B.C. The epidemiology of autoimmune diseases. *Autoimmun. Rev.* **2003**, *2*, 119–125. [CrossRef]
23. Tessier, F.J. The Maillard reaction in the human body. The main discoveries and factors that affect glycationLa réaction de Maillard dans le corps humain. Découvertes majeures et facteurs qui affectent la glycation. *Pathol. Biol.* **2010**, *58*, 214–219. [CrossRef] [PubMed]
24. Simm, A. Protein glycation during aging and in cardiovascular disease. *J. Proteom.* **2013**, *92*, 248–259. [CrossRef] [PubMed]
25. Harman, D. Aging: A theory based on free radical and radiation chemistry. *J. Gerontol.* **1956**, *11*, 298–300. [CrossRef] [PubMed]
26. Stadtman, E.R. Protein oxidation and aging. *Science* **1992**, *257*, 1220–1224. [CrossRef]
27. Agarwal, S.; Sohal, R.S. DNA oxidative damage and life expectancy in houseflies. *Proc. Natl. Acad. Sci. USA* **1994**, *91*, 12332–12335. [CrossRef]
28. Miyazawa, T. Lipid hydroperoxides in nutrition, health, and diseases. *Proc. Jpn. Acad. Ser. B Phys. Biol. Sci.* **2021**, *97*, 161–196. [CrossRef]
29. Cadenas, E.; Davies, K.J. Mitochondrial free radical generation, oxidative stress, and aging. *Free Radic. Biol. Med.* **2000**, *29*, 222–230. [CrossRef]
30. Kulinsky, V.I. Biochemical aspects of inflammation. *Biochemistry* **2007**, *72*, 595–607. [CrossRef] [PubMed]
31. Franceschi, C.; Garagnani, P.; Parini, P.; Giuliani, C.; Santoro, A. Inflammaging: A new immune-metabolic viewpoint for age-related diseases. *Nat. Rev. Endocrinol.* **2018**, *14*, 576–590. [CrossRef]
32. Fulop, T.; Larbi, A.; Witkowski, J.M. Human Inflammaging. *Gerontology* **2019**, *65*, 495–504. [CrossRef] [PubMed]
33. Santoro, A.; Martucci, M.; Conte, M.; Capri, M.; Franceschi, C.; Salvioli, S. Inflammaging, hormesis and the rationale for anti-aging strategies. *Ageing Res. Rev.* **2020**, *64*, 101142. [CrossRef] [PubMed]
34. Laberge, R.M.; Awad, P.; Campisi, J.; Desprez, P.Y. Epithelial-mesenchymal transition induced by senescent fibroblasts. *Cancer Microenviron.* **2012**, *5*, 39–44. [CrossRef] [PubMed]
35. Gasek, N.S.; Kuchel, G.A.; Kirkland, J.L.; Xu, M. Strategies for targeting senescent cells in human disease. *Nat. Aging* **2021**, *1*, 870–879. [CrossRef]
36. Colchero, F.; Aburto, J.M.; Archie, E.A.; Boesch, C.; Breuer, T.; Campos, F.A.; Collins, A.; Conde, D.A.; Cords, M.; Crockford, C.; et al. The long lives of primates and the 'invariant rate of ageing' hypothesis. *Nat. Commun.* **2021**, *12*, 3666. [CrossRef] [PubMed]
37. Robert, J.H. Successful Aging. *Gerontologist* **1961**, *1*, 8–13.
38. Cumming, E.; Henry, W. Growing Old: The Process of Disengagement. Basic Books, New York, 1961. (Reprint: Arno, New York, 1979, ISBN 0405 118147). *Ageing Soc.* **1991**, *11*, 217–220.
39. Atchley, R.C. Activity theory. In *The Encyclopedia of Aging*, 2nd ed.; Maddox, G.L., Ed.; Springer: Berlin/Heidelberg, Germany, 1995; pp. 9–12.
40. Elder, G.H., Jr. Life Course and Human Development. In *Handbook of Child Psychology*; Damon, W., Ed.; Wiley: New York, NY, USA, 1998; pp. 939–991.
41. Cheval, B.; Sieber, S.; Guessous, I.; Orsholits, D.; Courvoisier, D.S.; Kliegel, M.; Stringhini, S.; Swinnen, S.P.; Burton-Jeangros, C.; Cullati, S.; et al. Effect of early-and adult-life socioeconomic circumstances on physical inactivity. *Med. Sci. Sports Exerc.* **2018**, *50*, 476–485. [CrossRef]
42. Selvamani, Y.; Arokiasamy, P. Association of life course socioeconomic status and adult height with cognitive functioning of older adults in India and China. *BMC Geriatr.* **2021**, *21*, 354. [CrossRef]
43. Atchley, R.C. Continuity Theory. In *The Encyclopedia of Aging*, 2nd ed.; Maddox, G.L., Ed.; Springer: Berlin/Heidelberg, Germany, 1995; pp. 227–230.
44. Dodig, S.; Cepelak, I.; Pavic, I. Hallmarks of senescence and aging. *Biochem. Med.* **2019**, *29*, 030501. [CrossRef] [PubMed]
45. Cheng, W.-H.; Bohr, V.A.; de Cabo, R. Nutrition and aging. *Mech. Ageing Dev.* **2010**, *131*, 223–224. [CrossRef] [PubMed]
46. Flatt, T.; Partridge, L. Horizons in the evolution of aging. *BMC Biol.* **2018**, *16*, 93. [CrossRef] [PubMed]
47. Trichopoulou, A.; Costacou, T.; Bamia, C.; Trichopoulos, D. Adherence to a Mediterranean diet and survival in a Greek population. *N. Engl. J. Med.* **2003**, *348*, 2599–2608. [PubMed]
48. Levitan, E.B.; Lewis, C.E.; Tinker, L.F.; Eaton, C.B.; Ahmed, A.; Manson, J.E.; Snetselaar, L.G.; Martin, L.W.; Trevisan, M.; Howard, B.V.; et al. Mediterranean and DASH diet scores and mortality in women with heart failure: The Women's Health Initiative. *Circ. Heart Fail.* **2013**, *6*, 1116–1123. [CrossRef] [PubMed]
49. Olsen, A.; Egeberg, R.; Halkjær, J.; Christensen, J.; Overvad, K.; Tjønneland, A. Healthy aspects of the Nordic diet are related to lower total mortality. *J. Nutr.* **2011**, *141*, 639–644. [CrossRef]
50. Roswall, N.; Sandin, S.; Lof, M.; Skeie, G.; Olsen, A.; Adami, H.O.; Weiderpass, E. Adherence to the Healthy Nordic Food Index and total and cause-specific mortality among Swedish women. *Eur. J. Epidemiol.* **2015**, *30*, 509–517. [CrossRef]
51. Abe, S.; Zhang, S.; Tomata, Y.; Tsuduki, T.; Sugawara, Y.; Tsuji, I. Japanese diet and survival time: The Ohsaki Cohort 1994 study. *Clin. Nutr.* **2020**, *39*, 298–303. [CrossRef] [PubMed]
52. Okada, E.; Nakamura, K.; Ukawa, S.; Wakai, K.; Date, C.; Iso, H.; Tamakoshi, A. The Japanese food score and risk of all-cause, CVD and cancer mortality: The Japan Collaborative Cohort Study. *Br. J. Nutr.* **2018**, *120*, 464–471. [CrossRef]

53. Bazzano, L.A.; He, J.; Ogden, L.G.; Loria, C.M.; Vupputuri, S.; Myers, L.; Whelton, P.K. Fruit and vegetable intake and risk of cardiovascular disease in US adults: The first National Health and Nutrition Examination Survey Epidemiologic Follow-up Study. *Am. J. Clin. Nutr.* **2002**, *76*, 93–99. [CrossRef]
54. Leenders, M.; Sluijs, I.; Ros, M.M.; Boshuizen, H.C.; Siersema, P.D.; Ferrari, P.; Weikert, C.; Tjønneland, A.; Olsen, A.; Boutron-Ruault, M.C.; et al. Fruit and vegetable consumption and mortality: European prospective investigation into cancer and nutrition. *Am. J. Epidemiol.* **2013**, *178*, 590–602. [CrossRef] [PubMed]
55. Stefler, D.; Pikhart, H.; Kubinova, R.; Pajak, A.; Stepaniak, U.; Malyutina, S.; Simonova, G.; Peasey, A.; Marmot, M.G.; Bobak, M. Fruit and vegetable consumption and mortality in Eastern Europe: Longitudinal results from the Health, Alcohol and Psychosocial Factors in Eastern Europe study. *Eur. J. Prev. Cardiol.* **2016**, *23*, 493–501. [CrossRef]
56. Zhang, X.; Shu, X.O.; Xiang, Y.B.; Yang, G.; Li, H.; Gao, J.; Cai, H.; Gao, Y.T.; Zheng, W. Cruciferous vegetable consumption is associated with a reduced risk of total and cardiovascular disease mortality. *Am. J. Clin. Nutr.* **2011**, *94*, 240–246. [CrossRef] [PubMed]
57. Saglimbene, V.M.; Wong, G.; Ruospo, P.; Palmer, S.C.; Garcia-Larsen, V.; Natale, P.; Teixeira-Pinto, A.; Campbell, K.L.; Carrero, J.-J.; Stenvinkel, P.; et al. Fruit and vegetable intake and mortality in adults undergoing maintenance hemodialysis. *Clin. J. Am. Soc. Nephrol.* **2019**, *14*, 250–260. [CrossRef] [PubMed]
58. Appleby, P.N.; Crowe, F.L.; Bradbury, K.E.; Travis, R.C.; Key, T.J. Mortality in vegetarians and comparable nonvegetarians in the United Kingdom. *Am. J. Clin. Nutr.* **2016**, *103*, 218–230. [CrossRef] [PubMed]
59. Imran, T.F.; Kim, E.; Buring, J.E.; Lee, I.M.; Gaziano, J.M.; Djousse, L. Nut consumption, risk of cardiovascular mortality, and potential mediating mechanisms: The Women's Health Study. *J. Clin. Lipidol.* **2021**, *15*, 266–274. [CrossRef] [PubMed]
60. Wang, W.; Yang, M.; Kenfield, S.A.; Hu, F.B.; Stampfer, M.J.; Willett, W.C.; Fuchs, C.S.; Giovannucci, E.L.; Bao, Y. Nut consumption and prostate cancer risk and mortality. *Br. J. Cancer* **2016**, *115*, 371–374. [CrossRef] [PubMed]
61. Bonaccio, M.; Castelnuovo, A.D.; Curtis, D.A.; Costanzo, S.; Bracone, F.; Persichillo, M.; Donati, M.B.; Gaetano, G.; Iacoviello, L. Nut consumption is inversely associated with both cancer and total mortality in a Mediterranean population: Prospective results from the Moli-sani study. *Br. J. Nutr.* **2015**, *114*, 804–811. [CrossRef] [PubMed]
62. Yamakawa, M.; Wada, K.; Koda, S.; Uji, T.; Nakashima, Y.; Onuma, S.; Oba, S.; Nagata, C. Associations of total nut and peanut intakes with all-cause and cause-specific mortality in a Japanese community: The Takayama study. *Br. J. Nutr.* **2022**, *127*, 1378–1385. [CrossRef] [PubMed]
63. Eslamparast, T.; Sharafkhah, M.; Poustchi, H.; Hashemian, M.; Dawsey, S.M.; Freedman, N.D.; Boffetta, P.; Abnet, C.C.; Etemadi, A.; Pourshams, A.; et al. Nut consumption and total and cause-specific mortality: Results from the Golestan Cohort Study. *Int. J. Epidemiol.* **2017**, *46*, 75–85. [CrossRef] [PubMed]
64. Luo, C.; Zhang, Y.; Ding, Y.; Shan, Z.; Chen, S.; Yu, M.; Hu, F.B.; Liu, L. Nut consumption and risk of type 2 diabetes, cardiovascular disease, and all-cause mortality: A systematic review and meta-analysis. *Am. J. Clin. Nutr.* **2014**, *100*, 256–269. [CrossRef] [PubMed]
65. Guasch-Ferre, M.; Bullo, M.; Martinez-Gonzalez, M.A.; Ros, E.; Corella, D.; Estruch, R.; Fito, M.; Aros, F.; Warnberg, J.; Fiol, M.; et al. Frequency of nut consumption and mortality risk in the PREDIMED nutrition intervention trial. *BMC Med.* **2013**, *11*, 164. [CrossRef] [PubMed]
66. Wang, C.; Gu, K.; Wang, K.; Cai, H.; Zheng, W.; Bao, P.; Shu, X.-O. Nut consumption in association with overall mortality and recurrence/disease-specific mortality among long-term breast cancer survivors. *Int. J. Cancer* **2022**, *150*, 572–579. [CrossRef]
67. Abe, S.K.; Saito, E.; Sawada, N.; Tsugane, S.; Ito, H.; Lin, Y.; Tamakoshi, A.; Sado, J.; Kitamura, Y.; Sugawara, Y.; et al. Green tea consumption and mortality in Japanese men and women: A pooled analysis of eight population-based cohort studies in Japan. *Eur. J. Epidemiol.* **2019**, *34*, 917–926. [CrossRef] [PubMed]
68. Unno, K.; Nakamura, Y. Green tea suppresses brain aging. *Molecules* **2021**, *26*, 4897. [CrossRef] [PubMed]
69. Hao, Z.; Liu, Y.; Li, Y.; Song, W.; Yu, J.; Li, H.; Wang, W. Association between longevity and element levels in food and drinking water of typical Chinese longevity area. *J. Nutr. Health Aging* **2016**, *20*, 897–903. [CrossRef]
70. Wang, X.; Chen, H.; Ouyang, Y.; Liu, J.; Zhao, G.; Bao, W.; Yan, M. Dietary calcium intake and mortality risk from cardiovascular disease and all causes: A meta-analysis of prospective cohort studies. *BMC Med.* **2014**, *12*, 158. [CrossRef] [PubMed]
71. Navarro, A.M.; Martinez-Gonzalez, M.A.; Gea, A.; Grosso, G.; Martín-Moreno, J.M.; Lopez-Garcia, E.; Martin-Calvo, N.; Toledo, E. Coffee consumption and total mortality in a Mediterranean prospective cohort. *Am. J. Clin. Nutr.* **2018**, *108*, 1113–1120. [CrossRef]
72. Shadyab, A.H.; Manson, J.E.; Luo, J.; Haring, B.; Saquib, N.; Snetselaar, L.G.; Chen, J.C.; Groessl, E.J.; Wassertheil-Smoller, S.; Sun, Y.; et al. Associations of coffee and tea consumption with survival to age 90 years among older women. *J. Am. Geriatr. Soc.* **2020**, *68*, 1970–1978. [CrossRef] [PubMed]
73. Takata, Y.; Shu, X.O.; Gao, Y.T.; Li, H.; Zhang, X.; Gao, J.; Cai, H.; Yang, G.; Xiang, Y.B.; Zheng, W. Red meat and poultry intakes and risk of total and cause-specific mortality: Results from cohort studies of Chinese adults in Shanghai. *PLoS ONE* **2013**, *8*, e56963.
74. Lv, Y.; Kraus, V.B.; Gao, X.; Yin, Z.; Zhou, J.; Mao, C.; Duan, J.; Zeng, Y.; Brasher, M.S.; Shi, W.; et al. Higher dietary diversity scores and protein-rich food consumption were associated with lower risk of all-cause mortality in the oldest old. *Clin. Nutr.* **2020**, *39*, 2246–2254. [CrossRef]

75. Stefler, D.; Brett, D.; Sarkadi-Nagy, E.; Kopczynska, E.; Detchev, S.; Bati, A.; Scrob, M.; Koenker, D.; Aleksov, B.; Douarin, E.; et al. Traditional Eastern European diet and mortality: Prospective evidence from the HAPIEE study. *Eur. J. Nutr.* **2021**, *60*, 1091–1100. [CrossRef]
76. Schnabel, L.; Kesse-Guyot, E.; Alles, B.; Touvier, M.; Srour, B.; Hercberg, S.; Buscail, C.; Julia, C. Association between ultraprocessed food consumption and risk of mortality among middle-aged adults in France. *JAMA Intern. Med.* **2019**, *179*, 490–498. [CrossRef]
77. Bonaccio, M.; Di Castelnuovo, A.; Costanzo, S.; De Curtis, A.; Persichillo, M.; Sofi, F.; Cerletti, C.; Donati, M.B.; de Gaetano, G.; Iacoviello, L. Ultra-processed food consumption is associated with increased risk of all-cause and cardiovascular mortality in the Moli-sani Study. *Am. J. Clin. Nutr.* **2021**, *113*, 446–455. [CrossRef] [PubMed]
78. Blanco-Rojo, R.; Sandoval-Insausti, H.; Lopez-Garcia, E.; Graciani, A.; Ordovas, J.M.; Banegas, J.R.; Rodriguez-Artalejo, F.; Guallar-Castillon, P. Consumption of ultra-processed foods and mortality: A national prospective cohort in Spain. *Mayo Clin. Proc.* **2019**, *94*, 2178–2188. [CrossRef] [PubMed]
79. Sun, Y.; Liu, B.; Snetselaar, L.G.; Robinson, J.G.; Wallace, R.B.; Peterson, L.L.; Bao, W. Association of fried food consumption with all cause, cardiovascular, and cancer mortality: Prospective cohort study. *BMJ* **2019**, *364*, k5420. [CrossRef] [PubMed]
80. Veronese, N.; Stubbs, B.; Noale, M.; Solmi, M.; Vaona, A.; Demurtas, J.; Nicetto, D.; Crepaldi, G.; Schofield, P.; Koyanagi, A.; et al. Fried potato consumption is associated with elevated mortality: An 8-y longitudinal cohort study. *Am. J. Clin. Nutr.* **2017**, *106*, 162–167. [CrossRef]
81. Trichopoulou, A.; Martínez-González, M.A.; Tong, T.Y.N.; Forouhi, N.G.; Khandelwal, S.; Prabhakaran, D.; Mozaffarian, D.; de Lorgeril, M. Definitions and potential health benefits of the Mediterranean diet: Views from experts around the world. *BMC Med.* **2014**, *12*, 112. [CrossRef]
82. Crous-Bou, M.; Fung, T.T.; Prescott, J.; Julin, B.; Du, M.; Sun, Q.; Rexrode, K.M.; Hu, F.B.; De Vivo, I. Mediterranean diet and telomere length in Nurses' Health Study: Population based cohort study. *BMJ* **2014**, *349*, g6674. [CrossRef] [PubMed]
83. Sasaki, S. What is the scientific definition of the Japanese diet from the viewpoint of nutrition and health? *Nutr. Rev.* **2020**, *78*, 18–26. [CrossRef]
84. Colman, R.J.; Anderson, R.M.; Johnson, S.C.; Kastman, E.K.; Kosmatka, K.J.; Beasley, T.M.; Allison, D.B.; Cruzen, C.; Simmons, H.A.; Kemnitz, J.W.; et al. Caloric restriction delays disease onset and mortality in rhesus monkeys. *Science* **2009**, *325*, 201–204. [CrossRef] [PubMed]
85. Fontana, L.; Partridge, L. Promoting health and longevity through diet: From model organisms to humans. *Cell* **2015**, *161*, 106–118. [CrossRef] [PubMed]
86. Gourd, E. Ultra-processed foods might increase cancer risk. *Lancet Oncol.* **2018**, *19*, e186. [CrossRef]
87. Monteiro, C.A.; Cannon, G.; Lawrence, M.; Costa Louzada, M.D.; Pereira Machado, P. *Ultra-Processed Foods, Diet Quality, and Health Using the NOVA Classification System*; FAO: Rome, Italy, 2019.
88. Monteiro, C.A.; Cannon, G.; Levy, R.; Moubarac, J.-C.; Jaime, P.; Martins, A.P.; Canella, D.; Louzada, M.; Parra, D. NOVA. The star shines bright. *World Nutr.* **2016**, *7*, 28–38.
89. Fiolet, T.; Srour, B.; Sellem, L.; Kesse-Guyot, E.; Alles, B.; Mejean, C.; Deschasaux, M.; Fassier, P.; Latino-Martel, P.; Beslay, M.; et al. Consumption of ultra-processed foods and cancer risk: Results from NutriNet-Sante prospective cohort. *BMJ* **2018**, *360*, k322. [CrossRef]
90. da Costa, J.P.; Vitorino, R.; Silva, G.M.; Vogel, C.; Duarte, A.C.; Rocha-Santos, T. A synopsis on aging-Theories, mechanisms and future prospects. *Ageing Res. Rev.* **2016**, *29*, 90–112. [CrossRef]
91. Jalel, A.; Soumaya, G.S.; Hamdaoui, M.H. Vitiligo treatment with vitamins, minerals and polyphenol supplementation. *Indian J. Dermatol.* **2009**, *54*, 357–360. [CrossRef] [PubMed]
92. Kim, J.; Jeong, I.H.; Kim, C.S.; Lee, Y.M.; Kim, J.M.; Kim, J.S. Chlorogenic acid inhibits the formation of advanced glycation end products and associated protein cross-linking. *Arch. Pharm. Res.* **2011**, *34*, 495–500. [CrossRef]
93. Najjar, F.M.; Taghavi, F.; Ghadari, R.; Sheibani, N.; Moosavi-Movahedi, A.A. Destructive effect of non-enzymatic glycation on catalase and remediation via curcumin. *Arch. Biochem. Biophys.* **2017**, *630*, 81–90. [CrossRef]
94. Matsumaru, D.; Motohashi, H. The KEAP1-NRF2 system in healthy aging and longevity. *Antioxidants* **2021**, *10*, 1929. [CrossRef] [PubMed]
95. Tapia, P.C. Sublethal mitochondrial stress with an attendant stoichiometric augmentation of reactive oxygen species may precipitate many of the beneficial alterations in cellular physiology produced by caloric restriction, intermittent fasting, exercise and dietary phytonutrients: "Mitohormesis" for health and vitality. *Med. Hypotheses* **2006**, *66*, 832–843. [PubMed]
96. Miyazawa, T.; Burdeos, G.C.; Itaya, M.; Nakagawa, K.; Miyazawa, T. Vitamin E: Regulatory redox interactions. *IUBMB Life* **2019**, *71*, 430–441. [CrossRef] [PubMed]
97. Ristow, M.; Schmeisser, K. Mitohormesis: Promoting health and lifespan by increased levels of reactive oxygen species (ROS). *Dose Response* **2014**, *12*, 288–341. [CrossRef] [PubMed]
98. Santos, M.A.; Franco, F.N.; Caldeira, C.A.; de Araujo, G.R.; Vieira, A.; Chaves, M.M.; Lara, R.C. Antioxidant effect of resveratrol: Change in MAPK cell signaling pathway during the aging process. *Arch. Gerontol. Geriatr.* **2021**, *92*, 104266. [CrossRef] [PubMed]
99. Chen, H.; Dong, L.; Chen, X.; Ding, C.; Hao, M.; Peng, X.; Zhang, Y.; Zhu, H.; Liu, W. Anti-aging effect of phlorizin on D-galactose-induced aging in mice through antioxidant and anti-inflammatory activity, prevention of apoptosis, and regulation of the gut microbiota. *Exp. Gerontol.* **2022**, *163*, 111769. [CrossRef] [PubMed]

100. Tian, Y.; Wen, Z.; Lei, L.; Li, F.; Zhao, J.; Zhi, Q.; Li, F.; Yin, R.; Ming, J. Coreopsis tinctoria flowers extract ameliorates D-galactose induced aging in mice via regulation of Sirt1-Nrf2 signaling pathway. *J. Funct. Foods.* **2019**, *60*, 103464. [CrossRef]
101. Wang, L.; Lee, W.; Cui, Y.R.; Ahn, G.; Jeon, Y.-J. Protective effect of green tea catechin against urban fine dust particle-induced skin aging by regulation of NF-κB, AP-1, and MAPKs signaling pathways. *Environ. Pollut.* **2019**, *252*, 1318–1324. [CrossRef]
102. Wang, Y.; Xiong, Y.; Zhang, A.; Zhao, N.; Zhang, J.; Zhao, D.; Yu, Z.; Xu, N.; Yin, Y.; Luan, X.; et al. Oligosaccharide attenuates aging-related liver dysfunction by activating Nrf2 antioxidant signaling. *Food Sci. Nutr.* **2020**, *8*, 3872–3881. [CrossRef]
103. Maleki, M.; Khelghati, N.; Alemi, F.; Bazdar, M.; Asemi, Z.; Majidinia, M.; Sadeghpoor, A.; Mahmoodpoor, A.; Jadidi-Niaragh, F.; Targhazeh, N.; et al. Stabilization of telomere by the antioxidant property of polyphenols: Anti-aging potential. *Life Sci.* **2020**, *259*, 118341. [CrossRef] [PubMed]
104. Luo, J.; Si, H.; Jia, Z.; Liu, D. Dietary anti-aging polyphenols and potential mechanisms. *Antioxidants* **2021**, *10*, 283. [CrossRef]
105. Ozawa, H.; Miyazawa, T.; Miyazawa, T. Effects of dietary food components on cognitive functions in older adults. *Nutrients* **2021**, *13*, 2804. [CrossRef] [PubMed]
106. Lorenzon dos Santos, J.; Schaan de Quadros, A.; Weschenfelder, C.; Bueno Garofallo, S.; Marcadenti, A. Oxidative stress biomarkers, nut-related antioxidants, and cardiovascular disease. *Nutrients* **2020**, *12*, 682. [CrossRef] [PubMed]
107. The Dictionary by Merriam-Webster. Available online: https://www.merriam-webster.com/dictionary/vitamin (accessed on 27 January 2022).
108. Cambridge Dictionary. Available online: https://dictionary.cambridge.org/dictionary/english/vitamin (accessed on 27 January 2022).
109. Meyers, D.G.; Maloley, P.A.; Weeks, D. Safety of Antioxidant Vitamins. *Arch. Intern. Med.* **1996**, *156*, 925–935. [CrossRef] [PubMed]
110. Abe, C.; Higuchi, O.; Matsumoto, A.; Miyazawa, T. Determination of intracellular ascorbic acid using tandem mass spectrometry. *Analyst* **2022**, *147*, 2640–2643. [CrossRef] [PubMed]
111. Miyazawa, T.; Matsumoto, A.; Miyahara, Y. Determination of cellular vitamin C dynamics by HPLC-DAD. *Analyst* **2019**, *144*, 3483–3487. [CrossRef] [PubMed]
112. Lykkesfeldt, J.; Tveden-Nyborg, P. The pharmacokinetics of vitamin C. *Nutrients* **2019**, *11*, 2412. [CrossRef]
113. Lewis, L.N.; Hayhoe, R.P.G.; Mulligan, A.A.; Luben, R.N.; Khaw, K.T.; Welch, A.A. Lower dietary and circulating vitamin C in middle-and older-aged men and women are associated with lower estimated skeletal muscle mass. *J. Nutr.* **2020**, *150*, 2789–2798. [CrossRef]
114. Qu, Y.N.; Zhang, L.; Wang, T.; Zhang, H.Y.; Yang, Z.J.; Yuan, F.F.; Wang, Y.; Li, S.W.; Jiang, X.X.; Xie, X.H. Vitamin C Treatment rescues prelamin A-induced premature senescence of subchondral bone mesenchymal stem cells. *Stem Cells Int.* **2020**, *2020*, 3150716. [CrossRef]
115. Aumailley, L.; Warren, A.; Garand, C.; Dubois, M.J.; Paquet, E.R.; Le Couteur, D.G.; Marette, A.; Cogger, V.C.; Lebel, M. Vitamin C modulates the metabolic and cytokine profiles, alleviates hepatic endoplasmic reticulum stress, and increases the life span of Gulo−/− mice. *Aging* **2016**, *8*, 458–483. [CrossRef]
116. Dixit, S.; Bernardo, A.; Walker, J.M.; Kennard, J.A.; Kim, G.Y.; Kessler, E.S.; Harrison, F.E. Vitamin C deficiency in the brain impairs cognition, increases amyloid accumulation and deposition, and oxidative stress in APP/PSEN1 and normally-aging mice. *ACS Chem. Neurosci.* **2015**, *6*, 570–581. [CrossRef]
117. Kaźmierczak-Barańska, J.; Boguszewska, K.; Adamus-Grabicka, A.; Karwowski, B.T. Two faces of vitamin C—Antioxidative and pro-oxidative agent. *Nutrients* **2020**, *12*, 1501. [CrossRef]
118. Azzi, A. Tocopherols, tocotrienols and tocomonoenols: Many similar molecules but only one vitamin E. *Redox. Biol.* **2019**, *26*, 101259. [CrossRef]
119. Lai, G.Y.; Weinstein, S.J.; Taylor, P.R.; McGlynn, K.A.; Virtamo, J.; Gail, M.H.; Albanes, D.; Freedman, N.D. Effects of alpha-tocopherol and beta-carotene supplementation on liver cancer incidence and chronic liver disease mortality in the ATBC study. *Br. J. Cancer* **2014**, *111*, 2220–2223. [CrossRef]
120. Huang, J.; Weinstein, S.J.; Yu, K.; Mannisto, S.; Albanes, D. Relationship between serum alpha-tocopherol and overall and cause-specific mortality: A 30-year prospective cohort analysis. *Circ. Res.* **2019**, *125*, 29–40. [CrossRef] [PubMed]
121. Mangialasche, F.; Xu, W.; Kivipelto, M.; Costanzi, E.; Ercolani, S.; Pigliautile, M.; Cecchetti, R.; Baglioni, M.; Simmons, A.; Soininen, H.; et al. Tocopherols and tocotrienols plasma levels are associated with cognitive impairment. *Neurobiol. Aging* **2012**, *33*, 2282–2290. [CrossRef]
122. Guan, J.Z.; Guan, W.P.; Maeda, T.; Makino, N. Effect of vitamin E administration on the elevated oxygen stress and the telomeric and subtelomeric status in Alzheimer's disease. *Gerontology* **2012**, *58*, 62–69. [CrossRef] [PubMed]
123. Tucker, L.A. Alpha-and gamma-tocopherol and telomere length in 5768 US men and women: A NHANES study. *Nutrients* **2017**, *9*, 601. [CrossRef]
124. Hanson, C.; Lyden, E.; Furtado, J.; Campos, H.; Sparrow, D.; Vokonas, P.; Litonjua, A.A. Serum tocopherol levels and vitamin E intake are associated with lung function in the normative aging study. *Clin. Nutr.* **2016**, *35*, 169–174. [CrossRef]
125. Boccardi, V.; Arosio, B.; Cari, L.; Bastiani, P.; Scamosci, M.; Casati, M.; Ferri, E.; Bertagnoli, L.; Ciccone, S.; Rossi, P.D.; et al. Beta-carotene, telomerase activity and Alzheimer's disease in old age subjects. *Eur. J. Nutr.* **2020**, *59*, 119–126. [CrossRef]
126. Huang, J.; Weinstein, S.J.; Yu, K.; Mannisto, S.; Albanes, D. Serum beta carotene and overall and cause-specific mortality: A prospective cohort study. *Circ. Res.* **2018**, *123*, 1339–1349. [CrossRef]
127. Min, K.B.; Min, J.Y. Association between leukocyte telomere length and serum carotenoid in US adults. *Eur. J. Nutr.* **2017**, *56*, 1045–1052. [CrossRef]

128. Yazaki, K.; Yoshikoshi, C.; Oshiro, S.; Yanase, S. Supplemental cellular protection by a carotenoid extends lifespan via Ins/IGF-1 signaling in Caenorhabditis elegans. *Oxid. Med. Cell Longev.* **2011**, *2011*, 596240. [CrossRef]
129. Wu, W.; Wang, X.; Xiang, Q.; Meng, X.; Peng, Y.; Du, N.; Liu, Z.; Sun, Q.; Wang, C.; Liu, X. Astaxanthin alleviates brain aging in rats by attenuating oxidative stress and increasing BDNF levels. *Food Funct.* **2014**, *5*, 158–166. [CrossRef] [PubMed]
130. El-Far, A.H.; Lebda, M.A.; Noreldin, A.E.; Atta, M.S.; Elewa, Y.H.A.; Elfeky, M.; Mousa, S.A. Quercetin attenuates pancreatic and renal D-galactose-induced aging-related oxidative alterations in rats. *Int. J. Mol. Sci.* **2020**, *21*, 4348. [CrossRef]
131. Wang, H.; Jo, Y.-J.; Oh, J.S.; Kim, N.-H. Quercetin delays postovulatory aging of mouse oocytes by regulating SIRT expression and MPF activity. *Oncotarget* **2017**, *8*, 38631–38641. [CrossRef]
132. Geng, L.; Liu, Z.; Zhang, W.; Li, W.; Wu, Z.; Wang, W.; Ren, R.; Su, Y.; Wang, P.; Sun, L.; et al. Chemical screen identifies a geroprotective role of quercetin in premature aging. *Protein Cell* **2019**, *10*, 417–435. [CrossRef] [PubMed]
133. Li, J.; Zhao, R.; Zhao, H.; Chen, G.; Jiang, Y.; Lyu, X.; Wu, T. Reduction of aging-induced oxidative stress and activation of autophagy by bilberry anthocyanin supplementation via the AMPK-mTOR signaling pathway in aged female rats. *J. Agric. Food Chem.* **2019**, *67*, 7832–7843. [CrossRef]
134. Miyazawa, T.; Nakagawa, K.; Kudo, M.; Muraishi, K.; Someya, K. Direct intestinal absorption of red fruit anthocyanins, cyanidin-3-glucoside and cyanidin-3,5-diglucoside, into rats and humans. *J. Agric. Food Chem.* **1999**, *47*, 1083–1091. [CrossRef]
135. de Ferrars, R.M.; Czank, C.; Zhang, Q.; Botting, N.P.; Kroon, P.A.; Cassidy, A.; Kay, C.D. The pharmacokinetics of anthocyanins and their metabolites in humans. *Br. J. Pharmacol.* **2014**, *171*, 3268–3282. [CrossRef]
136. Alonso, A.; Gonzalez-Pardo, H.; Garrido, P.; Conejo, N.M.; Llaneza, P.; Diaz, F.; Rey, C.G.D.; Gonzalez, C. Acute effects of 17 β-estradiol and genistein on insulin sensitivity and spatial memory in aged ovariectomized female rats. *Age* **2010**, *32*, 421–434. [CrossRef]
137. Li, Y.; Ren, X.; Lio, C.; Sun, W.; Lai, K.; Liu, Y.; Zhang, Z.; Liang, J.; Zhou, H.; Liu, L.; et al. A chlorogenic acid-phospholipid complex ameliorates post-myocardial infarction inflammatory response mediated by mitochondrial reactive oxygen species in SAMP8 mice. *Pharmacol. Res.* **2018**, *130*, 110–122. [CrossRef]
138. Gines, C.; Cuesta, S.; Kireev, R.; Garcia, C.; Rancan, L.; Paredes, S.D.; Vara, E.; Tresguerres, J.A.F. Protective effect of resveratrol against inflammation, oxidative stress and apoptosis in pancreas of aged SAMP8 mice. *Exp. Gerontol.* **2017**, *90*, 61–70. [CrossRef]
139. Porquet, D.; Casadesus, G.; Bayod, S.; Vicente, A.; Canudas, A.M.; Vilaplana, J.; Pelegri, C.; Sanfeliu, C.; Camins, A.; Pallas, M.; et al. Dietary resveratrol prevents Alzheimer's markers and increases life span in SAMP8. *Age* **2013**, *35*, 1851–1865. [CrossRef]
140. Navarro-Cruz, A.R.; Ramirez, Y.; Ayala, R.; Ochoa-Velasco, C.; Brambila, E.; Avila-Sosa, R.; Perez-Fernandez, S.; Morales-Medina, J.C.; Aguilar-Alonso, P. Effect of chronic administration of resveratrol on cognitive performance during aging process in rats. *Oxid. Med. Cell Longev.* **2017**, *2017*, 8510761. [CrossRef] [PubMed]
141. Caldeira, C.A.; Santos, M.A.; Araujo, G.R.; Lara, R.C.; Franco, F.N.; Chaves, M.M. Resveratrol: Change of SIRT 1 and AMPK signaling pattern during the aging process. *Exp. Gerontol.* **2021**, *146*, 111226. [CrossRef]
142. Semba, R.D.; Ferrucci, L.; Bartali, B.; Urpi-Sarda, M.; Zamora-Ros, R.; Sun, K.; Cherubini, A.; Bandinelli, S.; Andres-Lacueva, C. Resveratrol levels and all-cause mortality in older community-dwelling adults. *JAMA Intern. Med.* **2014**, *174*, 1077–1084. [CrossRef] [PubMed]
143. Gliemann, L.; Nyberg, M.; Hellsten, Y. Effects of exercise training and resveratrol on vascular health in aging. *Free Radic. Biol. Med.* **2016**, *98*, 165–176. [CrossRef]
144. Shen, L.R.; Xiao, F.; Yuan, P.; Chen, Y.; Gao, Q.K.; Parnell, L.D.; Meydani, M.; Ordovas, J.M.; Li, D.; Lai, C.Q. Curcumin-supplemented diets increase superoxide dismutase activity and mean lifespan in Drosophila. *Age* **2013**, *35*, 1133–1142. [CrossRef]
145. Miyazawa, T.; Nakagawa, K.; Kim, S.H.; Thomas, M.J.; Paul, L.; Zingg, J.-M.; Dolnikowski, G.G.; Roberts, S.B.; Kimura, F.; Miyazawa, T.; et al. Curcumin and piperine supplementation of obese mice under caloric restriction modulates body fat and interleukin-1β. *Nutr. Metab.* **2018**, *15*, 12. [CrossRef]
146. Shailaja, M.; Gowda, K.M.D.; Vishakh, K.; Kumari, N.S. Anti-aging role of curcumin by modulating the inflammatory markers in albino wistar rats. *J. Natl. Med. Assoc.* **2017**, *109*, 9–13. [CrossRef]
147. Sun, Y.; Hu, X.; Hu, G.; Xu, C.; Jiang, H. Curcumin attenuates hydrogen peroxide-induced premature senescence via the activation of SIRT1 in human umbilical vein endothelial cells. *Biol. Pharm. Bull.* **2015**, *38*, 1134–1141. [CrossRef]
148. Hasani, A.S.; Hamid, N.; Amin, A.M.; Fatemeh, E.; Allahbakhshian, F.M.; Ghaffari, N.M. The antioxidant curcumin postpones ovarian aging in young and middle-aged mice. *Reprod. Fertil. Dev.* **2020**, *32*, 292–303.
149. Hagl, S.; Kocher, A.; Schiborr, C.; Kolesova, N.; Frank, J.; Eckert, G.P. Curcumin micelles improve mitochondrial function in neuronal PC12 cells and brains of NMRI mice—Impact on bioavailability. *Neurochem. Int.* **2015**, *89*, 234–242. [CrossRef] [PubMed]
150. Sarker, M.R.; Franks, S.; Sumien, N.; Thangthaeng, N.; Filipetto, F.; Forster, M. Curcumin mimics the neurocognitive and anti-inflammatory effects of caloric restriction in a mouse model of midlife obesity. *PLoS ONE* **2015**, *10*, e0140431. [CrossRef] [PubMed]
151. Rahman, M.A.; Shuvo, A.A.; Bepari, A.K.; Hasan, A.M.; Shill, M.C.; Hossain, M.; Uddin, M.; Islam, M.R.; Bakshi, M.K.; Hasan, J.; et al. Curcumin improves D-galactose and normal-aging associated memory impairment in mice: In vivo and in silico-based studies. *PLoS ONE* **2022**, *17*, e0270123. [CrossRef] [PubMed]

152. Moore, T.L.; Bowley, B.; Shultz, P.; Calderazzo, S.; Shobin, E.; Killiany, R.J.; Rosene, D.L.; Moss, M.B. Chronic curcumin treatment improves spatial working memory but not recognition memory in middle-aged rhesus monkeys. *Geroscience* **2017**, *39*, 571–584. [CrossRef]
153. Gutierrez-Mariscal, F.M.; Perez-Martinez, P.; Delgado-Lista, J.; Yubero-Serrano, E.M.; Camargo, A.; Delgado-Casado, N.; Cruz-Teno, C.; Santos-Gonzalez, M.; Rodriguez-Cantalejo, F.; Castano, J.P.; et al. Mediterranean diet supplemented with coenzyme Q10 induces postprandial changes in p53 in response to oxidative DNA damage in elderly subjects. *Age* **2012**, *34*, 389–403. [CrossRef]
154. Ben-Meir, A.; Burstein, E.; Borrego-Alvarez, A.; Chong, J.; Wong, E.; Yavorska, T.; Naranian, T.; Chi, M.; Wang, Y.; Bentov, Y.; et al. Coenzyme Q10 restores oocyte mitochondrial function and fertility during reproductive aging. *Aging Cell* **2015**, *14*, 887–895. [CrossRef]
155. Zhang, D.; Yan, B.; Yu, S.; Zhang, C.; Wang, B.; Wang, Y.; Wang, J.; Yuan, Z.; Zhang, L.; Pan, J. Coenzyme Q10 inhibits the aging of mesenchymal stem cells induced by D-galactose through Akt/mTOR signaling. *Oxid. Med. Cell Longev.* **2015**, *2015*, 867293. [CrossRef]
156. Huo, J.; Xu, Z.; Hosoe, K.; Kubo, H.; Miyahara, H.; Dai, J.; Mori, M.; Sawashita, J.; Higuchi, K. Coenzyme Q10 prevents senescence and dysfunction caused by oxidative stress in vascular endothelial cells. *Oxid. Med. Cell Longev.* **2018**, *2018*, 3181759. [CrossRef]
157. Miyazawa, T.; Hiratsuka, Y.; Toda, M.; Hatakeyama, N.; Ozawa, H.; Abe, C.; Cheng, T.Y.; Matsushima, Y.; Miyawaki, Y.; Ashida, K.; et al. Artificial intelligence in food science and nutrition: A narrative review. *Nutr. Rev.* **2022**, nuac033, *epub ahead of print*. [CrossRef]
158. Mezgec, S.; Seljak, B.K. NutriNet: A deep learning food and drink image recognition system for dietary assessment. *Nutrients* **2017**, *9*, 657. [CrossRef] [PubMed]
159. Lemay, D.G.; Baldiviez, L.M.; Chin, E.L.; Spearman, S.S.; Cervantes, E.; Woodhouse, L.R.; Keim, N.L.; Stephensen, C.B.; Laugero, K.D. Technician-scored stool consistency spans the full range of the bristol scale in a healthy US population and differs by diet and chronic stress load. *J. Nutr.* **2021**, *151*, 1443–1452. [CrossRef] [PubMed]
160. Miyazawa, T.; Itaya, M.; Burdeos, G.C.; Nakagawa, K.; Miyazawa, T. A critical review of the use of surfactant-coated nanoparticles in nanomedicine and food nanotechnology. *Int. J. Nanomed.* **2021**, *16*, 3937–3999. [CrossRef] [PubMed]
161. Plagg, B.; Zerbe, S. How does the environment affect human ageing? An interdisciplinary review. *J. Gerontol. Geriatr.* **2020**, *61*, 53–67. [CrossRef]
162. Trzeciak, A.R.; Barnes, J.; Ejiogu, N.; Foster, K.; Brant, L.J.; Zonderman, A.B.; Evans, M.K. Age, sex, and race influence single-strand break repair capacity in a human population. *Free Radic. Biol. Med.* **2008**, *45*, 1631–1641. [CrossRef]
163. Cuervo, A.M.; Macian, F. Autophagy and the immune function in aging. *Curr. Opin. Immunol.* **2014**, *29*, 97–104. [CrossRef]
164. Rando, T.A.; Chang, H.Y. Aging, rejuvenation, and epigenetic reprogramming: Resetting the aging clock. *Cell* **2012**, *148*, 46–57. [CrossRef] [PubMed]
165. Dikalov, S.I.; Harrison, D.G. Methods for detection of mitochondrial and cellular reactive oxygen species. *Antioxid. Redox Signal.* **2014**, *20*, 372–382. [CrossRef]
166. Gladyshev, V.N. The free radical theory of aging is dead. Long live the damage theory! *Antioxid. Redox Signal.* **2014**, *20*, 727–731. [CrossRef]
167. Perez, V.I.; Van Remmen, H.; Bokov, A.; Epstein, C.J.; Vijg, J.; Richardson, A. The overexpression of major antioxidant enzymes does not extend the lifespan of mice. *Aging Cell* **2009**, *8*, 73–75. [CrossRef]
168. Perez-Estrada, J.R.; Hernandez-Garcia, D.; Leyva-Castro, F.; Ramos-Leon, J.; Cuevas-Benítez, O.; Diaz-Munoz, M.; Castro-Obregon, S.; Ramirez-Solis, R.; Garcia, C.; Covarrubias, L. Reduced lifespan of mice lacking catalase correlates with altered lipid metabolism without oxidative damage or premature aging. *Free Radic. Biol. Med.* **2019**, *135*, 102–115. [CrossRef]
169. Van Raamsdonk, J.M.; Hekimi, S. Superoxide dismutase is dispensable for normal animal lifespan. *Proc. Natl. Acad. Sci. USA* **2012**, *109*, 5785–5790. [CrossRef] [PubMed]

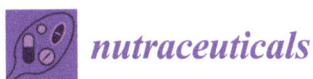

Review

Goji Berry: Health Promoting Properties

Prodromos Skenderidis *, Stefanos Leontopoulos and Dimitrios Lampakis

Laboratory of Food and Biosystems Engineering, Department of Agrotechnology, University of Thessaly, 41110 Larissa, Greece; sleontopoulos@uth.gr (S.L.); dlampakis@uth.gr (D.L.)
* Correspondence: pskenderidis@uth.gr; Tel.: +30-697-331-3565

Abstract: Since ancient times, it has been noticed that Goji berry fruit juice, roots and leaves consist of ingredients that contain a wide variety of bioactive substances. The consumption of goji berry fruits results in properties which improve the subjective feeling of general well-being. The aim of this work is to present the information from the existing literature on the possible role of goji berry plant parts and their extracts as a functional food. *Lycium barbarum* Polysaccharides (LBP) and polyphenols are the most researched aspects of fruits associated with the promotion of human health. Goji berry fruits demonstrated anti-oxidative properties that are associated with age-related diseases such as diabetes, atherosclerosis and antitumor and immunoregulatory activities. Bioactive secondary metabolites contained in fruit lead to positive effects for human vision, while other biochemicals contained in the root bark have shown hepatoprotective and inhibitory actions on the rennin/angiotensin system. The results presented so far in the literature verify their use in traditional medicine.

Keywords: goji berry; functional foods; antioxidant; health; antibacterial; health promotion

Citation: Skenderidis, P.; Leontopoulos, S.; Lampakis, D. Goji Berry: Health Promoting Properties. *Nutraceuticals* **2022**, *2*, 32–48. https://doi.org/10.3390/nutraceuticals2010003

Academic Editors: Ivan Cruz-Chamorro and Mario Allegra

Received: 8 February 2022
Accepted: 9 March 2022
Published: 14 March 2022

Publisher's Note: MDPI stays neutral with regard to jurisdictional claims in published maps and institutional affiliations.

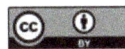

Copyright: © 2022 by the authors. Licensee MDPI, Basel, Switzerland. This article is an open access article distributed under the terms and conditions of the Creative Commons Attribution (CC BY) license (https://creativecommons.org/licenses/by/4.0/).

1. Introduction

Modern life-styles and dietary habits are the main cause of several human modern diseases such as diabetes, hepatitis and cardiovascular issues [1–3]. About 1/5 of the known plant species [4] that have participated in pharmaceutical studies cover a wide range of beneficial effects on human health, animal welfare and crop protection by enhancing human health against free radical damage [5–13]. The high concentrations of phytochemicals found in plants are accumulated mainly in their fruits and vegetables. Among beneficial phytochemicals, antioxidant compounds including phenolics, anthocyanins, carotenoids, and tocopherols may be used as a supplement for the human body by acting as natural antioxidants [14]. Thus, the consumption of fruit and vegetables has been linked with several health benefits, as a result of medicinal properties and high nutritional value [15] and is recommended by many scientists throughout the world [16]. In more detail, many studies mention the antioxidant and pharmacological activities of different plant extracts [17–20].

Among important plant species with significant biomedical issues is the Goji berry where fruit juice, roots and leaves contain ingredients that have a variety of bioactive properties [21–24].

The objective of this paper is to provide a review of phytochemical studies that have addressed the beneficial effects for human health of bioactive compounds contained in Goji berries.

Search Strategy

An electronic literature search was conducted using PubMed, Medline (OvidSP), and Google Scholar for the period between 1992 to 2022. Additional articles were identified from references in the retrieved articles. Search terms included combinations of the following: "goji berry", "*Lycium barbarum*", "health promoting effects", "phytochemical", "antioxidant", "*Lycium barbarum* polysaccharides" and "pharmacological". The search was restricted to articles in English that addressed the phytochemical constituents and pharmacological properties of goji berries.

2. Bioactivities

2.1. Antioxidant Activity

The most studied molecular mechanism of the oxidation of cellular components is that of lipid peroxidation. This is a circular feedback chain process, which, if started and not suspended in time, can oxidize all the biological material. DNA can tolerate a large number of different oxidative lesions, depending on the factors that cause them. Unlike oxidized proteins, which are usually fragmented and their amino acids reused, the oxidized DNA can be repaired in situ. Insufficient DNA repair can result in mutation and, ultimately, cell death by either necrosis or apoptosis.

The amino acids cysteine, methionine, tyrosine, phenylalanine, tryptophan and histidine are more susceptible to oxidative modifications. Relatively recent research results in this field commented on the fact that oxidative modifications of amino acid residues in proteins, besides the negative effects, may also play a positive role by participating in the redox signaling process.

Goji berries have been shown to possess antioxidant properties, neutralizing the oxidative action of free radicals and activating antioxidant mechanisms (Figure 1), such as an increase in superoxide dismutase (SOD), glutathione (GSH), glutathione peroxidase (GPx), catalase (CAT), and erythroid-derived 2-like 2 (Nrf2) expression of several antioxidant and cytoprotective enzymes [25]. Thus, *L. barbarum* extracts exhibited the binding of peroxide anion radicals and the subsequent reduction of their activity [26].

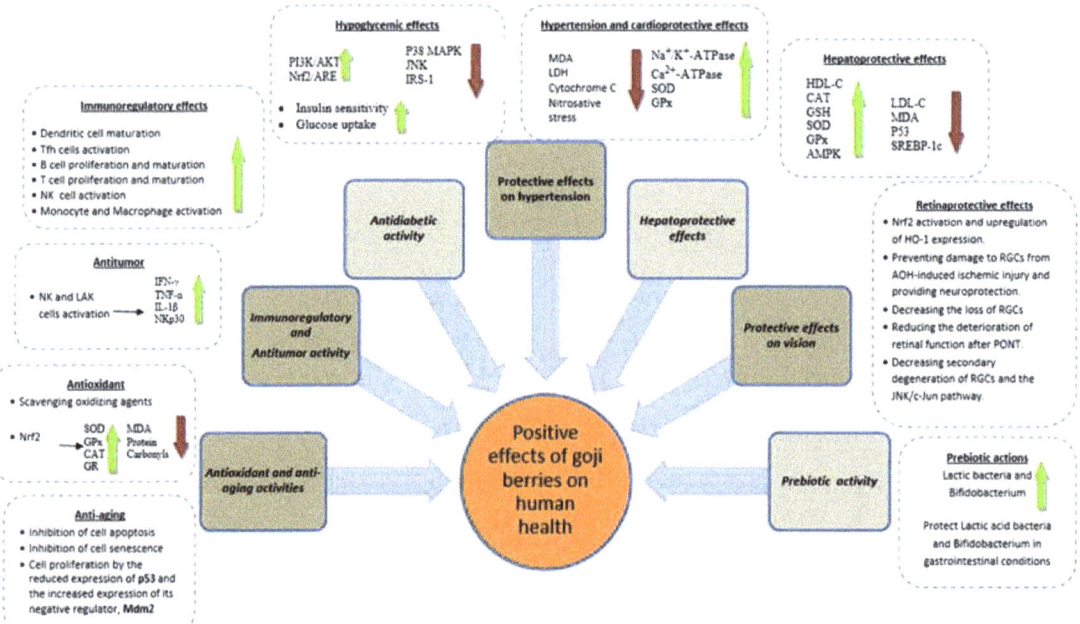

Figure 1. Health-promoting properties of goji berry fruits and extracts.

The protective effect on the inhibition of lipid peroxidation by goji berry extracts is probably due to the polyphenols of goji berry fruit (Figure 2) [27]. Caffeic acid, which is the main hydroxycinnamic acid in goji berries, not only has potent antioxidant effects but also has anti-inflammatory and anti-cancer effects, while recent studies have shown that caffeic acid in its free form or conjugated to other groups, such as quinic acid and sugars, has a protective effect against Alzheimer's disease [28].

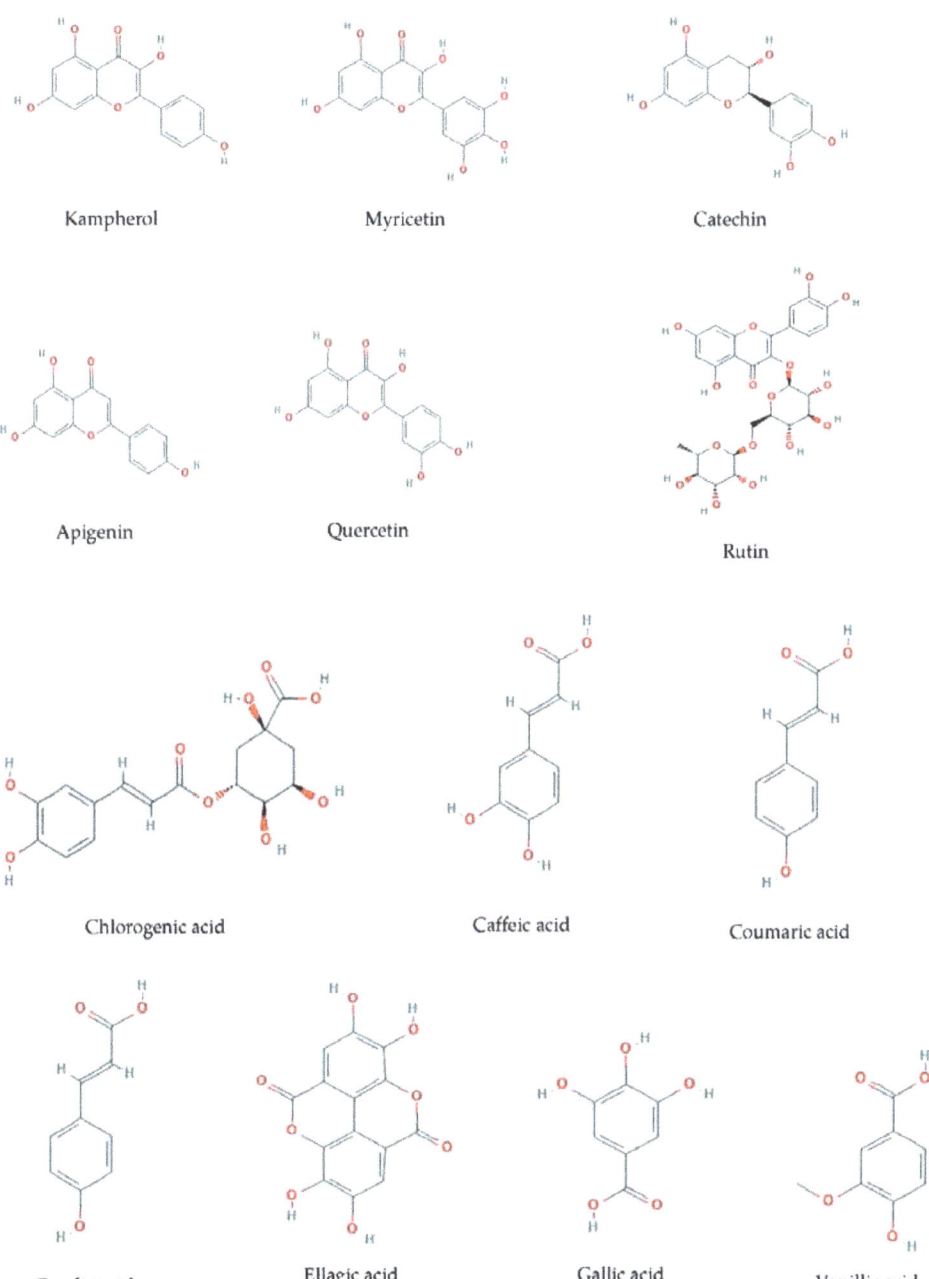

Figure 2. The chemical structure of the polyphenols contained in "Goji berries".

Moreover, ethanol extract (70% w/v) of *L. chinense* protects hepatic cells against oxidative stress-induced cell damage by removing intracellular ROS, SOD recovery, CAT and glutathione action, reducing lipid oxidation, DNA destruction and protein carbonyl values [29]. Further, Changbo et al. [30] have shown that the administration of LBP in mice can reduce the oxidative stress caused after exercise in swimming, increasing the antioxidant enzymes SOD, CAT and GPx.

An important ingredient that contributes to the antioxidant activity of fruits is also AA-2βG, which has similar antioxidant properties to vitamin C. Studies focusing on its effects showed that it exhibits strong binding activity against DPPH and H_2O_2 and inhibits H_2O_2-mediated hemolysis better than vitamin C. Studies have also demonstrated similar effects in the binding of OH radicals. Although the in vitro antioxidant capacity has shown that AA-2βG presented lower activity compared to vitamin C; on the contrary, in vivo studies demonstrated that AA-2βG protected mice liver from carbon tetrachloride-induced acute liver injury better than vitamin C [31].

Furthermore, several studies have identified the protective mechanisms of the biochemical action of goji berries in relation to the induction of the Nrf2 nuclear factor [25,32]. A recent study, suggested that goji berry aqueous extracts exhibit antimutagenic activity, protecting DNA against peroxyl and hydroxyl radicals [33]. In the context of the same study, substantial antioxidant activity of goji berry aqueous extracts in C_2C_{12} muscle cells was also observed, indicated by increased glutathione (GSH) levels up to 189.5% and a decrease of protein carbonyls and lipid peroxidation by 29.1% and 21.8%, respectively [33].

2.2. Antiaging Activity

Aging is defined as the accumulation of various deleterious changes in cells and tissues [34], especially for elderly people [35].

Several studies have shown that genetic and environmental factors regulate specific pathways involved in hormone signaling, nutritional signaling and the detection of mitochondrial and ROS signaling and genomic survival. It is a common belief that the accumulation of the effects of oxidative stress contributes to the aging process [36–38]. For this reason, many of the experimental aging models use the pouring of D-galactose into mouse or rat tissues for a period of 6–8 weeks as a toxin in order to produce free radicals [39]. According to Deng et al. [40], the addition on a daily basis of 100 mg LBP/kg to the diet of mice reduced serum advanced glycation end products (AGE), retrieving the memory pointer back to experimental animals, increasing superoxide dismutase levels in erythrocytes and finally helping them to restore kinetic activity.

The life cycle of *Drosophila melanogaster* (fruit-fly) has been used as an alternative model for aging studies. Based on this model, the addition of 16 mg LBP/kg shows a statistically significant increase of the average life span of male insects [41].

Furthermore, studies conducted on elderly mice have shown that the consumption of 200–500 mg/kg of LBP promotes oxidative stress reduction, as it reduces the oxidative stress markers associated with the aging process [42]. It has also been reported that LBP activates the antioxidative pathways Nrf2/ARE and Nrf2/HO-1 by activating antioxidants and detoxifying enzymes. One of these enzymes is heme oxygenase-1 (HO-1), which is regulated by the factor associated with the nuclear factor erythroid 2–related factor 2 (Nrf2) [43].

In vivo studies on Factor Nrf2 have shown that it plays an important role in the endogenous antioxidant system by regulating the expression of important antioxidant enzymes, such as oxygenase-1 (HO-1), SOD and CAT. In particular, in oxidative stress or exogenous (pharmacological) activation, Nrf2 moves into the cell nucleus and induces the expression of antioxidant enzymes by blocking the antioxidant response (ARE) [44]. It has also been commented that activation of PI3K/AKT/Nrf2 not only prevents the development of oxidative stress but also prevents metabolic glucose abnormalities such as the occurrence of insulin resistance. Activation of Nrf2 by LBP offers a new alternative therapeutic approach to the prevention of insulin resistance caused by a long-term high-fat diet [45].

The effect of ultraviolet radiation (UVB) causes skin damage by inducing oxidative and inflammatory lesions and thus causes aging and carcinogenicity of the skin. The protective effect of LBPs through the induction of Nrf2 is likely to exert a protective effect against the negative effect of ultraviolet radiation on the skin by binding to the active radicals and reducing DNA damage, resulting in the suppression of the ultraviolet-induced P38 MAP pathway. Based on the previous beneficial effects, LBP could potentially be used as an ingredient in products intended to protect the skin against oxidative damage from environmental conditions [32].

A recent study investigating retinal protection from damage caused by I/R radiation showed that activation of the Nrf2/HO-1 antioxidant pathway was adapted to neutralize damage to the retina. The use of LBP not only reduced the production of ROS but also enhanced the activation of the Nrf2/HO-1 antioxidant pathway in retinas under the influence of I/R [46].

All of the previous studies support that LBP has positive anti-aging effects, while a clinical study indicates that dietary intake of a total of 500 mg of L. barbarum over 10 days can significantly reduce plasma triglyceride levels and increase levels of cyclic adenosine monophosphate (cAMP) and SOD [47].

As the anti-aging effects of L. barbarum display a wide range of target tissues, it is believed that it can overall protect cells from oxidative, hyperglycemic and hyperlipidemic conditions. According to the results of a previous clinical study conducted in alloxan-treated rabbits, the LBP group reduced the blood glucose levels [48].

In addition to polysaccharides, the presence of components in fruits, such as carotenes, betaine, polyphenols and vitamin C in the precursor form of 2-O-β-D-glucopyranosyl-L- ascorbic acid, contributes to antioxidant and anti-aging properties of the goji berry fruit. Thus, betaine has been shown to have a protective effect against skin aging by ultraviolet radiation by mouse-assisted research. Betaine's protective effect is mediated by inhibition of the extracellular kinase signal transducer (ERP), protein kinase (MEK) and metalloproteinase 9 (MMP-9), resulting in a reduction in collagen wrinkles and damage caused by UVB [49].

Finally, the regulation of the operation of a basic organ, such as the liver or kidneys, results in the regulation of other organs or even of the entire body, according to the traditional Chinese medicine theory. Based on this theory, in traditional Chinese medicine, the use and consumption of L. barbarum fruits is recommended for the treatment of aging-related diseases due to the appearance of a wide range of positive effects, reducing all risk factors in aging-related diseases.

2.3. Antitumor and Immunoregulatory Activity

The defensive mechanisms of vertebrates are also known as the immune system. The immune system recognizes and destroys foreign invaders and toxic substances by a process known as an immune response. The molecule that causes the immune response is called an antigen. In addition, these mechanisms are involved in the body's effort to remove aged or damaged cells, as well as destroying cancer cells, while sometimes they cause damage against the tissues of the organism itself.

The two main groups of cells in the immune system are the cells of the medullary line and the lymphocytes. Lymphocytes include B-lymphocytes and T-lymphocytes as well as a large granular cell, NK (or natural killer cells). The medullary cells consist of monocytes/macrophages, dendritic cells, neutrophils, eosinophils and basophils. B lymphocytes have an antibody molecule in their membrane, whereas T lymphocytes have an antigen-binding receptor in their membrane. When a B cell encounters an antigen, it quickly divides and differentiates into a B-cell memory and a B-cell effector or plasmid cell. Plasmocytes produce a large number of antibodies (antibody, Ab) or immunoglobulin (immunoglobulin, Ig) that act on the antigen and destroy it. T-lymphocytes, when they meet an antigen or tumor, secrete cytokines (growth factors), directly killing the infected target cell (CD8 killer T cells) and also activating B-cells to make antibody responses and macrophages to destroy microorganisms that either invaded the macrophage or were ingested by it (CD4 helper T cell). There are two types of immunity—humoral and cellular. Humoral immunity is mediated by antibodies produced by B cells and is the main defensive mechanism against extracellular microbes and their toxins, with secreted antibodies binding to them by inducing their elimination. Cellular immunity is mediated by T cells, with dendritic cells playing an important role against antigens.

A clinical study completed by Cao et al. [50] examined the effect of a combination of lymphokine-activated killer (LAK)/IL-2 and LBP on advanced cancer patients (79 patients). The results of this study showed that the response rate and duration of mean tumor regression of patients treated with LAK/IL-2 plus LBPs was higher than those of patients receiving only LAK/IL-2. LAK/IL-2 plus LBP therapy resulted in a more pronounced increase in NK and LAK activity than LAK/IL-2 alone. Furthermore, a study carried out by Gan et al. [51] showed that the administration of LBP3p polysaccharide enhanced the immune system in S180-bearing mice by increasing spleen lymphocyte proliferation and cytotoxic T-lymphocyte activity (CTL).

However, results published by Zhang et al. [52] showed that LBP therapy inhibited growth of hepatoma cell line QGY7703, phase S, phase interruption and induction of apoptosis, as well as a simultaneous increase in the amount of cellular RNA and Ca^{2+} concentration in human tissues.

Clinical studies demonstrated the immunomodulatory effects of standardized *L. barbarum* (GoChi) fruit juice on elderly healthy people in China. The results showed that the GoChi group differed, statistically increasing the number of lymphocytes and levels of interleukin-2 and immunoglobulin G. This study concludes that daily consumption of GoChi significantly increases several immune responses and subjective feelings of general well-being without any undesirable effects [21,22].

Follicular helper CD4 T helper cells (Tfh) are the specialized help providers in B lymphocytes since they are necessary for their maintenance and for differentiation into plasmocytes and memory B cells. For this reason, the correlation of Tfh with the production of antibodies from B lymphocytes was studied. Su et al. [53] investigated whether LBP upregulated expression in such molecules on Tfh cells. BALB/c mice were administered 5 mg/kg, 25 mg/kg and 50 mg/kg LBP daily for 7 days, and the enhancement of the humoral immune response by the activation of Tfh cells using LBP was confirmed by the increase of the expression of numerous molecules, including CXCR5 and PD-1 surface markers. Furthermore, Yang et al. [54] showed in their study that LBPs can enhance the immune system against antigenic infection by enhancing phagocytosis in RAW264.7 phagocytes.

He et al. [55], by observing intracellular ROS production and DNA damage, reported a stimulation effect of LBB on the apoptosis of MCF-7 human breast carcinoma cells and the inhibition of the cell cycle in the G0/G1 phase.

Moreover, Huang et al. [56] investigated the mechanisms of LBP suppressive action against breast cancer in MCF-7 cells in vitro. The results of their study showed that LBP therapy can inhibit the proliferation of MCF-7 cells with insulin-like growth factor 1 (IGF-1) in a dose- and time-dependent manner to suppress phosphatidylinositol 3-kinase activity (PI3 K) and phosphorylated-PI3 K (p-PL3 K) inhibit protein-1 (HIF-1) accumulation caused by hypoxia and suppress the expression of vascular endothelial growth factor (VEGF) mRNA and protein production. These results indicated that LBPs could inhibit tumor cell growth by suppressing IGF-1-induced angiogenesis via the PI3 K/HIF-1/VEGF signaling pathways. In a recent study completed by Deng et al. [57] it was presented that LBP3 polysaccharide could reduce immune toxicity and enhance the antitumor activity of doxorubicin in mice. The results of the aforementioned study showed that LBP3 did not offer protection against body weight loss caused by dox, but it promoted the recovery of body weight starting 5 days after dox treatment in tumor-free mice. Furthermore, LBP3 was found to promote cell cycle recovery in bone marrow cells, improve peripheral blood lymphocyte counts, and restored the cytotoxicity of natural killer cells. Moreover, the antitumor activity of dox, peripheral blood and lymphocyte counts has been improved.

Apart from polysaccharides, phytochemical compounds mentioned previously contribute to the anti-aging activity exerting a protective effect against cancer cells. For example, betaine has been shown to have an inhibitory effect on colorectal cancer because of its anti-inflammatory action. Kim et al. [58] showed that adding betaine to a mouse diet could achieve a reduction of the incidence of colitis associated with cancer by reducing the levels of ROS and its ratio with oxidized glutathione (GSSG), related to the inflammation of cytokines such as IL-6, IL-1β and IL-22 and protein levels of COX-2 and iNOS with azoxymethane-induced colitis. In addition, Hsu et al. [22] demonstrated that the inhibition of colonic HT29 cancer cells from a mixture of nanoparticle and carotenoid extracts from *L. barbarum* was activated by increasing expression of P53 and P21, reducing the expression of CDK1, CDK2, cyclin A and cyclin B arresting cell cycle at G2/M.

The antitumor activity of goji berry extracts (primarily LBP-based studies) is mainly due to their ability to induce the disruption of cell cycle apoptosis and the inhibition of some important signaling pathways that act as carcinogenic protective agents by eliminating cancerous cells.

2.4. Antidiabetic Activity

The number of patients with diabetes worldwide has quadrupled over the last 30 years, and it is the ninth leading cause of death. One in 11 adults today has type II diabetes, accounting for 90% of diabetes cases, and the prediction is that by 2050, one in three will suffer from diabetes. The majority of people suffering from diabetes are aged between 45 and 64.

Sugar, a common constituent of diet, is also a major factor often responsible for elevating the glucose level in diabetic patients [59]. Diabetes mellitus is a metabolic disease characterized by an increase in blood sugar (hyperglycemia) and a metabolic disorder of glucose ($C_6H_{12}O_6$), either as a result of decreased insulin secretion or due to a decrease in the sensitivity of cells to insulin. Insulin is a hormone produced in the pancreas that forces the liver and muscle cells to absorb blood glucose and store it as glycogen for future body energy needs. In case the insulin concentration in the body is low or zero and glucose absorption cannot take place, the body begins to use fat as a source of energy by transporting lipids from adipose tissue to the liver [60]. Nowadays, there are known various types of diabetes. The main diabetes types are type I and type II. In general, diabetes is associated with the risk of serious health complications, including myocardial infarction, stroke, kidney failure, vision loss and premature death. So required care for diabetics is likely to be needed for many years [61].

The effect of the antidiabetic action of goji berry extracts has been investigated in various studies. Goji berries may have a positive effect on blood glucose control, as documented in relevant studies described in a study published by Silva et al. [62]. Furthermore, in a study completed by Wu et al. [63] feeding of type 2 diabetic mice with goji berry extract for 4 weeks showed a decrease in blood glucose levels by 35%. Moreover, Zhang et al. [64] suggested that the fraction LBPF4-OL of the LBP promotes lymphocyte proliferation secreting TNF-α and IL-1β. Luo et al. [48] also showed that *L. barbarum* extracts have hypoglycemic and hypolipidemic effects as well as strong antioxidant activity in rabbits with diabetes and hyperlipidemia from aloxane.

One of the causative factors for insulin resistance development is oxidative stress. Oxidative stress is one of the factors that can activate the JNK pathway under the diabetes condition. Recent research presented that under an oxidative status, the nuclear factor Nrf2 plays a role in insulin-mediated glucose uptake [33]. The positive effects on insulin resistance from Nrf2 activation caused from the enhancement of insulin sensitivity due to the decrease of ROS production are presented in a study completed by Bagul et al. [65]. Nakatani et al. [66] showed also that activation of c-jun N-terminal kinase (JNK) leads to a decrease of insulin sensibility due to the increase of IRS-1 serine phosphorylation insulin target tissues, while insulin resistance status was improved in the JNK-KO of mice. Furthermore, studies done by Kaneto [67] commented that the activation of p38 mitogen-activated protein kinase (MAPK) and JNK signaling can directly or indirectly promote diabetes. It has been reported that the JNK pathway plays a crucial role in the progression of insulin resistance [68].

Another positive finding regarding the use of LBP was reported by Yang et al. [69]. According to the authors, there is a link between oxidative stress, Nrf2 activity and insulin resistance. According to the above-mentioned study, in vivo and in vitro studies demonstrated that high-fat induced-insulin resistance could be ameliorated by LBP by the upregulation of the PI3K/AKT/Nrf2 signaling pathway. Due to this reaction, it was suggested that LBP may have a promising role in managing insulin resistance-associated oxidative stress in acute or chronic liver damage. Furthermore, Cai et al. [70] studied 67 patients in vivo for three months and found protective effects against the two types of hypoglycemia, lowering the glucose levels in the blood and increasing insulin. Finally, Zhao et al. [71] researched the prophylactic effects of LBP using 25 Japanese male diabetic rabbits induced by Alloxan. Results of this study showed improvement in renal function and inflammation in diabetic rabbits. However, the effect was more effective in preventing disease rather than treating it.

2.5. Hypertension and Heart Protective Effects

Hypertension is today one of the major public health problems due to its high incidence, its importance in cardiovascular disease and its correlation with a large number of health problems leading to death. Nearly one in two adults (about 103 million people) suffer from hypertension in the United States only [72]. Hypertension is influenced by factors such as genetics, lack of exercise and dietary intake of sodium, which is one of the most common causes of hypertension. It has been reported that the dietary sodium intake has been correlated with blood pressure, confirming the sensitivity of blood pressure to salt [73].

Regarding LBP's protective positive effects on myocardial I/R damage Shao Ping and Pin-Ting [74] used in their study of Wistar adult male rats. In their study, it was presented that LBPs protected rat hearts from I/R injury via upregulation of heart Na^+/K^+-ATPase and inhibition of cardiomyocyte apoptosis concluding the cardioprotective effect of LBP stems caused by their antioxidant, anti-inflammatory and anti-apoptotic activities.

Prophylactic activity of LBP against cardiotoxic side effects of doxorubicin (DOX), which is a potent antitumor agent, has been also demonstrated in acute DOX-induced cardiotoxicity in rats [75,76] and beagle dogs [77]. Data of previous studies indicated that *L. barbarum* fruits and extracts may exert a potent protective effect on DOX-induced cardiomyocyte damage, mainly via antioxidative and free radical-scavenging pathways. Zhang et al. [78] in their study, related the anti-hypertensive effect of *L. barbarum* to down regulated expression of renal endothelial lncRNAs ONE in a rat model of salt-sensitive hypertension. In conclusion, their study commented that *L. barbarum* treatment can restore blood pressure to normal levels. At the same time, the expression of long noncoding RNA (lncRNA) was found to be reduced by the suppression of the antisense mRNA (sONE). Moreover, the improvement of endothelial nitric oxide synthase (eNOS) levels in the hypertensive model rats treated with *L. barbarum* compared with that receiving a high-salt diet was also observed. In addition, Guo et al. [79], using a meta-analysis of randomized controlled trials, presented that *L. barbarum* treatment significantly reduced fasting glucose concentrations while marginally reducing concentrations of total cholesterol and yielded no benefit in terms of bodyweight and blood pressure.

2.6. Hepatoprotective Activity

Alcohol use is the third leading risk factor contributing to the global burden of disease, after high blood pressure and tobacco smoking. According to a WHO report published in September 2018, alcohol causes 3 million annual deaths globally and accounts for 5.3% of all deaths. Despite the three above mentioned factors affecting liver Demori and Voci [80] commented that modern eating habits involving high-calorie diets that lead to obesity also can cause liver diseases such as hepatic steatosis. Chronic alcohol overdrinking (CAO) typically progresses through the stages of fatty liver or simple steatosis, alcoholic hepatitis and chronic hepatitis with hepatic fibrosis or cirrhosis [81].

The use of *L. barbarum* was originally proposed in traditional Chinese medicine for the treatment of liver diseases. Nowadays, studies done by Xiao et al. [82] have proved that feeding alcohol-induced liver injury rats with 300 mg/kg LBP for 30 days showed positive reverse effects, reducing liver injury, preventing the progression of alcohol-induced fatty liver and improving antioxidant function, in contrast with the ethanol group.

Pretreatment with 50 µg/mL LBP of rat normal hepatocyte line BRL-3A cells has shown a significant reduction of 24-hour ethanol-induced over expression of thioredoxin-interacting protein (TXNIP) increasing cellular apoptosis. Xiao et al. [83] also observed an activation of NOD-like receptor 3 (NLRP3) inflammasome and reduction of the antioxidant enzyme expression and ROS. Non-alcoholic fatty liver disease is an important factor in causing hepatocarcinoma and is associated with obesity, insulin resistance and metabolic syndrome. As mentioned previously, obesity leads to a decrease in insulin sensitivity (IR), a decrease in the antioxidant enzymes SOD, CAT and GSH-Px but also an increase in ROS, leading to liver dysfunction, hepatic steatosis and depletion of the hepatocyte population [80,84,85].

Cui et al. [27] examined the effects of *L. barbarum* aqueous (LBAE) and ethanol (LBEE) extracts on oxidative stress and antioxidant enzymes in the liver of rats fed with a high-fat diet (HFD). They concluded that LBAE and especially LBEE have strong antioxidant activities and can prevent or reduce the effects of HFD on several parameters of toxicity in HF rats. LBEE displayed stronger antioxidant and hepatoprotective effects than the aqueous extract of *L. barbarum*, a fact that probably has to do with the higher concentration of polyphenolic content that led to higher antioxidant activity and lipid peroxidation inhibition.

Protection against hepatotoxic effects of CCl4 has been documented by Kim et al. [86] using two cerebrosides isolated from *L. chinense* fruits (1-O-β-D-glucopyranosyl- (2S, 3R, 4E, 8Z)-2-N-palmitoyloctadecasphinga-4,8-dienine and 1-D-glucopyranosyl-(2S, 3R, 4E, 8Z)-2-N-(2′-hydroxypalmitoyl) octadecasphinga-4,8-dienine) in the culture of rat hepatocytes. Xiao et al. [87] also tested the effects of LBP on oxidative stress and liver necrosis of mice. Both studies showed significant sub-protective action, while in the second, it was shown that LBP reduced hepatic necrosis and alanine aminotransferase (ALT) levels in serum caused by CCl4, indicating that the beneficial effect on hepatotoxicity ought partly to reduce the activity of the kappa-B nuclear factor. Additionally, the use of LBP reduced hepatic inflammation by reducing pro-inflammatory mediators and chemokines.

2.7. Eye and Vision Activity

Zeaxanthin and lutein are two common carotenoids found in plants and are constituents of the yellow macular pigment in human retina [88]. Biological functions of these macular pigments include the absorption of spectra. The function of these pigments is to absorb the blue light that can cause harm to the retina, but this chronic process of absorption may affect these macular pigments [89].

Glaucoma is the second most common cause of blindness and is a degenerative disease of retinal ganglion cells (RGCs) and the optic nerve and is expected to affect about 111.8 million people between 40 and 80 years by 2040 [90]. The most common types of glaucoma are primary open angle glaucoma (POAG) and primary angle closure glaucoma (PACG) [91]. The appearance of glaucoma caused mainly by the progressive disruption of RGC axonal transport or with retinal ischemia. Pathologically, glaucoma is characterized by the death of RGCs and increased intraocular pressure (IOP) [92]. Increased IOP is an important contributor to POAG. Elevation of IOP could cause many changes that are involved in the pathogenesis of glaucoma, such as oxidative stress, glutamate toxicity and ischemia [91].

The positive effects of goji berries on eye diseases such as glaucoma, cataract and rhinitis pigmentosa (RP) have been proposed by Chinese herbalists due to their high concentration of zeaxanthin and their esters, which are ready absorbed into serum, resulting in protection of the retina against free radicals and blue light damage. Leung et al. [93] reported that the levels of these two carotenoids in the serum and tissues of rhesus monkeys after feeding with *L. barbarum* fruits were significantly higher against the control group. Furthermore, clinical studies focused on *L. barbarum* as a therapy for retinal diseases in humans exist in the scientific literature. Chan et al. [94], in a study involving retinitis pigmentosa patients, showed that *L. barbarum* treatment can provide a neuroprotective effect for the retina and could help delay or minimize cone degeneration in RP. The positive effect of goji berries on glaucoma is due to the activation of the microglia at a moderate level resulting RGCs protection against IOP regulating important intracellular pathways that stimulate the body's defense under stress situations.

Chu et al. [95] studied the positive effects of LBP on preserving retinal function by multifocal electroretinogram (mfERG) analysis of 30 eyes of 30 Sprague-Dawley rats using a partial optic nerve transection (PONT) model in order to study secondary degeneration of retinal ganglion cells. The experimental results demonstrated that the feeding for 4 weeks with LBP, altered the functional reduction caused by PONT by regulating the signal from the outer retina. Li et al. [96] also suggested that LBP can reduce the loss of axons in the central optic nerves (ONs). Preservation of the g-ratio (axon diameter/fiber diameter) in the ventral Ons activates the microglia/macrophages in the Ons 12 h after PONT and finally decreases the magnitude response of microglia/macrophages 4 weeks after PONT. When the supply of blood to the retina is inadequate, the appearance of retinal ischemia due to lack of oxygen results in an altered metabolic function that eventually leads to irreversible cell death. An LBP diet of mice with acute ocular hypertension showed that it reduces the loss of RGC, protecting nerve fiber density, reducing immunoglobulin leakage and increasing blood vessel density [97–99]. Furthermore, similar studies in rats completed by He et al. [100] and Chu et al. [95] confirmed the protection of RGCs, commenting on the importance of Nrf2 activation that leads to an increase of heme oxygenase-1 (HO-1) expression. Thus, the induction of the antioxidant pathway plays an important role in maintaining the redox status of the retina.

The blood-retinal barrier (BRB) is a protective barrier that consists of the outer and inner BRB. The role of the BRB is to maintain the homeostatic condition of the retinal microenvironment and prevent harmful substances from getting into the retina. It has been presented that mice administered with LBP a week before retinal ischemia showed protection against neuronal cell death and to retinal oxidative stress by inhibition of lipid peroxidation and against disruption of the BRB 48 h after reperfusion [99].

Age-related macular degeneration may occur gradually over a period of years (dry AMD) or suddenly in weeks or months (wet AMD). The macula has a large number of light detection cells that provide acute central vision. It is located at the back of the eye and is the most sensitive part of the retina. These cells convert light into electrical signals, sending them through the optic nerve to the brain, where they are "translated" into the images we see. Any damage to the macula leads to a blurred, distorted or dark representation of the center of the field of vision [101]. Studies by Bucheli et al. [102] in elderly people have shown that daily goji berry consumption for a period of 90 days increases plasma zeoxanthine and antioxidant levels. In addition, it protects against hypopigmentation and soft drusen accumulation in the macula of elderly people. The deposition of extracellular amyloid beta (Aβ), oxidative stress, and inflammation have all been implicated in AMD. Yoshida et al. [103] has commented that retinal ganglion cells and retinal pigment epithelium also synthesize Aβ, which are secreted in the posterior eye. Age-related changes in the composition of Aβ as well as its degradative enzymes lead to an increase in the amount of deposition in the retina [104]. The protective effect of LBPs on macular neurons during the pathogenesis of AMD is due to the protection of these cell neurons from the stress caused by Aβ [97,98,105].

Finally, Chien et al. [106] examined goji berry effects on dry eye disease in a male Sprague-Dawley rat model. Their study indicated that in the group treated with goji berries, the severity of the kerato conjunctival staining decreased significantly and ameliorated dry eye disease symptoms appeared in a dose-dependent manner.

According to the above-mentioned studies it is believed that Goji berry consumption positively affects eye and vision activity in many ways.

2.8. Pre-Biotic Activity

The term probiotic originates from the Greek words pre + bios and has been used with many different meanings in recent decades. Initially, the term "probiotic" was used to describe compounds produced by a protozoan that stimulated the growth of another [107]. Finally, experts from the Food and Agriculture Organization/World Health Organization have identified probiotics as "living microorganisms, which when consumed in sufficient quantities as part of the feed contribute to the beneficial effect of the host" [108].

The use of probiotics extends back to a time before the discovery of microbes. Fermented dairy products were depicted in Egyptian hieroglyphics, and buffalo milk fermentation was traditionally used by Mongolian nomads to preserve their milk during their long journeys [109]. So far, many microorganisms such as fungi, yeasts, bacteria or their mixed combination have been considered or used as probiotics. The two main bacterial genera mainly referred to as probiotics are those of *Lactobacillus* and *Bifidobacterium* [110].

Historically, during the 1800s, the positive effect on human health of the consumption of fermented dairy products was observed by scientists. Although Louis Pasteur identified bacteria and yeasts that were responsible for the fermentation process did not associate these microbes with any apparent health effects. In 1905, Elie Metchnikoff, who had worked with Pasteur in the 1860s, observed that Bulgarian shepherd's longevity was mainly due to the lactobacilli used for yogurt fermentation and the presence of these lactobacilli in the sheep intestine in Bulgaria not with the yogurt they consumed but with [111]. In particular, Metchnikoff, in his study, "The Prologue of Life" in 1908, assumed that lactic acid bacteria detected in Bulgarian yogurts, the so-called Balkan Bulgarian, later known as *Lactobacillus bulgaricus* (now called *L. delbrueckii* subsp. *bulgaricus*) and *Streptococcus thermophilus*, are responsible for enhancing the intestinal system by inhibiting microbial fermentation, resulting in a reduction in unwanted by-products, such as amines and ammonia. Thus, for the first time, Metchnikoff highlighted the importance of specific micro-organisms and their contribution to human health and longevity.

Prebiotics are components of non-digestible foods that effectively affect the host by favoring growth and/or bacterial activity in the large intestine [112,113].

The term "symbiotic" is defined as a mixture of probiotics and prebiotics that beneficially affect the host by improving the survival of the beneficial microflora, enriching it with live beneficial bacteria found in dietary supplements in the gastrointestinal tract. These microorganisms promote health and thus improve welfare in the gastrointestinal tract. Symbiotics are aimed at enhancing the survival and activity of probiotics as proven in vivo, as well as stimulating *Bifidobacterium* species [111].

The prebiotic action of goji berries has been shown by its addition to yogurt [114], which resulted in maintenance the viability of lactic acid bacteria (LAB) at probiotic levels (106–107 log CFU/mL) during 21 days of storage compared to classic yogurt control. Similar results were presented in the study of Baba et al. [115], where the addition of aqueous extracts of *L. barbarum* to yogurt significantly improved the bioavailability of probiotic bacteria *Lactobacillus* spp. and *Streptococcus thermophilus*.

Furthermore, Liao et al. [116] demonstrated the beneficial prebiotic effect of the addition of *L. barbarum* to fermentation in Sichuan pickle (traditional Chinese pickle). According to the results presented in this study, *L. barbarum* addition not only increased the amount of LAB but also improved considerably the organoleptic quality and reduced the nitrite content of the pickle. Additionally, the results of a recent study completed by Zhou et al. [117] demonstrated that LBP improved the tolerance of *B. longum* subsp. *infantis* Bi-26 and *L. acidophilus* NCFM to the gastrointestinal environment. These results were also found to be in line with the study completed by Skenderidis et al. [19] that indices that LBP promotes the proliferation protecting *Bifidobacterium* and *Lactobacillus* strains by enhancing carbon and energy metabolism. These results also reported that the viability of *L. casei* was less affected, followed by *B. lactis* Bb12, which showed the greatest tolerance in the acidic environment, while the survival of *B. longum* 42 was low. Similar results were also confirmed by González-Rodríguez et al. [118], where *B. longum* 42 showed lower resistance in low pH conditions compared to *B. lactis* Bb12.

To confer a health benefit on the host, the LAB must be able to overcome the physical and chemical barriers of the gastrointestinal tract, especially acidic and proteolytic enzymes and bile stresses [119]. Consequently, the LAB should be resistant to the gastrointestinal environment.

The existence of an extracellular polysaccharide film produced by certain lactic bacteria or *Bifidobacterium* has also been reported in the literature [120,121]. This polysaccharide film protects probiotic bacterial cells from the environment and acts as a shield against the conditions prevailing in the gastrointestinal tract and helps them to survive. It has also been reported that *Bifidobacterium longum* strains produce larger amounts of this film than Bb12, resulting in higher bile strength [19]. This resistance is related to the binding of bile salts from the polysaccharide film, resulting in a reduction in its antimicrobial activity [116,120]. Finally, Skenderidis et al. [19] confirmed the increase of the Bb12 strain viability induced by goji berry extracts. This increase is probably related to goji berry polysaccharides, which consist of galactose, glucose, fructose, arabinose, mannose and xylose molecules, which are also the structural molecules of this extracellular polysaccharide antimicrobial [120–123].

2.9. Other Bioactivities

Additional bioactive effects of goji berries, such as skin protection and its synergistic potential within fertility treatment by inducing spermatogenesis, have been reported [25,33,124–126]. Studies carried out with phenolic compounds isolated from the fruits of *L. barbarum* showed that the extracts had a bactericidal effect against Gram positive and Gram-negative bacteria [10]. On the other hand, *L. chinense* leaf extracts were found to be more potent as antimicrobial agents than the fruit extracts, with the best microbiocidal activity exerted on *Bacillus subtilis* [127].

3. Conclusions

There are many scientific research results that support the positive effects of the consumption of goji berry fruits and their plant parts (bark, leaves) extracts. Their potential health benefits include protection against oxidative damage, antidiabetic, immunoregulatory, vision protective, hepatoprotective, and prebiotic activities that are associated with the promotion of risk reduction in the development of chronic diseases such as cancer, diabetes, cardiovascular disease, Alzheimer's disease, cataracts, and age-related diseases. Therefore, the screening of individual constituents of bioactive goji berries that exhibit health-promoting properties requires further investigation. This is because a cause–effect relationship between the intake of goji berries and its health effects can only be established when the composition of goji berries is properly characterized and standardized. Furthermore, extensive investigation is needed to examine the effects of adding these beneficial bioactive phytochemicals from goji berries, using advanced technologies, into food systems. Further research is also needed to evaluate the effectiveness of goji berry extracts in the food ecosystem and to establish their role as a functional agent in the design of new fortified foods.

Author Contributions: Conceptualization, P.S.; investigation, P.S. and S.L.; writing—original draft preparation, P.S.; writing—review and editing, P.S., S.L. and D.L.; visualization, P.S.; supervision, P.S.; All authors have read and agreed to the published version of the manuscript.

Funding: This research received no external funding.

Informed Consent Statement: Not applicable.

Data Availability Statement: Not applicable.

Conflicts of Interest: The authors declare no conflict of interest.

References

1. Knight, K.; Badamgarav, E.; Henning, J.M.; Hasselblad, V.; Anacleto, P.; Gano, P.; Ofman, J.J.; Weingarten, S.R. A Systematic review of diabetes disease management programs. *Am. J. Manag. Care* **2005**, *11*, 242–250. [PubMed]
2. Kannel, W.B. Diabetes and cardiovascular disease. The Framingham study. *JAMA* **1979**, *241*, 2035–2038. [CrossRef] [PubMed]
3. Sowers, J.R.; Epstein, M.; Frohlich, E.D. Diabetes, hypertension, and cardiovascular disease. *Hypertension* **2001**, *37*, 1053–1059. [CrossRef] [PubMed]
4. Naczk, M.; Shahidi, F. Phenolics in cereals, fruits and vegetables: Occurrence, extraction and analysis. *J. Pharm. Biomed. Anal.* **2006**, *41*, 1523–1542. [CrossRef] [PubMed]
5. Altemimi, A.; Lakhssassi, N.; Baharlouei, A.; Watson, D.G.; Lightfoot, D.A. Phytochemicals: Extraction, isolation, and identification of bioactive compounds from plant extracts. *Plants* **2017**, *6*, 42. [CrossRef] [PubMed]
6. Leontopoulos, S.; Skenderidis, P.; Kalorizou, H.; Petrotos, K. Bioactivity potential of polyphenolic compounds in human health and their effectiveness against various food borne and plant pathogens. A review. *J. Food Biosyst. Eng.* **2017**, *7*, 1–19.
7. Lampakis, D.; Skenderidis, P.; Leontopoulos, S. Technologies and extraction methods of polyphenolic compounds derived from pomegranate (*Punica granatum*) peels. A mini review. *Processes* **2021**, *9*, 236. [CrossRef]
8. Leontopoulos, S.; Skenderidis, P.; Vagelas, I.K. Potential use of polyphenolic compounds obtained from olive mill waste waters on plant pathogens and plant parasitic nematodes. In *Plant Defence: Biological Control*; Mérillon, J.-M., Ramawat, K.G., Eds.; Springer International Publishing: Cham, Switzerland, 2020; pp. 137–177, ISBN 978-3-030-51034-3.
9. Greathead, H. Plants and plant extracts for improving animal productivity. *Proc. Nutr. Soc.* **2003**, *62*, 279–290. [CrossRef]
10. Skenderidis, P.; Mitsagga, C.; Giavasis, I.; Petrotos, K.; Lampakis, D.; Leontopoulos, S.; Hadjichristodoulou, C.; Tsakalof, A. The in vitro antimicrobial activity assessment of ultrasound assisted *Lycium barbarum* fruit extracts and pomegranate fruit peels. *J. Food Meas. Charact.* **2019**, *13*, 2017–2031. [CrossRef]
11. Leontopoulos, S.; Skenderidis, P.; Petrotos, K.; Giavasis, I. Corn silage supplemented with pomegranate (*Punica granatum*) and avocado (*Persea americana*) pulp and seed wastes for improvement of meat characteristics in poultry production. *Molecules* **2021**, *26*, 5901. [CrossRef]
12. Zengin, Z.B.; Meza, L.; Pal, S.K.; Grivas, P. Chemoimmunotherapy in urothelial cancer: Concurrent or sequential? *Lancet Oncol.* **2021**, *22*, 894–896. [CrossRef]
13. Negi, G.; Kumar, A.; Joshi, R.P.; Sharma, S.S. Oxidative stress and Nrf2 in the pathophysiology of diabetic neuropathy: Old perspective with a new angle. *Biochem. Biophys. Res. Commun.* **2011**, *408*, 1–5. [CrossRef]
14. Boots, A.W.; Haenen, G.R.; Bast, A. Health effects of quercetin: From antioxidant to nutraceutical. *Eur. J. Pharmacol.* **2008**, *585*, 325–337. [CrossRef] [PubMed]
15. Valko, M.; Rhodes, C.J.; Moncol, J.; Izakovic, M.; Mazur, M. Free radicals, metals and antioxidants in oxidative stress-induced cancer. *Chem. Biol. Interact.* **2006**, *160*, 1–40. [CrossRef] [PubMed]
16. Vivekananthan, D.P.; Penn, M.S.; Sapp, S.K.; Hsu, A.; Topol, E. Use of antioxidant vitamins for the prevention of cardiovascular disease: Meta-analysis of randomised trials. *Lancet* **2003**, *361*, 2017–2023. [CrossRef]
17. Rocchetti, G.; Senizza, B.; Putnik, P.; Kovačević, D.B.; Barba, F.J.; Trevisan, M.; Lucini, L. Untargeted screening of the bound/free phenolic composition in tomato cultivars for industrial transformation. *J. Sci. Food Agric.* **2019**, *99*, 6173–6181. [CrossRef]
18. Rocchetti, G.; Lucini, L.; Corrado, G.; Colla, G.; Cardarelli, M.; De Pascale, S.; Rouphael, Y. Phytochemical profile, mineral content, and bioactive compounds in leaves of seed-propagated artichoke hybrid cultivars. *Molecules* **2020**, *25*, 3795. [CrossRef]
19. Skenderidis, P.; Mitsagga, C.; Lampakis, D.; Petrotos, K.; Giavasis, I. The effect of encapsulated powder of goji berry (*Lycium barbarum*) on growth and survival of probiotic bacteria. *Microorganisms* **2020**, *8*, 57. [CrossRef]
20. Skenderidis, P.; Leontopoulos, S.; Petrotos, K.; Giavasis, I. Vacuum microwave-assisted aqueous extraction of polyphenolic compounds from avocado (*Persea Americana*) solid waste. *Sustainability* **2021**, *13*, 2166. [CrossRef]
21. Amagase, H.; Sun, B.; Borek, C. *Lycium barbarum* (goji) juice improves in vivo antioxidant biomarkers in serum of healthy adults. *Nutr. Res.* **2009**, *29*, 19–25. [CrossRef]
22. Hsu, C.-H.; Nance, D.M.; Amagase, H. A meta-analysis of clinical improvements of general well-being by a standardized *Lycium barbarum*. *J. Med. Food* **2012**, *15*, 1006–1014. [CrossRef]
23. Yao, R.; Heinrich, M.; Zou, Y.; Reich, E.; Zhang, X.; Chen, Y.; Weckerle, C. Quality variation of goji (Fruits of *Lycium* spp.) in China: A comparative morphological and metabolomic analysis. *Front. Pharmacol.* **2018**, *9*, 151. [CrossRef] [PubMed]
24. Skenderidis, P.; Lampakis, D.; Giavasis, I.; Leontopoulos, S.; Petrotos, K.; Hadjichristodoulou, C.; Tsakalof, A. Chemical properties, fatty-acid composition, and antioxidant activity of goji berry (*Lycium barbarum* L. and *Lycium chinense* Mill.) Fruits. *Antioxidants* **2019**, *8*, 60. [CrossRef]
25. Cao, S.; Du, J.; Hei, Q. *Lycium barbarum* polysaccharide protects against neurotoxicity via the Nrf2-HO-1 pathway. *Exp. Ther. Med.* **2017**, *14*, 4919–4927. [CrossRef] [PubMed]
26. Ahmed, N.; Wang, M.; Shu, S. Effect of commercial *Bacillus thuringiensis* toxins on *Tyrophagus putrescentiae* (Schrank) fed on wolfberry (*Lycium barbarum* L.). *Int. J. Acarol.* **2016**, *42*, 1–5. [CrossRef]
27. Cui, B.; Liu, S.; Lin, X.; Wang, J.; Li, S.; Wang, Q.; Li, S. Effects of *Lycium barbarum* aqueous and ethanol extracts on high-fat-diet induced oxidative stress in rat liver tissue. *Molecules* **2011**, *16*, 9116–9128. [CrossRef] [PubMed]
28. Habtemariam, S. Protective effects of caffeic acid and the Alzheimer's brain: An update. *Mini-Rev. Med. Chem.* **2017**, *17*, 667–674. [CrossRef]

29. Zhang, R.; Kang, K.A.; Piao, M.J.; Kim, K.C.; Kim, A.D.; Chae, S.; Park, J.S.; Youn, U.J.; Hyun, J.W. Cytoprotective effect of the fruits of *Lycium chinense* Miller against oxidative stress-induced hepatotoxicity. *J. Ethnopharmacol.* **2010**, *130*, 299–306. [CrossRef]
30. Changbo, D. Supplementation of *Lycium barbarum* polysaccharides protection of skeletal muscle from exercise-induced oxidant stress in mice. *Afr. J. Pharm. Pharmacol.* **2012**, *6*, 643–647. [CrossRef]
31. Zhang, Z.; Liu, X.; Zhang, X.; Liu, J.; Hao, Y.; Yang, X.; Wang, Y. Comparative evaluation of the antioxidant effects of the natural vitamin C analog 2-O-β-D-glucopyranosyl-L-ascorbic acid isolated from Goji berry fruit. *Arch. Pharmacal. Res.* **2011**, *34*, 801–810. [CrossRef]
32. Li, H.; Li, Z.; Peng, L.; Jiang, N.; Liu, Q.; Zhang, E.; Liang, B.; Li, R.; Zhu, H. *Lycium barbarum* polysaccharide protects human keratinocytes against UVB-induced photo-damage. *Free Radic. Res.* **2017**, *51*, 200–210. [CrossRef] [PubMed]
33. Skenderidis, P.; Kerasioti, E.; Karkanta, E.; Stagos, D.; Kouretas, D.; Konstantinos, P.; Hadjichristodoulou, C. Assessment of the antioxidant and antimutagenic activity of extracts from goji berry of Greek cultivation. *Toxicol. Rep.* **2018**, *5*, 251–257. [CrossRef]
34. Bucheli, P.; Gao, Q.; Redgwell, R.; Karine, V.; Wang, J.; Zhang, W.; Nong, S.; Cao, B. Chapter 14 Wolfberry biomolecular and clinical aspects of Chinese. In *Herbal Medicine: Biomolecular and Clinical Aspects*; CRC Press: Boca Raton, FL, USA, 2013; pp. 1–17.
35. Kaur, D.; Rasane, P.; Singh, J.; Kaur, S.; Kumar, V.; Mahato, D.K.; Dey, A.; Dhawan, K.; Kumar, S. Nutritional interventions for elderly and considerations for the development of geriatric Foods. *Curr. Aging Sci.* **2019**, *12*, 15–27. [CrossRef] [PubMed]
36. Li, X.; Zhou, A. Evaluation of antioxidant activity of the polysaccharides extracted from *Lycium barbarum* fruits in vitro. *Eur. Polym. J.* **2007**, *43*, 488–497. [CrossRef]
37. Yi, R.; Liu, X.-M.; Dong, Q. A study of *Lycium barbarum* polysaccharides (LBP) extraction technology and its anti-aging effect. *Afr. J. Tradit. Complement. Altern. Med.* **2013**, *10*, 171–174. [CrossRef] [PubMed]
38. Xia, G.; Xin, N.; Liu, W.; Yao, H.; Hou, Y.; Qi, J. Inhibitory effect of *Lycium barbarum* polysaccharides on cell apoptosis and senescence is potentially mediated by the p53 signaling pathway. *Mol. Med. Rep.* **2014**, *9*, 1237–1241. [CrossRef] [PubMed]
39. Ho, S.-C.; Liu, J.-H.; Wu, R.-Y. Establishment of the mimetic aging effect in mice caused by D-galactose. *Biogerontology* **2003**, *4*, 15–18. [CrossRef]
40. Deng, H.-B.; Cui, D.-P.; Jiang, J.-M.; Feng, Y.-C.; Cai, N.-S.; Li, D.-D. Inhibiting effects of Achyranthes bidentata polysaccharide and *Lycium barbarum* polysaccharide on non-enzyme glycation in D-galactose induced mouse aging model. *Biomed. Environ. Sci.* **2003**, *16*, 267–275.
41. Wang, Y.; Zhao, H.; Sheng, X.; Gambino, P.E.; Costello, B.; Bojanowski, K. Protective effect of *Fructus lycii* polysaccharides against time and hyperthermia-induced damage in cultured seminiferous epithelium. *J. Ethnopharmacol.* **2002**, *82*, 169–175. [CrossRef]
42. Ji, L.L. Antioxidant signaling in skeletal muscle: A brief review. *Exp. Gerontol.* **2007**, *42*, 582–593. [CrossRef]
43. Ma, Q. Role of Nrf2 in Oxidative stress and toxicity. *Annu. Rev. Pharmacol. Toxicol.* **2013**, *53*, 401–426. [CrossRef]
44. David, J.A.; Rifkin, W.J.; Rabbani, P.S.; Ceradini, D.J. The Nrf2/Keap1/ARE Pathway and oxidative stress as a therapeutic target in type II diabetes mellitus. *J. Diabetes Res.* **2017**, *2017*, 4826724. [CrossRef] [PubMed]
45. Yang, P.; Li, D.; Jin, S.; Ding, J.; Guo, J.; Shi, W.; Wang, C. Stimuli-responsive biodegradable poly (methacrylic acid) based nano-capsules for ultrasound traced and triggered drug delivery system. *Biomaterials* **2014**, *35*, 2079–2088. [CrossRef]
46. Gao, Y.; Wei, Y.; Wang, Y.; Gao, F.; Chen, Z. *Lycium barbarum*: A traditional Chinese herb and a promising anti-aging agent. *Aging Dis.* **2017**, *8*, 778–791. [CrossRef] [PubMed]
47. Ming, M.; Guanhua, L.; Zhanhai, Y.; Guang, C.; Xuan, Z. Effect of the *Lycium barbarum* polysaccharides administration on blood lipid metabolism and oxidative stress of mice fed high-fat diet in vivo. *Food Chem.* **2009**, *113*, 872–877. [CrossRef]
48. Luo, Q.; Cai, Y.; Yan, J.; Sun, M.; Corke, H. Hypoglycemic and hypolipidemic effects and antioxidant activity of fruit extracts from *Lycium barbarum*. *Life Sci.* **2004**, *76*, 137–149. [CrossRef] [PubMed]
49. Im, A.-R.; Lee, H.J.; Youn, U.J.; Hyun, J.W.; Chae, S. Orally administered betaine reduces photodamage caused by UVB irradiation through the regulation of matrix metalloproteinase-9 activity in hairless mice. *Mol. Med. Rep.* **2016**, *13*, 823–828. [CrossRef]
50. Cao, G.; Yang, W.; Du, P. Observation of the effects of LAK/IL-2 Therapy combining with *Lycium barbarium* polysaccharides in the treatment of 75 cancer patients. *Chin. J. Oncol.* **1994**, *16*, 428–431.
51. Gan, L.; Zhang, S.H.; Yang, X.L.; Xu, H.B. Immunomodulation and antitumor activity by a polysaccharide À protein complex from *Lycium barbarum*. *Int. Immunopharmacol.* **2004**, *4*, 563. [CrossRef]
52. Zhang, M.; Chen, H.; Huang, J.; Li, Z.; Zhu, C.; Zhang, S. Effect of *Lycium barbarum* polysaccharide on human hepatoma QGY7703 cells: Inhibition of proliferation and induction of apoptosis. *Life Sci.* **2005**, *76*, 2115–2124. [CrossRef]
53. Su, C.-X.; Duan, X.-G.; Liang, L.-J.; Wang, F.; Zheng, J.; Fu, X.-Y.; Yan, Y.-M.; Huang, L.; Wang, N.-P. *Lycium barbarum* polysaccharides as an adjuvant for recombinant vaccine through enhancement of humoral immunity by activating Tfh cells. *Veter-Immunol. Immunopathol.* **2014**, *158*, 98–104. [CrossRef] [PubMed]
54. Yang, R.-F.; Zhao, C.; Chen, X.; Chan, S.-W.; Wu, J.-Y. Chemical properties and bioactivities of Goji (*Lycium barbarum*) polysaccharides extracted by different methods. *J. Funct. Foods* **2015**, *17*, 903–909. [CrossRef]
55. He, N.; Yang, X.; Jiao, Y.; Tian, L.; Zhao, Y. Characterisation of antioxidant and antiproliferative acidic polysaccharides from Chinese wolfberry fruits. *Food Chem.* **2012**, *133*, 978–989. [CrossRef]
56. Huang, X.; Zhang, Q.-Y.; Jiang, Q.-Y.; Kang, X.-M.; Zhao, L. Polysaccharides derived from *Lycium barbarum* suppress IGF-1-induced angiogenesis via PI3K/HIF-1α/VEGF signalling pathways in MCF-7 cells. *Food Chem.* **2012**, *131*, 1479–1484. [CrossRef]
57. Deng, X.; Luo, S.; Luo, X.; Hu, M.; Ma, F.; Wang, Y.; Zhou, L.; Huang, R. Fraction From *Lycium barbarum* Polysaccharides Reduces Immunotoxicity and Enhances Antitumor Activity of Doxorubicin in Mice. *Integr. Cancer Ther.* **2018**, *17*, 860–866. [CrossRef]

58. Kim, N.H.; Sung, B.; Kang, Y.J.; Jang, J.Y.; Hwang, S.Y.; Lee, Y.; Kim, M.; Im, E.; Yoon, J.-H.; Kim, C.M.; et al. Anti-inflammatory effects of betaine on AOM/DSS-induced colon tumorigenesis in ICR male mice. *Int. J. Oncol.* **2014**, *45*, 1250–1256. [CrossRef] [PubMed]
59. Singh, J.; Rasane, P.; Kaur, S.; Kumar, V.; Dhawan, K.; Mahato, D.K.; Malhotra, S.; Sarma, C.; Kaur, D.; Bhattacharya, J. Nutritional interventions and considerations for the development of low calorie or sugar free foods. *Curr. Diabetes Rev.* **2020**, *16*, 301–312. [CrossRef]
60. Zheng, Y.; Ley, S.H.; Hu, F.B. Global aetiology and epidemiology of type 2 diabetes mellitus and its complications. *Nat. Rev. Endocrinol.* **2018**, *14*, 88–98. [CrossRef]
61. Wild, S.; Roglic, G.; Green, A.; Sicree, R.; King, H. Global prevalence of diabetes: Estimates for the Year 2000 and projections for 2030. *Diabetes Care* **2004**, *27*, 1047–1053. [CrossRef]
62. Silva, C.; Alves, B.; Azzalis, L.; Junqueira, V.; Fonseca, R.; Fonseca, A.; Fonseca, F. Goji Berry (*Lycium Barbarum*) in the treatment of diabetes melitus: A systematic review. *Food Res.* **2017**, *1*, 221–224. [CrossRef]
63. Wu, H.; Guo, H.; Zhao, R. Effect of *Lycium barbarum* Polysaccharide on the improvement of antioxidant ability and DNA damage in NIDDM Rats. *Yakugaku Zasshi* **2006**, *126*, 365–371. [CrossRef] [PubMed]
64. Zhang, M.; Tang, X.; Wang, F.; Zhang, Q.; Zhang, Z. Characterization of *Lycium barbarum* polysaccharide and its effect on human hepatoma cells. *Int. J. Biol. Macromol.* **2013**, *61*, 270–275. [CrossRef] [PubMed]
65. Bagul, P.K.; Middela, H.; Matapally, S.; Padiya, R.; Bastia, T.; Madhusudana, K.; Reddy, B.R.; Chakravarty, S.; Banerjee, S.K. Attenuation of insulin resistance, metabolic syndrome and hepatic oxidative stress by resveratrol in fructose-fed rats. *Pharmacol. Res.* **2012**, *66*, 260–268. [CrossRef] [PubMed]
66. Nakatani, Y.; Kaneto, H.; Kawamori, D.; Hatazaki, M.; Miyatsuka, T.; Matsuoka, T.-A.; Kajimoto, Y.; Matsuhisa, M.; Yamasaki, Y.; Hori, M. Modulation of the JNK pathway in liver affects insulin resistance status. *J. Biol. Chem.* **2004**, *279*, 45803–45809. [CrossRef] [PubMed]
67. Kaneto, H. The JNK pathway as a therapeutic target for diabetes. *Expert Opin. Ther. Targets* **2005**, *9*, 581–592. [CrossRef]
68. Kaneto, H.; Matsuoka, T.-A.; Nakatani, Y.; Kawamori, D.; Miyatsuka, T.; Matsuhisa, M.; Yamasaki, Y. Oxidative stress, ER stress, and the JNK pathway in type 2 diabetes. *Klin. Wochenschr.* **2005**, *83*, 429–439. [CrossRef] [PubMed]
69. Yang, Y.; Li, W.; Li, Y.; Wang, Q.; Gao, L.; Zhao, J. Dietary *Lycium barbarum* Polysaccharide induces Nrf2/ARE pathway and ameliorates insulin resistance induced by high-fat via activation of PI3K/AKT signaling. *Oxidative Med. Cell. Longev.* **2014**, *2014*, 1–10. [CrossRef]
70. Cai, H.; Liu, F.; Zuo, P.; Huang, G.; Song, Z.; Wang, T.; Lu, H.; Guo, F.; Han, C.; Sun, G. Practical application of antidiabetic efficacy of *Lycium barbarum* polysaccharide in patients with Type 2 diabetes. *Med. Chem.* **2015**, *11*, 383–390. [CrossRef] [PubMed]
71. Zhao, R.; Gao, X.; Zhang, T.; Li, X. Effects of *Lycium barbarum*. polysaccharide on type 2 diabetes mellitus rats by regulating biological rhythms. *Iran. J. Basic Med. Sci.* **2016**, *19*, 1024–1030. [CrossRef]
72. Finegold, J.A.; Asaria, P.; Francis, D.P. Mortality from ischaemic heart disease by country, region, and age: Statistics from World Health Organisation and United Nations. *Int. J. Cardiol.* **2013**, *168*, 934–945. [CrossRef]
73. Levy, D.; Ehret, G.B.; Rice, K.; Verwoert, G.C.; Launer, L.J.; Dehghan, A.; Glazer, N.L.; Morrison, A.C.; Johnson, A.D.; Aspelund, T.; et al. Genome-wide association study of blood pressure and hypertension. *Nat. Genet.* **2009**, *41*, 677–687. [CrossRef] [PubMed]
74. Lu, S.-P.; Zhao, P.-T. Chemical characterization of *Lycium barbarum* polysaccharides and their reducing myocardial injury in ischemia/reperfusion of rat heart. *Int. J. Biol. Macromol.* **2010**, *47*, 681–684. [CrossRef] [PubMed]
75. Xin, Y.-F.; Zhou, G.-L.; Deng, Z.-Y.; Chen, Y.-X.; Wu, Y.-G.; Xu, P.-S.; Xuan, Y.-X. Protective effect of *Lycium barbarum* on doxorubicin-induced cardiotoxicity. *Phytother. Res.* **2007**, *21*, 1020–1024. [CrossRef]
76. Xin, Y.-F.; Wan, L.-L.; Peng, J.-L.; Guo, C. Alleviation of the acute doxorubicin-induced cardiotoxicity by *Lycium barbarum* polysaccharides through the suppression of oxidative stress. *Food Chem. Toxicol.* **2011**, *49*, 259–264. [CrossRef]
77. Xin, Y.; Zhang, S.; Gu, L.; Liu, S.; Gao, H.; You, Z.; Zhou, G.; Wen, L.; Yu, J.; Xuan, Y. Electrocardiographic and Biochemical evidence for the cardioprotective effect of antioxidants in acute doxorubicin-induced cardiotoxicity in the beagle dogs. *Biol. Pharm. Bull.* **2011**, *34*, 1523–1526. [CrossRef]
78. Zhang, X.; Yang, X.; Lin, Y.; Suo, M.; Gong, L.; Chen, J.; Hui, R. Anti-hypertensive effect of *Lycium barbarum* L. with down-regulated expression of renal endothelial lncRNA sONE in a rat model of salt-sensitive hypertension. *Int. J. Clin. Exp. Pathol.* **2015**, *8*, 6981–6987.
79. Guo, X.F.; Li, Z.H.; Cai, H.; Li, D. The Effects of *Lycium Barbarum* L. (*L. Barbarum*) on cardiometabolic risk factors: A me-ta-analysis of randomized controlled trials. *Food Funct.* **2017**, *8*, 1741–1748. [CrossRef] [PubMed]
80. Demori, I.; Voci, A.; Fugassa, E.; Burlando, B. Combined effects of high-fat diet and ethanol induce oxidative stress in rat liver. *Alcohol* **2006**, *40*, 185–191. [CrossRef] [PubMed]
81. Orman, E.S.; Odena, G.; Bataller, R. Alcoholic liver disease: Pathogenesis, management, and novel targets for therapy. *J. Gastroenterol. Hepatol. (Aust.)* **2013**, *28*, 77–84. [CrossRef]
82. Xiao, J.; Wang, J.; Xing, F.; Han, T.; Jiao, R.; Liong, E.C.; Fung, M.-L.; So, K.-F.; Tipoe, G.L. Zeaxanthin Dipalmitate therapeutically improves hepatic functions in an alcoholic fatty liver disease model through modulating MAPK pathway. *PLoS ONE* **2014**, *9*, e95214. [CrossRef]
83. Xiao, J.; Zhu, Y.; Liu, Y.; Tipoe, G.L.; Xing, F.; So, K.-F. *Lycium barbarum* polysaccharide attenuates alcoholic cellular injury through TXNIP-NLRP3 inflammasome pathway. *Int. J. Biol. Macromol.* **2014**, *69*, 73–78. [CrossRef]

84. Assy, N.; Kaita, K.; Mymin, D.; Levy, C.; Rosser, B.; Minuk, G. Fatty infiltration of liver in hyperlipidemic patients. *Am. J. Dig. Dis. Sci.* **2000**, *45*, 1929–1934. [CrossRef] [PubMed]
85. Lee, Y.M.; Choi, J.S.; Kim, M.H.; Jung, M.H.; Lee, Y.S.; Song, J. Effects of dietary genistein on hepatic lipid metabolism and mitochondrial function in mice fed high-fat diets. *Nutrition* **2006**, *22*, 956–964. [CrossRef] [PubMed]
86. Kim, S.Y.; Lee, E.J.; Kim, H.P.; Kim, Y.C.; Moon, A. A novel cerebroside from *Lycii fructus* preserves the hepatic glutathione redox system in primary cultures of rat hepatocytes. *Biol. Pharm. Bull.* **1999**, *22*, 873–875. [CrossRef]
87. Xiao, J.; Liong, E.C.; Ching, Y.P.; Chang, R.C.C.; So, K.F.; Fung, M.L.; Tipoe, G.L. *Lycium barbarum* polysaccharides protect mice liver from carbon tetrachloride-induced oxidative stress and necroinflammation. *J. Ethnopharmacol.* **2012**, *139*, 462–470. [CrossRef] [PubMed]
88. Krinsky, N.I.; Landrum, J.T.; Bone, R.A. Biologic mechanisms of the protective role of lutein and Zeaxanthin in the eye. *Annu. Rev. Nutr.* **2003**, *23*, 171. [CrossRef] [PubMed]
89. Taylor, H.R.; West, S.; Muñoz, B.; Rosenthal, F.S.; Bressler, S.B.; Bressler, N.M. The Long-term effects of visible light on the eye. *Arch. Ophthalmol.* **1992**, *110*, 99–104. [CrossRef]
90. Tham, Y.-C.; Li, X.; Wong, T.Y.; Quigley, H.A.; Aung, T.; Cheng, C.-Y. Global prevalence of glaucoma and projections of glaucoma burden through 2040: A systematic review and meta-analysis. *Ophthalmology* **2014**, *121*, 2081–2090. [CrossRef]
91. Quigley, H.; Broman, A.T. The number of people with glaucoma worldwide in 2010 and 2020. *Br. J. Ophthalmol.* **2006**, *90*, 262–267. [CrossRef]
92. Prasanna, G.; Hulet, C.; Desai, D.; Krishnamoorthy, R.R.; Narayan, S.; Brun, A.-M.; Suburo, A.M.; Yorio, T. Effect of elevated intraocular pressure on endothelin-1 in a rat model of glaucoma. *Pharmacol. Res.* **2005**, *51*, 41–50. [CrossRef]
93. Leung, I.; Tso, M.; Li, W.; Lam, T. Absorption and tissue distribution of Zeaxanthin and lutein in rhesus monkeys after taking *Fructus lycii* (Gou Qi Zi) extract. *Investig. Ophthalmol. Vis. Sci.* **2001**, *42*, 466.
94. Chan, H.H.-L.; Lam, C.H.-I.; Choi, K.-Y.; Li, S.Z.-C.; Lakshmanan, Y.; Yu, W.-Y.; Chang, R.C.-C.; Lai, J.S.-M.; So, K.-F. Delay of cone degeneration in retinitis pigmentosa using a 12-month treatment with *Lycium barbarum* supplement. *J. Ethnopharmacol.* **2019**, *236*, 336–344. [CrossRef] [PubMed]
95. Chu, P.H.W.; Li, H.-Y.; Chin, M.-P.; So, K.-F.; Chan, H.H.L. Effect of *Lycium barbarum* (Wolfberry) polysaccharides on preserving retinal function after partial optic nerve transection. *PLoS ONE* **2013**, *8*, e81339. [CrossRef]
96. Li, H.-Y.; Ruan, Y.-W.; Kau, P.W.-F.; Chiu, K.; Chang, R.C.-C.; Chan, H.H.L.; So, K.-F. Effect of *Lycium barbarum* (Wolfberry) on alleviating axonal degeneration after partial optic nerve transection. *Cell Transplant.* **2015**, *24*, 403–417. [CrossRef]
97. Mi, X.-S.; Feng, Q.; Lo, A.C.Y.; Chang, R.C.-C.; Lin, B.; Chung, S.K.; So, K.-F. Protection of retinal ganglion cells and retinal vasculature by *Lycium barbarum* polysaccharides in a mouse model of acute ocular hypertension. *PLoS ONE* **2012**, *7*, e45469. [CrossRef]
98. Mi, X.S.; Chiu, K.; Van, G.; Leung, J.W.; Lo, A.C.; Chung, S.K.; Chang, R.C.; So, K.F. Effect of *Lycium barbarum* polysaccharides on the expression of endothelin-1 and its receptors in an ocular hypertension model of rat glaucoma. *Neural Regen. Res.* **2012**, *7*, 645–651. [CrossRef] [PubMed]
99. Li, S.-Y.; Yang, D.; Yeung, C.-M.; Yu, W.Y.; Chang, R.C.-C.; So, K.-F.; Wong, D.; Lo, A.C.Y. *Lycium barbarum* polysaccharides reduce neuronal damage, blood-retinal barrier disruption and oxidative stress in retinal ischemia/reperfusion injury. *PLoS ONE* **2011**, *6*, e16380. [CrossRef]
100. He, M.; Pan, H.; Chang, R.C.-C.; So, K.-F.; Brecha, N.C.; Pu, M. Activation of the Nrf2/HO-1 antioxidant pathway contributes to the protective effects of *Lycium barbarum* polysaccharides in the rodent retina after ischemia-reperfusion-induced damage. *PLoS ONE* **2014**, *9*, e84800. [CrossRef]
101. Flammer, J.; Mozaffarieh, M. What is the present pathogenetic concept of glaucomatous optic neuropathy? *Surv. Ophthalmol.* **2007**, *52*, S162–S173. [CrossRef] [PubMed]
102. Bucheli, P.; Vidal, K.; Shen, L.; Gu, Z.; Zhang, C.; Miller, L.; Wang, J. Goji berry effects on macular characteristics and plasma antioxidant levels. *Optom. Vis. Sci.* **2011**, *88*, 257–262. [CrossRef] [PubMed]
103. Yoshida, A.; Ishiko, S.; Akiba, J.; Kitaya, N.; Nagaoka, T. Radiating retinal folds detected by scanning laser ophthalmoscopy using a diode laser in a dark-field mode in idiopathic macular holes. *Graefe's Arch. Clin. Exp. Ophthalmol.* **1998**, *236*, 445–450. [CrossRef] [PubMed]
104. Prasad, T.; Zhu, P.; Verma, A.; Chakrabarty, P.; Rosario, A.M.; Golde, T.E.; Li, Q. Amyloid β peptides overexpression in retinal pigment epithelial cells via AAV-mediated gene transfer mimics AMD-like pathology in mice. *Sci. Rep.* **2017**, *7*, 3222. [CrossRef] [PubMed]
105. Ho, Y.-S.; Yu, M.-S.; Lai, C.S.-W.; So, K.-F.; Yuen, W.-H.; Chang, R.C.-C. Characterizing the neuroprotective effects of alkaline extract of *Lycium barbarum* on β-amyloid peptide neurotoxicity. *Brain Res.* **2007**, *1158*, 123–134. [CrossRef] [PubMed]
106. Chien, K.; Horng, C.; Huang, Y.; Hsieh, Y.; Wang, C.; Yang, J.; Lu, C.; Chen, F. Effects of *Lycium barbarum* (goji berry) on dry eye disease in rats. *Mol. Med. Rep.* **2018**, *17*, 809–818. [CrossRef] [PubMed]
107. Lilly, D.M.; Stillwell, R.H. Probiotics: Growth-promoting factors produced by microorganisms. *Science* **1965**, *147*, 747–748. [CrossRef] [PubMed]
108. FAO/WHO. *Probiotics in Food Health and Nutritional Properties and Guidelines for Evaluation*; Food and Nutrition Paper; FAO: Rome, Italy, 2001; Volume 85.

109. Guo, L.; Li, T.; Tang, Y.; Yang, L.; Huo, G. Probiotic properties of *Enterococcus* strains isolated from traditional naturally fermented cream in China. *Microb. Biotechnol.* **2015**, *9*, 737–745. [CrossRef] [PubMed]
110. Ohimain, E.I.; Ofongo, R.T.S. The Effect of probiotic and prebiotic feed supplementation on chicken health and gut microflora: A Review. *Int. J. Anim. Vet. Adv.* **2012**, *4*, 135–143.
111. Gibson, G.R.; Roberfroid, M.B. Dietary modulation of the human colonic microbiota: Introducing the concept of prebiotics. *J. Nutr.* **1995**, *125*, 1401–1412. [CrossRef]
112. Gibson, G.R.; Scott, K.P.; Rastall, R.A.; Tuohy, K.M.; Hotchkiss, A.; Dubert-Ferrandon, A.; Gareau, M.; Murphy, E.F.; Saulnier, D.; Loh, G.; et al. Dietary prebiotics: Current status and new definition. *Food Sci. Technol. Bull. Funct. Foods* **2010**, *7*, 1–19. [CrossRef]
113. Trowell, H.; Southgate, D.A.T.; Wolever, T.M.S.; Leeds, A.R.; Gassull, M.A.; Jenkins, D.J.A. Dietary fibre redefined. *Lancet* **1976**, *307*, 967. [CrossRef]
114. Schweizer, T.F.; Würsch, P. The physiological and nutritional importance of dietary fibre. *Experientia* **1991**, *47*, 181–186. [CrossRef] [PubMed]
115. Baba, A.S.; Najarian, A.; Shori, A.B.; Lit, K.W.; Keng, G.A. Viability of lactic acid bacteria, Antioxidant activity and in vitro inhibition of angiotensin-I-converting enzyme of *Lycium barbarum* yogurt. *Arab. J. Sci. Eng.* **2014**, *39*, 5355–5362. [CrossRef]
116. Liao, M.; Wu, Z.Y.; Yu, G.H.; Zhang, W.X. Improving the quality of Sichuan pickle by adding a traditional Chinese medicinal herb *Lycium barbarum* in its fermentation. *Int. J. Food Sci. Technol.* **2017**, *52*, 936–943. [CrossRef]
117. Zhou, F.; Jiang, X.; Wang, T.; Zhang, B.; Zhao, H. *Lycium barbarum* polysaccharide (LBP): A novel prebiotics candidate for Bifidobacterium and Lactobacillus. *Front. Microbiol.* **2018**, *9*, 1034. [CrossRef]
118. González-Rodríguez, I.; Sánchez, B.; Ruiz, L.; Turroni, F.; Ventura, M.; Ruas-Madiedo, P.; Gueimonde, M.; Margolles, A. Role of extracellular transaldolase from *Bifidobacterium bifidum* in mucin adhesion and aggregation. *Appl. Environ. Microbiol.* **2012**, *78*, 3992–3998. [CrossRef]
119. Nami, Y.; Abdullah, N.; Haghshenas, B.; Radiah, D.; Rosli, R.; Khosroushahi, A.Y. Probiotic potential and biotherapeutic effects of newly isolated vaginal *Lactobacillus acidophilus* 36YL strain on cancer cells. *Anaerobe* **2014**, *28*, 29–36. [CrossRef]
120. Alp, G.; Aslim, B.; Suludere, Z.; Akca, G. The role of hemagglutination and effect of exopolysaccharide production on bifidobacteria adhesion to Caco-2 cells in vitro. *Microbiol. Immunol.* **2010**, *54*, 658–665. [CrossRef]
121. Al-Sheraji, S.H.; Ismail, A.; Manap, M.Y.; Mustafa, S.; Yusof, R.M. Viability and activity of Bifidobacteria during refrigerated storage of yoghurt containing *Mangifera pajang* fibrous polysaccharides. *J. Food Sci.* **2012**, *77*, 624–630. [CrossRef] [PubMed]
122. Redgwell, R.J.; Curti, D.; Wang, J.; Dobruchowska, J.M.; Gerwig, G.J.; Kamerling, J.P.; Bucheli, P. Cell wall polysaccharides of Chinese Wolfberry (*Lycium barbarum*): Part Characterisation of arabinogalactan-proteins. *Carbohydr. Polym.* **2011**, *84*, 1075–1083. [CrossRef]
123. Redgwell, R.J.; Curti, D.; Wang, J.; Dobruchowska, J.M.; Gerwig, G.J.; Kamerling, J.P.; Bucheli, P. Cell wall polysaccharides of Chinese Wolfberry (*Lycium barbarum*): Part Characterization of soluble and insoluble polymer fractions. *Carbohydr. Polym.* **2011**, *84*, 1344–1349. [CrossRef]
124. Reeve, V.E.; Allanson, M.; Arun, S.J.; Domanski, D.; Painter, N. Mice drinking goji berry juice (*Lycium barbarum*) are protected from UV radiation-induced skin damage via antioxidant pathways. *Photochem. Photobiol. Sci.* **2010**, *9*, 601–607. [CrossRef] [PubMed]
125. Shi, G.-J.; Zheng, J.; Wu, J.; Qiao, H.-Q.; Chang, Q.; Niu, Y.; Sun, T.; Li, Y.-X.; Yu, J.-Q. Beneficial effects of *Lycium barbarum* polysaccharide on spermatogenesis by improving antioxidant activity and inhibiting apoptosis in streptozotocin-induced diabetic male mice. *Food Funct.* **2017**, *8*, 1215–1226. [CrossRef] [PubMed]
126. Vidović, B.B.; Milinčić, D.D.; Marčetić, M.D.; Djuriš, J.D.; Ilić, T.D.; Kostić, A.Ž.; Pešić, M.B. Health benefits and applications of goji berries in functional food products development: A review. *Antioxidants* **2022**, *11*, 248. [CrossRef] [PubMed]
127. Mocan, A.; Vlase, L.; Vodnar, D.C.; Bischin, C.; Hanganu, D.; Gheldiu, A.-M.; Oprean, R.; Silaghi-Dumitrescu, R.; Crișan, G. Polyphenolic content, antioxidant and antimicrobial activities of *Lycium barbarum* L. and *Lycium chinense* Mill. leaves. *Molecules* **2014**, *19*, 10056–10073. [CrossRef] [PubMed]

MDPI
St. Alban-Anlage 66
4052 Basel
Switzerland
Tel. +41 61 683 77 34
Fax +41 61 302 89 18
www.mdpi.com

Nutraceuticals Editorial Office
E-mail: nutraceuticals@mdpi.com
www.mdpi.com/journal/nutraceuticals

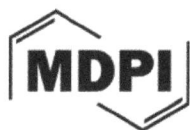

www.ingramcontent.com/pod-product-compliance
Lightning Source LLC
LaVergne TN
LVHW070423100526
838202LV00014B/1513